Diabetes For Canadians For Dummies®

Cheat Sheet

Screening to Determine if You Have Diabetes

The Canadian Diabetes Association recommends that you be tested for diabetes:

✔ Every 3 years once you reach 40 years of age; more frequently and/or earlier if you have risk factors including:

- Having a parent, sibling, or child with diabetes

- Being a member of a high-risk population (such as people of Aboriginal, Hispanic, Asian, South Asian, or African descent)

- Having a history of prediabetes, gestational diabetes, or have given birth to a large baby

- Being overweight

- Having hardening of the arteries (atherosclerosis), high blood pressure, abnormal lipids (cholesterol and triglycerides), schizophrenia, polycystic ovary syndrome, or a type of skin rash called acanthosis nigricans

✔ Immediately, if you are having symptoms of high blood glucose (such as thirst, frequent urination, and weight loss)

Target Test Results

The Canadian Diabetes Association recommends the following targets:

✔ Blood glucose before meals: 4.0 to 7.0 mmol/L (4.0 to 6.0 if it can be safely achieved). (See Chapter 9.)

✔ Blood glucose 2 hours after meals: 5.0 to 10.0 mmol/L (5.0 to 8.0 if it can be safely achieved). (See Chapter 9.)

✔ A1C level of 7 percent or less (6 percent or less if it can be safely achieved). (See Chapter 9.)

✔ LDL cholesterol less than 2.5 mmol/L (less than 3.5 if you are not at high risk of vascular disease). (See Chapter 6.)

✔ Total cholesterol (TC)/HDL cholesterol less than 4.0 (less than 5.0 if you are not at high risk of vascular disease). (See Chapter 6.)

✔ Urine albumin/creatinine ratio ("ACR") less than 2.0 (men) or less than 2.8 (women). (See Chapter 6.)

✔ Blood pressure less than or equal to 130/80. (See Chapter 6.)

Your Personal Test Results Record

Ideal	My Personal Target	Date:	Date:	Date:	Date:
Blood Pressure ≤ 130/80					
A1C ≤ 6					
TC/HDL < 4					
LDL < 2.5					
ACR < 2.0 (men)					
< 2.8 (women)					

For Dummies: Bestselling Book Series for Beginners

Diabetes For Canadians For Dummies®

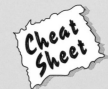

Frequency of Tests

The Canadian Diabetes Association recommends the following testing schedule (*for adults*, except as noted):

- **A1C:** every 3 months (see Chapter 9)
- **Blood glucose meter** (see Chapter 9):
  - Type 1 diabetes: *at least* three times daily
  - Type 2 diabetes: *at least* once daily
- **Lipids:** total cholesterol (TC), HDL cholesterol, TC/HDL ratio, LDL cholesterol, triglycerides (TG) at time of diagnosis and then every 1 to 3 years (more frequently if treatment has been initiated or changed. See Chapter 6)
- **Urine albumin/creatinine ratio ("ACR")** (see Chapter 6):
  - Type 1 diabetes: annually beginning 5 years after the onset of diabetes
  - Type 2 diabetes: at the time of diagnosis then annually
- **Blood creatinine level and calculation of creatinine clearance:** annually (unless kidney damage is present in which case these tests should be done at least every 6 months. See Chapter 6)

- **Blood pressure:** at every diabetes visit (see Chapter 6)
- **Screening for peripheral neuropathy** (with a 10-gram monofilament or tuning fork. See Chapter 6):
  - Type 1 diabetes: annually beginning 5 years after the onset of diabetes
  - Type 2 diabetes: at the time of diagnosis then annually
- **Foot examination** (see Chapter 6):
  - By your doctor: *at least* annually
  - By you: daily (see Chapter 6)
- **Eye exam** (by an experienced eye specialist. See Chapter 6):
  - Type 1 diabetes: annually, beginning 5 years after the onset of diabetes if you are 15 years of age or older
  - Type 2 diabetes: at the time of diagnosis and then every 1 to 2 years (more often if you have anything more than minimal retinopathy)

Top Ten Ways to Prevent Diabetes Complications

- Eating earnestly
- Exercising enthusiastically
- Learning for life
- Giving the heave-ho to harmful habits
- Going for great glucose

- Containing cholesterol and taming triglycerides
- Beating back blood pressure
- Eyeing your eye doctor
- Fussing over your feet
- Mastering medicines

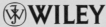

WILEY

Copyright © 2004 John Wiley & Sons Canada, Ltd. All rights reserved.
Cheat Sheet $2.99 value. Item 3360-2.
For more information about John Wiley & Sons Canada, Ltd. call 1-800-567-4797

For Dummies: Bestselling Book Series for Beginners

Diabetes
For Canadians

FOR

DUMMIES®

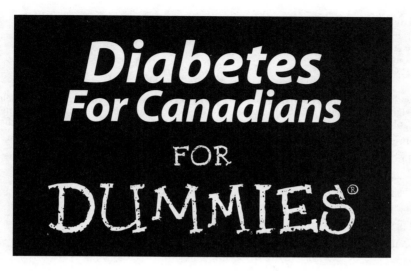

Diabetes
For Canadians
FOR
DUMMIES®

by Ian Blumer, M.D., F.R.C.P.(C)
Alan L. Rubin, M.D.

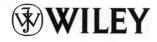

John Wiley & Sons Canada, Ltd

Diabetes For Canadians For Dummies®

Published by
John Wiley & Sons Canada, Ltd
6045 Freemont Boulevard
Mississauga, ON L5R 4J3
www.wiley.ca

National Library of Canada Cataloguing in Publication

Diabetes For Canadians For Dummies / Ian Blumer.

Includes index.

ISBN 0-470-83370-X

1. Diabetes–Popular works. I. Title.

RA645.D5B48 2003   616.4'62   C2003-905489-6

Printed in Canada

4 5 TRI 07 06

Distributed in Canada by John Wiley & Sons Canada, Ltd.

For general information on John Wiley & Sons Canada, Ltd., including all books published by Wiley Publishing, Inc., please call our warehouse, Tel 1-800-567-4797. For reseller information, including discounts and premium sales, please call our sales department, Tel 416-646-7992. For press review copies, author interviews, or other publicity information, please contact our marketing department, Tel: 416-646-4584, Fax 416-236-4448.

For authorization to photocopy items for corporate, personal, or educational use, please contact Cancopy, The Canadian Copyright Licensing Agency, One Yonge Street, Suite 1900, Toronto, ON, M5E 1E5 Tel 416-868-1620 Fax 416-868-1621; www.cancopy.com.

About the Authors

Ian Blumer, M.D., F.R.C.P.(C), is a diabetes specialist with a community practice in the Durham region of Ontario. He has a teaching appointment as a medical associate with Mount Sinai Hospital (part of the University of Toronto) and is actively involved in diabetes research. An enthusiastic lecturer, he has spoken about diabetes to numerous professional and lay audiences and has appeared regularly in the Canadian media. He is a member of the Clinical and Scientific Section of the Canadian Diabetes Association, the American Diabetes Association, and the European Association for the Study of Diabetes. Ian is the author of *What Your Doctor* Really *Thinks* (Dundurn, 1999) and the medical advisor for the *Everything Diabetes Book* (Adams Media, 2003). His popular Web site (www.ianblumer.com) offers practical advice on how to manage diabetes. Ian is married to a rheumatologist and has three children, the eldest of which, to Ian's astonishment, is now old enough that she is attending university. In his spare time, Ian can be found skiing down mogul runs and battling wind and waves during a sailing race. One day he hopes to emulate lucky Vancouverites who get to do both on the same day, though not necessarily at the same time. Ian welcomes your comments about this book at diabetes@ianblumer.com.

Alan L. Rubin, M.D., is a professional member of the American Diabetes Association and the Endocrine Society and has been in private practice specializing in diabetes and thyroid disease for more than 28 years. Dr. Rubin was Assistant Clinical Professor of Medicine at University of California Medical Center in San Francisco for 20 years. He has spoken about diabetes to professional medical audiences and non-medical audiences around the world. He has been a consultant to many pharmaceutical companies and companies that make diabetes products.

Dedication

This book is dedicated to Ian's parents, Rhoda and Jack, whose love, generosity, and wisdom are as cherished today as they were way back when.

This book is also dedicated to Alan's wife, Enid, and to Alan's children, Renee and Larry. Their patience, enthusiasm, and encouragement helped to make Alan's writing a real pleasure.

Acknowledgments

Ian Blumer would like to let his wonderful wife, Heather, know that now this book is completed, he promises to once again spend leisurely Sunday breakfasts with her instead of with his laptop.

Ian would like to express his appreciation to Marian Barltrop, a superb diabetes educator and his research assistant on this project. Without her immensely helpful footwork, Ian would still be writing Chapter 1. Ian would also like to thank Bin Chin, a terrific dietitian and Ian's nutrition teacher, for her invaluable help with the Food Groups Appendix. Thanks also to the dietitians from across Canada that contributed recipes to the book. Marlene Grass, R.N., the epitome of selfless dedication and a pioneer in childhood and young adult diabetes education, cannot be thanked enough, not only for her helpful suggestions but moreover for her guidance by way of example. Drs. Amir Hanna, Stewart Harris, Ralph Kern, and Bernard Zinman are all to be thanked for their helpful tips. A special thanks to Dr. Anne Kenshole for her keen insights and thoughtful suggestions. Randall McDonald (Omni Insurance) and Wayne Redford (Allstate) were kind enough to provide assurance about insurance. Jeff Hirst, BPHE, PFLC, a former Canadian Olympian who is now a fitness consultant (Training Zone Inc.), has been an invaluable resource in all matters relating to the role of exercise in good diabetes health. Thanks, Jeff.

To all the nurse educators and dietitians in Durham and Northumberland counties that have worked with Ian over the past 20 years, thanks for your tireless efforts. Your unwavering commitment to the patients we serve is a constant reminder of the importance and value of working as a diabetes health care team. Ian hopes this book carries that message to all who read it.

Not a day goes by that Ian does not marvel at the skills of his greatest mentor, Dr. Barney Berris. Dr. Berris, "a physician's physician," is the epitome of all that is admirable in a doctor. Ian's choice of a career in internal medicine is in no small measure a result of the example set by this fine man.

Ian would like to thank his colleague, Alan Rubin, whose book, *Diabetes For Dummies*, created a wonderful foundation upon which this book could be created.

One group of teachers — our patients — deserves special attention. Their trials and tribulations have been our raison d'être.

Lastly, Ian wishes to thank Lisa Berland and Allyson Latta, whose skillful editing of this book has reminded Ian why he should have paid much more attention to his English teachers and much less attention to the Habs.

Alan Rubin thanks the great acquisitions editor and midwife, Tami Booth; she deserves great appreciation for helping to deliver this new baby. Her optimism and her ideas actually made this book possible. Alan's project editor, Kelly Ewing, has made sure that this book follows the laws of grammar and is readable and understandable in the great *For Dummies* tradition. Thanks to Dr. Seymour Levin for the technical editing of this book.

Dietitian Nancy Bennett evaluated all the recipes in the original edition, cooked them, tasted them, and put them into a form that readers could follow. She also provided great food for thought about the role of the dietitian in diabetes care.

Alan wants to thank ophthalmologist Dr. John Norris of Pacific Eye Associates in San Francisco for helping him to see the place of the eye physician in diabetes care. He also wants to thank podiatrist Dr. Mark Pinter for helping him get a leg up on his specialty.

Librarians Mary Ann Zaremska and Nancy Phelps at St. Francis Memorial Hospital were tremendously helpful in providing the articles and books upon which the information in the book is based.

Alan wants to thank Dr. Richard Bernstein of Marin County, California, for the many years of learning, collaboration, and enjoyment together.

Ronnie and Michael Goldfield should definitely be considered the godparents of this book.

Alan's friends in the Dawn Patrol kept him laughing throughout the production of this book. Their willingness to follow him convinced him that others would be willing to read what he wrote.

Alan's teachers are too numerous to mention, but one group deserves special attention. They are his patients over the last 28 years, the people whose trials and tribulations caused him to seek the knowledge that you will find in this book.

This book is written on the shoulders of thousands of men and women who made the discoveries and held the committee meetings. Their accomplishments cannot possibly be given adequate acclaim. We owe them big time.

Publisher's Acknowledgments

We're proud of this book; please send us your comments at canadapt@wiley.com. Some of the people who helped bring this book to market include the following:

Acquisitions and Editorial

Associate Editor: Michelle Marchetti

Developmental Editor: Lisa Berland

Copy Editor: Allyson Latta

Production

Publishing Services Director: Karen Bryan

Project Manager: Elizabeth McCurdy

Project Coordinator: Robert Hickey

Layout and Graphics: Pat Loi

Proofreader: Susan Gaines

Indexer: Belle Wong

John Wiley & Sons Canada, Ltd.

    Bill Zerter, Chief Operating Officer

    Robert Harris, General Manager, Professional and Trade Division

Publishing and Editorial for Consumer Dummies

    Diane Graves Steele, Vice President and Publisher, Consumer Dummies

    Joyce Pepple, Acquisitions Director, Consumer Dummies

    Kristin A. Cocks, Product Development Director, Consumer Dummies

    Michael Spring, Vice President and Publisher, Travel

    Suzanne Jannetta, Editorial Director, Travel

Publishing for Technology Dummies

    Andy Cummings, Acquisitions Director

Composition Services

    Gerry Fahey, Executive Director of Production Services

    Debbie Stailey, Director of Composition Services

Contents at a Glance

Table of Contents

· ·

Introduction

*I*s there ever a good time to have diabetes? No, of course there isn't. But at the beginning of the 21st century, people with diabetes are better off than at any other time in history. A hundred years ago, people with diabetes did not live very long. As recently as 30 years ago, most people with diabetes were destined to suffer all sorts of complications often including blindness and amputations. But now we have the means to protect ourselves. We can lead not only long lives, but full, active, and healthy lives. And it all starts with knowledge. Because when it comes to diabetes, knowledge is power and the key to success.

Alan Rubin (one of the co-authors of this book you're holding) tells the funny story (in a black-humour sort of way) about the doctor who called his patient to give him the results of his blood tests):

"I have bad news and worse news," said the doctor.

"My gosh," said the patient. "What's the bad news?"

"Your lab tests indicate that you have only 24 hours to live," said the doctor.

"What could be worse than that?" said the patient.

"I've been trying to reach you since yesterday," said the doctor.

Diabetes is also good news/bad news. It's bad news to be told you have a health problem you could do without, thank you very much. But it can be good news if you see it as an opportunity to have a look at your lifestyle and make those changes that may have been due anyhow. It's never too late to start leading a healthier life!

As for humour, at times you will feel like doing anything but laughing about your diabetes. But scientific studies are clear about the benefits of a positive attitude. In a very few words: He who laughs, lasts. Also, people learn more and retain more when humour is part of the process. Our goal is not to trivialize human suffering by being comic about it, but to lighten the burden of a chronic disease by showing that it is not all doom and gloom.

About This Book

Diabetes For Canadians For Dummies is not meant to be read from cover to cover, although if you know nothing about diabetes, it might be a good approach to do so. This book is to serve as a source for information about diabetes, what causes it, how it affects you, and, most importantly, how to effectively deal with diabetes so that you can achieve and maintain good health.

Canada has a long and proud history of being in the forefront of diabetes research and therapy. *Diabetes For Canadians For Dummies* looks at the special issues that Canadians with diabetes have to face (like Ian's patient who returned to his car one February morning after his son's hockey practice, only to find his insulin frozen solid!) and uses the most recent Canadian Diabetes Association recommendations ("2003 Clinical Practice Guidelines for the Prevention and Management of Diabetes in Canada").

In addition to discussing the latest facts about diabetes, this book tells you about the best sources you can access to discover any information that comes out after the publication of this edition. You will find frequent reference to Web sites that offer excellent information. If you do not have Internet access yourself, you can still get online at your neighbourhood library. As Internet addresses change frequently, we generally will refer to the "home page" of a site, from where you can follow the links to the appropriate Web page.

As you may have already noticed, this book was co-written by Ian (that would be me) and Alan (that would be me). Fortunately, we share the same perspectives on diabetes management. (Thank goodness! Sure would have been hard to write this book otherwise.)

Conventions Used in This Book

Diabetes, as you know, is associated with sugar problems. But sugars come in many types, so doctors avoid using the words *sugar* and *glucose* interchangeably. In this book (unless we slip up), we use the word *glucose* rather than *sugar*. As well, because it gets to be redundant to keep adding *mmol/L* after every blood glucose value to which we refer, you can safely assume that when we say, for example, that a normal fasting blood glucose is under 6.1, we mean 6.1 *mmol/L*.

What You Don't Have to Read

Throughout the book, you will find shaded areas, which are called sidebars. These sidebars contain material that is interesting but not essential. We hereby give you permission to skip them if the material inside them is of no particular interest to you. You will still understand everything else.

Foolish Assumptions

This book assumes that you know nothing about diabetes. You will not suddenly have to face a term that is not explained and that you never heard of before. For those who already know a lot about diabetes, you can find more in-depth explanations. You can pick and choose how much you want to know about a subject. The key points are clearly marked.

How This Book Is Organized

This book is divided into six parts to help you find out all you can about the topic of diabetes.

Part I: Dealing with the Diagnosis of Diabetes

To slay the dragon, you have to be able to identify it. This part sorts out the different types of diabetes and looks at how you get diabetes and how you can help protect your family from developing it.

In this part, you will also find out how to deal with the emotional and psychological consequences of the diagnosis and what all those big words mean.

Part II: How Diabetes Affects Your Body

Diabetes may be *associated* with "sugar," but to say that it is the *same* as sugar is like saying that a car is the same as a spark plug. Diabetes is far more than that and can affect every part of you. If you understand diabetes, you will understand how your body works both when it is healthy and when it is not.

In this part, you find out what you need to know about both the acute and long-term problems that diabetes can cause. You also find out about sexual problems related to diabetes and about how diabetes can affect pregnancy.

Part III: Rule Your Diabetes: Don't Let It Rule You!

In this part, you discover all the tools available to treat diabetes. You find out about the health care team that is there to assist you and you learn about the ways that you can make effective use of good nutrition and exercise to keep yourself healthy. You also discover the medications that may assist you with controlling your blood glucose.

We also take a look at alternative and complementary therapies, including natural products that people with diabetes often take.

Part IV: Special Considerations for Living with Diabetes

Diabetes affects people differently depending on their age group. In this part, you hear about those differences and how to manage them. You also find out about diabetes in Aboriginal peoples.

We look at employment and insurance difficulties that people with diabetes can face and how to address them. This part also discusses diabetes and driving and offers suggestions to help you maintain a driver's licence and to obtain a commercial licence. Last, we look at the implications of having diabetes on one's ability to pilot an aircraft.

Part V: The Part of Tens

This part presents a concise summary of the most crucial stuff that people with diabetes should know. Find out not only the Top Ten Ways to Prevent Complications, but also the Top Ten Frequently Asked Questions. All that and more!

Part VI: Appendices

This part of the book takes you on a cross-Canada food trek as we present recipes submitted by dietitians from every province and territory. You will also find information on the Food Group System used in diabetes meal planning. In this part you will find out the best diabetes-oriented Internet sites. Last, we present a Glossary; we define words as we go along, but in case you forget what a term means, you can quickly flip to the back of the book.

Icons Used in This Book

The icons tell you what you must know, what you should know, and what you might find interesting but can live without.

This icon indicates a story about one of our patients.

This icon marks paragraphs where we define terms.

When you see this icon, it means the information is critical and is not to be missed.

This icon points out when you should contact your health care team (for example, if your blood glucose control is in need of improving or if you need a particular test done). Your health care team includes your family doctor, your diabetes specialist, your diabetes educator, your dietitian, your eye doctor, your pharmacist, and, when necessary, other specialists (such as a podiatrist, dentist, cardiologist, kidney specialist, neurologist, emergency room physician, and so forth). We will let you know which member of your team you should contact. (Incidentally, the most important member of your health care team is *you*.)

This icon is used when we share a practical, time-saving piece of advice, sometimes providing some additional detail on an important point.

Part I

Dealing with the Diagnosis of Diabetes

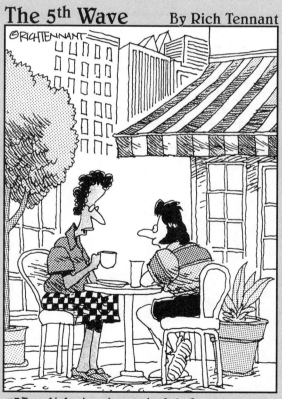

The 5th Wave   By Rich Tennant

"No, diabetes is not fatal, it's not contagious, and it doesn't mean you'll always get half my desserts."

In this part . . .

You have found out that you or a loved one has diabetes. What do you do now? This part looks at the cause of your diabetes and how it can make you feel — both mentally and physically.

Chapter 1

Membership in a Club You Didn't Ask to Join

As a person with diabetes, you already know that diabetes isn't "just a glucose problem." In fact, the moment you were told you had diabetes, many different thoughts may have run through your mind. You have feelings, and you have your own personal story. You are not the same person as your next-door neighbour or your sister or your friend, and your diabetes and the way that you respond to its challenges are unique to you.

And unless you live alone on a desert island, your diabetes doesn't affect just you. Your family, friends, and co-workers are influenced by your diabetes and by their desire to help you.

This chapter shows you some coping skills to help you deal with your diabetes and the way it affects your important relationships.

What Is Diabetes?

Since we are going to be spending so much time discussing diabetes, let's start by defining the condition. That should be a simple enough task — except that many dictionaries (including, sorry to say, Canadian ones) define it incorrectly. The simplest, *correct* definition is that diabetes is a disease in which there is too much glucose in the blood due to insufficient or ineffective insulin. Although that is technically correct, it misses out on so, so much, because diabetes is not just a problem of glucose; it is a *whole body* problem. To make this point, Ian has had a burst of creativity and has gone ahead and made up his own definition of diabetes: "a disease in which there are high blood glucose levels *and* an increased risk of damage to the body, much of which is preventable."

"Diabetes" is actually the short form for *diabetes mellitus*. The Romans had noticed that the urine of certain people was *mellitus*, the Latin word for *sweet*. The Greeks noticed that when people with sweet urine drank, fluids came out in the urine almost as fast as they went in the mouth, like a siphon. They called this by the Greek word for *siphon* — diabetes. Hence, diabetes mellitus, but we think this is much better captured by the 17th-century definition of diabetes: "the pissing evil." Talk about calling it the way you see it!

You Are Not Alone

Ian remembers encountering a huge lineup in front of one particular exhibit while attending a diabetes conference a few years back. There were so many people in line, in fact, that he figured there must have been some amazing new breakthrough product being demonstrated. Well, as it turns out, the big attraction was actually Nicole Johnson, the 1999 Miss America. She was there to talk about how she managed her diabetes.

Perhaps you have seen a movie staring the Academy-award winning actress Halle Berry. It's not likely that you noticed her diabetes affecting her acting, or her beauty for that matter. Similarly, you likely did not notice diabetes preventing the great success of athletes like Bobbie Clarke, Jackie Robinson or golf star Scott Verplank, authors like Ernest Hemingway or H. G. Wells, musicians like B. B. King and Jerry Garcia (of the Grateful Dead — which came long before Cherry Garcia ice cream!) or inventors like Thomas Edison, to name but a few famous people with diabetes.

John Dennis is a Canadian who likes to sail. That he also has diabetes does not make him unique in the sailing community. Oh; did we happen to mention where he sails? That would be circumnavigating the globe. Alone!

You may not have spoken to Stephen Steele, but it is quite possible he has spoken to you. Stephen is a commercial pilot with a major Canadian airline. (You'll get to know Stephen better in Chapter 18.) And in the event that you have the bad luck to be in dire straits on some sinking vessel off the Atlantic coast, it is quite possible that the hero plucking you from the ocean will be none other than Major Chuck Grenkow, a Medal of Bravery–winning Canadian Forces pilot and aircraft commander performing search and rescue operations with the Canadian military. Oh, by the way, they both have insulin-treated diabetes.

Diabetes is a common disease, so it's bound to occur in some very uncommon people. Have a look at the Famous Diabetics Web site (`www.angelarose.com/FamousDiabetics/index.html`). But one does not have to be famous to be considered exceptional. Indeed, every day of the week we see special people, people who have diabetes yet look after families, work in automotive plants or office buildings, write exams, go to movies, and do their best to live life to the fullest. People just like you.

The point is, diabetes should not define your life. You are the same person the day after you found out you had diabetes as you were the day before. It just happens that you have been given an additional issue to deal with. Diabetes should not stop you from doing what you want to do with your life. Certainly, it does complicate things in some ways, but if you follow the rules of good diabetes care that are discussed in this book, you may actually be *healthier* than people without diabetes who smoke, overeat, under-exercise, or engage in other, unhealthy activities.

Handling the News

Do you remember what you were doing when you found out that you or a loved one had diabetes? Unless you were too young to understand, the news was likely quite a shock. Suddenly you had a condition from which people get sick and can die. The following sections describe the normal stages of reacting to a diagnosis of a major medical condition such as diabetes.

The stage of denial

You may have begun by denying that you had diabetes, despite all the evidence to the contrary. Your doctor may have inadvertently helped you to deny by saying that you had "just a bit of sugar" or "borderline diabetes," which is an impossibility equivalent to having "a touch of pregnancy." You probably looked for any evidence that the whole thing was a mistake, and you may not have followed the advice you were given. But ultimately, you had to accept the diagnosis and begin to gather the information needed to start to help yourself.

Hopefully, you not only came to accept the diabetes diagnosis yourself, but also shared the news with your family and other people close to you. Having diabetes isn't something to be ashamed of, and it isn't something that you should have to hide from anyone.

Your diabetes isn't your fault. You didn't want to have diabetes. You didn't try to get diabetes. And no one can catch it from you. It is estimated that about seven and a half percent of Canadians have diabetes. That's well over 2 million Canadians with diabetes. You have joined a very, very large club! Next time you are out shopping, take a look around you. The likelihood is very high that some of the people you are looking at also have diabetes.

When you and others are accepting and open about having diabetes, you'll find that you're far from alone in your situation. (If you don't believe us, read the section "You Are Not Alone" earlier in this chapter.) And you will likely find it comforting to know there are others with whom you can relate and from whom you can draw support. For example, one of Alan's patients told him about an uplifting experience that she had. She arrived at work one morning and was very worried when she realized that she had forgotten her insulin. But she remembered that a co-worker had diabetes and was able to borrow some insulin. Another time, at a party, she left the crowd and stepped into a friend's bedroom to give herself an injection of insulin — and found a man there doing the same thing. She recalls their camaraderie at discovering one another.

The stage of anger

When you've passed the stage of denying that you or a loved one has diabetes, you may become angry that you're saddled with this "terrible" diagnosis. But you'll quickly find that diabetes isn't so terrible, and that you can't rid yourself of the disease. Your anger only worsens your situation, and it's detrimental in the following ways:

- If you aim your anger at a person, you hurt him or her.
- You will often feel guilt if your anger harms you and those close to you.
- Anger will often keep you from successfully managing your diabetes.

As long as you're angry, you are not in a problem-solving mode. Diabetes requires your focus and attention. Channel your anger into creative ways of managing your diabetes. (For ways to manage your diabetes, see Part III.)

The stage of bargaining

The anger that you experience may lead to a stage where you or your loved ones become increasingly aware of your mortality and bargain for more time. At this point, most people with diabetes realize that they have plenty of life ahead of them, but they start to feel overwhelmed by the talk of complications, blood tests, and pills or insulin. You may experience depression, which makes good diabetes care all the more difficult.

Studies have shown that people with diabetes suffer from depression at a rate that is two to four times higher than the rate for the general population. Those with diabetes are also more likely to experience feelings of anxiety.

If you suffer from depression, you may feel that your diabetes situation creates problems for you that justify your being depressed. You may rationalize your depression by saying that it's caused by the following reasons:

- You don't have the freedom to eat whatever you want whenever you want.
- You have to adjust your leisure activities.
- You may feel that you're too tired to overcome difficulties.
- You may dread the future and possible diabetic complications.
- You may feel that diabetes hinders you as you try to form new relationships.
- You may feel annoyed over all the minor inconveniences of dealing with diabetes.

All of the preceding concerns are legitimate, but also they are all surmountable. How do you handle your many concerns and fend off depression? The following are a few important methods:

- Try to achieve excellent blood glucose control.
- Begin a regular exercise program.
- Recognize that not every abnormal blip in your blood glucose is your fault.

The final stage: Moving on

If you can't overcome the depression brought on by your diabetes concerns, you may need to consider therapy. But you probably won't reach that point. You may experience the various stages of reacting to your diabetes in a different order than we describe in the previous sections. Some stages may be more prominent; others may be hardly noticeable.

Almost everyone with diabetes goes through periods when they pay less attention to their health, do less blood glucose testing, fall off their lifestyle treatment program, and even start missing some of their medicines. That is a fact of diabetes life and there is no need to feel guilty. By the time you recognize that this is happening to you, you will probably also discover that you are ready to get back on track. The trick is to not dwell on perceived "failure," but to refocus on future success.

Don't feel that any anger, denial, or sadness is wrong. These are natural coping mechanisms that serve a psychological purpose — for a brief time. Allow yourself to have these feelings, but then drop them. Move on and learn to live normally with your diabetes. You will be surprised how much more easily you can control your diabetes when your spirits improve.

When you're having trouble coping

You wouldn't hesitate to seek help for your physical ailments associated with diabetes, but you may be very reluctant to seek help when you can't adjust psychologically to diabetes. The problem is that sooner or later, depression or anxiety will prevent you from properly looking after your diabetes, and as a result your general health too will suffer. The following symptoms are indicators that it is time for you to seek professional help:

- You can't sleep.

- You have no energy.

- You can't think clearly.

- You can't find activities that interest or amuse you.

- You have no appetite.

- You find no humour in anything.

- You feel worthless.

- You have frequent thoughts of suicide.

Your sense of hopelessness may include the feeling that no one else can help you — but that simply isn't true. Your family physician is the first person to go to for advice. He or she may help you to see the need for some short-term or long-term therapy. Well-trained therapists can see solutions that you can't see in your current state. You need to find a therapist whom you can trust, so that when you're feeling low you can talk to this person and feel assured that he or she is very interested in your welfare.

Your therapist may decide that your situation is appropriate for medication to treat the anxiety or depression. Currently, many drugs are available that have been proven safe and effective. Sometimes a brief period of medication is enough to help you cope with your difficulties.

You can also find help in a support group. The huge and continually growing number of support groups shows their worth. In most support groups, participants share their stories and problems, which helps everyone involved to cope with their own feelings of isolation, futility, or depression. A good place to start is to contact a local chapter of the Canadian Diabetes Association (www.diabetes.ca). Another good place to seek out support is the online community. There are now many diabetes-oriented newsgroups (such as alt.support.diabetes) where people share their common concerns. The American Diabetes Association (www.diabetes.org) also has some excellent community forums.

Chapter 2

Glucose and You

• •

In This Chapter

▶ Diagnosing diabetes

▶ Recognizing how high glucose makes you feel

▶ Controlling glucose

▶ Losing control of glucose

▶ The financial impact of diabetes in Canada

• •

The ancient Greeks and Romans knew about diabetes. Fortunately, the way they tested for the condition — by tasting the urine — has gone by the wayside.

Most people with diabetes are diagnosed when they have their blood glucose level measured either as part of a routine check-up with their family doctor, or for some other coincidental reason (such as at the time of an insurance application or in preparation for surgery). Occasionally, a person with diabetes has the condition diagnosed after they develop symptoms that they recognize may be due to high blood glucose and they see their doctor asking to be tested for this.

Ian recently saw a 50-year-old businessman in the office. He had started to get up during the night to pass his urine. At first he blamed it on his prostate, but when he noticed that he was unexpectedly losing weight he recalled that a close relative had experienced similar symptoms and had been found to have diabetes. The businessman decided he should be tested for this too. His blood glucose turned out to be two times higher than normal. Ian had him meet up with a dietitian and a diabetes educator, and, with proper lifestyle measures, his glucose level was down to normal in a matter of weeks. He finally started to get a good night's sleep again, his energy improved, and his business took off. Now, his competitors may not have been too happy, but that's a different story.

You may have done some searching in books or on the Internet and come across another form of diabetes called *diabetes insipidus*. This term refers to an *entirely* different condition than diabetes mellitus. The only thing they have in common is a tendency to pass lots of urine. And now that we've clarified that, you will not see diabetes insipidus mentioned again in this book (unless you count the index at the back!).

What Is Glucose?

The sweetness of the urine with which the ancients had first-hand experience comes from *glucose*, also known as blood *sugar*. There are many different kinds of sugar, but the important one when it comes to diabetes is glucose. Glucose is the fuel that your body uses to provide instant energy so that muscles can move and important chemical reactions can take place. Sugar is a carbohydrate, one group of the three sources of energy in the body. The others are protein and fat, which we discuss in greater detail in Chapter 10.

Unlike in high school chemistry class, here we are going to let you off easy and, apart from our discussion about nutrition therapy, we won't talk about all the other sugars that are around. But just in case you are wondering, some examples of other sugars are fructose (the sugar found in fruits and vegetables) and sucrose (actually a combination of glucose and fructose).

How Diabetes Is Diagnosed

Diagnosing diabetes should be simple. You know by now that you have diabetes when your glucose level is too high. But what, exactly, is too high? One way to think of "too high" is to think of the level of blood glucose that can cause damage to your body. More difficult is attaching a specific number to that level. Different countries have different ways of deciding that, but in Canada we consider someone to have diabetes if they meet *any* one of the following three criteria:

- ✔ A **casual** blood glucose level ("casual" is defined as any time of day or night, without regard to the interval since the last time you ingested anything containing calories) equal to or greater than 11.1 millimoles per litre (mmol/L) with symptoms of high blood glucose (we discuss these symptoms in the next section).

- ✔ A **fasting** blood glucose level ("fasting" is defined as 8 or more hours without calorie intake) equal to or greater than 7.0 mmol/L.

- ✔ A blood glucose level equal to or greater than 11.1 mmol/L, when tested 2 hours after ingesting 75 grams of glucose as part of what is called a **"glucose tolerance test**." Doctors used to order this test quite often, but nowadays doctors have learned that it is usually unnecessary. The diagnosis of diabetes can generally be made more easily with one of the other two tests we just mentioned.

Testing positive for one of the above criteria is not enough to result in a diagnosis of diabetes. Any one of the tests must be positive on *another* day to establish the diagnosis. More than one patient has come to us with a diagnosis of diabetes after having been tested only once, and then when we retested their blood glucose it turned out to be normal. They didn't have diabetes after all. Remember that the diagnosis of diabetes should be based on a blood sample taken from a *vein*. If you borrow your friend's glucose meter (which you shouldn't do by the way; as we discuss in Chapter 9) and find your glucose level to be high, see your doctor to have a blood sample drawn at a laboratory. Don't diagnose yourself based on a glucose meter result.

The only time that a diagnosis of diabetes can be made without repeating a blood glucose test is if your blood glucose level is very high and you are clearly ill from it.

If you have visited U.S. Web sites you may have noticed that there (and nowhere else) they use different units — called milligrams per decilitre (abbreviated mg/dL). To convert mg/dL to mmol/L you divide mg/dL by 18: for example 200 mg/dL divided by 18 equals 11.1 mmol/L. And we promise that will be the last time we *ever* mention how they measure blood glucose outside of Canada!

How Having High Glucose Makes You Feel

To understand the symptoms of diabetes, it is helpful to know a bit about how your body normally handles glucose.

The pancreas makes a hormone called *insulin*. (We talk more about the pancreas in Chapter 3.) Insulin finely controls the level of glucose in your blood. A *hormone* is a chemical substance made in one part of the body that travels (usually through the bloodstream) to a distant part of the body where it performs its work. Insulin acts like a key to open the outside lining of a cell so that glucose can enter the cell. If glucose can't enter the cell, it cannot provide energy to the body.

Insulin is an amazing substance. Not only does it allow glucose to enter cells, but also it enables fat and muscle to form and allows for the storage of glucose in the liver (in a form called *glycogen*) for use when you may not be eating properly. How clever is that? Without insulin, the body's tissues start to break down. Perhaps you have seen a heart-rending photo of an ill-looking child with diabetes from before insulin was discovered, and the thrilling photo of that same child, now the picture of health, after starting insulin therapy. (We talk more about the discovery of insulin — and Canada's important contribution — in Chapter 3).

The pancreas normally functions like a precision tool; releasing just the right amount of insulin to keep your body's blood glucose in a remarkably tight range of about 3.3 to 6.1mmol/L. If the pancreas is not able to produce the proper amount of insulin, or if the insulin it makes is not working effectively, then your blood glucose level will start to rise. If it goes up just a bit, you will not have any symptoms, but if it reaches as high as 10.0 mmol/L or so, glucose begins to filter through the kidneys and spill into the urine (making it sweet). It is at that stage that you will begin to experience symptoms (see below). It's a shame that people don't get symptoms until the glucose level is almost twice the normal level, because by the time symptoms arise, damage may already have occurred to the body. We would be much better off if even slightly high glucose levels made our skin glow bright green; that way we would all know when there is a problem.

The following list contains the most common early symptoms of diabetes and how they occur. You may find that some of these remind you of what you were feeling when you found out you had diabetes:

- **Frequent urination and thirst:** High blood glucose makes more urine form, and the more urine you make, the more fluid you lose from your body. The large quantity of urine makes you feel the need to urinate more frequently during the day and to get up at night to empty your bladder, which keeps filling up. As the amount of water in your blood declines, you feel thirsty and drink much more frequently. Many people with newly diagnosed diabetes believe that they are urinating more often because they are drinking more, but it is actually the other way around.

- **Fatigue:** Because glucose can't enter most cells in the absence of insulin, if you have uncontrolled diabetes, glucose can't be used as a fuel to move muscles and help other tissues function properly. And just as you do when you try to pedal a bike with deflated tires, you get tired awfully quickly.

- **Weight loss:** Weight loss is common among people with newly diagnosed diabetes (especially if you have *type 1* diabetes, as we discuss in Chapter 4). People with diabetes either don't have enough insulin or the insulin they have is not working effectively. Insulin helps the body's tissues to be strong and healthy. Without proper insulin action, the body's tissues start to break down. You lose muscle tissue. You lose fat tissue. And as these tissues are lost, the body wastes away (again, this is especially true of type 1 diabetes). Your blood glucose level is high, but the glucose just can't work. It's as if your car has a full gas tank but the fuel line is blocked. The gauge reads "high" but the car stalls anyhow.

- **Persistent vaginal infections**: As blood glucose rises, all the fluids in your body contain higher levels of glucose. Women, therefore, have higher glucose levels in their vaginal secretions. Yeast organisms thrive in a high glucose environment and as a result women with elevated glucose levels are prone to vaginal yeast infections. Symptoms include vaginal itching or burning, an abnormal discharge from the vagina, and sometimes an odour.

- **Blurred vision:** When the blood glucose level changes substantially, it causes the amount of fluid in the eyeball to change also. This alters the way that light passes through your eye, making it bend more than usual and making things around you look blurry. Have you ever noticed how a knife in a glass of water looks bent? The same sort of thing is going on in your eye.

In the same way that your eyesight can become blurry as your blood glucose rises, it can become blurry as your blood glucose falls. Many people with diabetes become understandably alarmed when their vision gets *worse* after they first start diabetes therapy, but in fact this is often a *good* sign, as it means their treatment program is working. The visual blurring in this setting is caused by a change in the way that light is bending as it goes through the eye, and is not a result of damage to the eye. Your vision will return to its usual state within a few weeks. Do not waste your hard-earned money on expensive glasses. Buy inexpensive over-the-counter glasses at your neighbourhood drugstore, and you will likely find that within a month you can give them away.

Ian well remembers meeting Sam O'Reilly, a 60-year-old man who had just been diagnosed with diabetes. This was discovered shortly after he developed bothersome thirst and frequent passage of urine and had gone to the hospital to get checked out. His blood glucose level was found to be 25 mmol/L. He was immediately started on pills to reduce his glucose level and an appointment was arranged to see Ian 2 weeks thereafter. About 5 days before his appointment, Mr. O'Reilly called Ian's office in a near panic. He was sure he was going blind. Days after starting his new pills, his thirst and urine problems had improved, but now he could no longer read his daily newspaper or even see the television; everything had become one big blur. Ian had him come to the office right away, not because he was worried about Mr. O'Reilly but to reassure him. The only prescription Mr. O'Reilly needed turned out to be "tincture of time," and this worked perfectly. Indeed, within a week or so Mr. O'Reilly's eyesight was back to normal.

Controlling Glucose

Although there may never be a *good* time to have diabetes, far better to have it now than 100 years ago, when almost no therapy was available. Until insulin was discovered in the 1920s, little could be done to help people with diabetes. For years after that, insulin was the mainstay of therapy, but in the middle years of the last century a number of different drugs were discovered that combat high blood glucose (hyperglycemia). And in the later years of the 20th century, further discoveries made several entirely new types of medicine available. As Ian likes to say, it was about time that diabetes specialists were given more tools; we were getting very jealous of cardiologists who seemed to be getting all the neat drugs. Nowadays virtually anyone with diabetes can have excellent blood glucose control. It may not always be easy to achieve, but it *can* be achieved and, indeed, *must* be achieved if you are going to keep healthy.

Treatment is not just a matter of taking medicine, of course. In fact, medicine is often the least important of the diabetes treatments. The three key therapies are:

- Diet (more aptly called nutrition therapy; see Chapter 10)
- Exercise (see Chapter 10)
- Medication (see Chapters 11 and 12)

Most people with diabetes require a combination of all three of these strategies.

Losing Control of Glucose

You will find that once you improve your blood glucose control, you will feel better. You won't be running to the bathroom around the clock, your energy level will improve, and you will have a better sense of well-being. There will be times, however, when your blood glucose control worsens and some of your symptoms may start to return. You may find that things worsen if you are under greater stress, or if you have gotten off track with your nutrition plan, or if there has been yet another February blizzard and the idea of going out for your daily walk is just too daunting.

There are two main things to remember when your glucose control worsens:

- If you are feeling reasonably well, then even if your blood glucose levels climb up into the high teens (or even somewhat higher) there is no immediate danger to you. (The exception to this is if you have type 1 diabetes and are developing ketones. See Chapter 5 for a discussion of ketoacidosis). A few days of blood glucose readings of 20 will not damage your organs.
- Take it as a message that something is wrong and take corrective action. This may be as simple as adjusting your diet or restarting your exercise plan. Perhaps you have simply forgotten to refill a prescription for your oral hypoglycemic agent (see Chapter 11 for a discussion of these medicines), in which case a trip to the pharmacy is in order.

If your blood glucose readings have risen to the high teens or higher and you are feeling unwell (or if you have type 1 diabetes and you have developed ketones), then you need to seek immediate medical assistance. If you are very ill, proceed to the nearest emergency department. If you are not feeling all that badly, you may first contact your physician. (As we discuss in Chapter 5, some diabetes educators are trained and empowered to assist you with these situations also.)

Diabetes in Canada

Diabetes is a serious health problem, both for the individual with diabetes and for society as a whole. In Canada, there are more than 2 million people with diabetes (many of whom are not diagnosed). The older you get the more likely you are to have diabetes — some estimates suggest that as many as one out of every five people over the age of 60 in Canada has diabetes.

Canada is not unique in this realm. Indeed, virtually every country is experiencing alarming growth rates of diabetes and it is estimated that by the year 2010 there will be 300 million people world-wide with diabetes. Researchers once believed that the increasing numbers were a result of the advancing average age of the population, but recent evidence suggests that it may simply be the result of the fact that as we get older we tend to become overweight. Thus it may not be aging in itself that makes us more likely to get diabetes. (The moral: Eat properly and exercise whether you are 2 or 82.)

Interestingly, Japanese Sumo wrestlers — not exactly lightweights — have an extraordinarily high likelihood of getting diabetes. And it's even greater once they retire — as high as 40 percent!

The yearly economic costs of diabetes in Canada are estimated to be a staggering $12 billion. That is not a misprint. That's $12 billion! That works out to an average of $6,000 for every man, woman, and child with diabetes and even at that likely represents an underestimate. Can you just imagine the ways you could spend that money?

As a diabetes specialist practising in Canada, Ian has been terribly frustrated by the lack of attention that governments and hospital administrators have traditionally paid to diabetes. Diabetes is not a dramatic illness like heart disease. Diabetes usually does not draw on the emotional purse strings in the way that cancer (appropriately) does. And diabetes does not have the aura of glamour and mystique that surrounds complex procedures such as brain or heart surgery. Many people even think that with insulin and other therapies, diabetes is "just an inconvenience." Surely these people do not have diabetes themselves.

There has long been a tendency amongst health care policy-makers to address what are sometimes cynically called "sexy" problems, including the illnesses just mentioned. Diabetes simply hasn't been on the radar screen. Indeed, hospital administrators have reduced staff at diabetes education centres as they try to deal with their own fiscal restraints. Diabetes education is considered expendable because administrators and bureaucrats do not see short-term return on their economic investments. And that is a tragedy, because money spent on diabetes education would come back a hundredfold in savings, preventing complications and thus keeping people with diabetes healthy (and out of hospital!).

Thankfully, governments in Canada are finally coming to grips with the need to improve diabetes services and, in particular, working toward initiating preventive strategies. Hospitals are still lagging behind, though, and we can only hope that, working in concert with government and with the encouragement (read "pressure") of people like you and physicians like us, hospitals will not only stop cutting back on diabetes services but enhance them. Even better, let's get diabetes education centres out of hospitals and into the communities where they belong!

For a further discussion about the health care costs of diabetes in Canada, have a look at *Diabetes in Canada,* Second Edition, issued by Health Canada (www.hc-sc.gc.ca/ pphb-dgspsp/publicat/dic-dac2/ english/01cover_e.html).

Chapter 3

Figuring Out the Cause of Your Diabetes

*Y*ou may not think that having a personal relationship with one of your body organs is possible or even desirable. Then again, maybe it's just that you haven't had a chance to meet some of them up close and personal. In which case, this chapter is just for you.

When we think "diabetes," we (doctors and non-doctors alike) tend to think "pancreas," as if there is no other player. Well, that risks offending our fat cells and our muscle cells and, importantly, our liver. And we wouldn't want to do that, would we? Of course not. So let's take a look at the role each of these key participants has played in your diabetes. But please don't get mad at your organs; they didn't do this to you on purpose. In fact, in some ways it was beyond their control — their genetic destiny, in a sense. Which of course adds to the importance of picking your parents carefully, though that remains a little bit impractical, even with modern technology.

How Your Organs Make Music

You may not think of your organs as being music makers (singing and other, ruder noises notwithstanding), but when it comes to controlling glucose, your body is engaged in a wonderfully intricate symphony with each organ playing its part.

Glucose regulation starts the moment you begin to eat. When you ingest certain types of food, it gets broken down inside your gut into glucose, which is then absorbed across the lining of the small intestine into your blood. Once inside your blood, the glucose travels around your body looking for a nice place to go. Some of the glucose gets used by your brain and some gets taken up and stored in your liver and muscles (in a form called *glycogen*). Your muscles use some of the glucose straight away as they do their work. And fat cells store some of it as, well, fat (technically called *triglycerides*).

As you can see, there are several organs involved in glucose metabolism. So, with apologies to Raquel Welch and Hollywood, let's take a Fantastic Voyage inside our insides.

The pancreas

Unless you have diabetes, you probably don't ever think about that funny-looking organ tucked behind your stomach. Well, even if you do have diabetes, it's not likely that your dinnertime conversation centres around this tadpole-shaped (yuk!), 25.5-centimetre (10-inch) long, 80-gram (3-oz) organ. Figure 3-1 shows its location in your body.

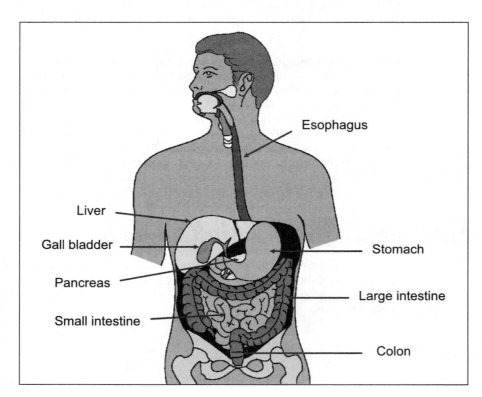

Figure 3-1:
The pancreas and liver.

The pancreas has two main functions. One is to produce enzymes, which are then released into your small intestine to assist with the breakdown of food. That is called the pancreas's *exocrine* function. The cells responsible for this take up 95 percent of the pancreas. People with diabetes seldom have this type of problem and we won't be discussing that part of things further.

Your pancreas's second task is called its *endocrine* function and that has everything to do with your diabetes. Within the pancreas are clusters of hormone-producing cells called *islet* cells. The most important of these islet cells when it comes to diabetes is the *beta* cell; it is the beta cell which produces and releases into the blood stream a hormone called *insulin*. A normal pancreas has about 1.5 million islet cells (which, if extracted and lumped together, could still fit inside a thimble. Note: Please do not try this at home!).

The pancreas also produces other hormones. We talk about one of those, *glucagon,* in Chapter 5. The others have little to do with diabetes.

The liver

Perhaps we are admitting our bias here, but we kind of feel bad for the liver. Apart from when people cook liver (and most people don't even like it), the only time it seems to get attention is when someone is suffering from hepatitis.

Your liver has many, many tasks to fulfill, including helping to rid your body of certain toxins and producing crucial proteins, such as clotting factors that prevent you from bleeding. The liver's role in glucose metabolism is to serve as a storage depot for excess glucose, removing it from or delivering it to the blood, depending on your body's needs at any given time.

The fat cells

You may know that if you are overweight you are more prone to getting type 2 diabetes. But not all fat tissue is the same. There is fat *inside* the abdomen (called *visceral fat*) and there is fat in the abdominal wall and legs and arms (called *non-visceral fat*; how creative is that?). Depending on how much of each of these types of fat you have, your risk for getting diabetes will vary. We discuss this further in the next section.

The fat cells' role in glucose metabolism is to store extra glucose (as fat). For this reason, even if you were to entirely avoid fats in your diet, you can still easily gain excess weight if you were eating excess calories (such as ingesting too many carbohydrates). Imagine eating 2 dozen apples and 1 pound of icing sugar a day. You wouldn't have seen an ounce of fat — not right away, that is. The fat would appear soon enough, though, but about a foot and a half lower than your lips!

The muscles

When you walked into the bookstore or library to pick up this book, you were using your muscles and, without even thinking about it, your muscles were actively using glucose to do their work. Some of this glucose comes from stores within muscle and some comes from actively extracting glucose from your blood. When we think "muscles" we tend to think "power" or "strength." We should also think "fuel," because glucose is a key energy source that your muscles need to work properly.

Hitting the right notes

When things are going right, as soon as your blood glucose level rises after eating, your pancreas releases insulin into the bloodstream. The insulin attaches to the lining of the cells and, as if a key has opened a door, the cells then allow the glucose to enter. As soon as the glucose level falls back to normal, the pancreas shuts off production of insulin (good thing too; otherwise we would always have low blood glucose; a condition called "hypoglycemia") and your glucose level immediately stabilizes.

If you haven't recently eaten, your body has to look elsewhere for glucose. Your insulin level will be low and this allows your liver to release some of its stored glucose into the blood stream and to actually make glucose out of protein, which it then releases into the blood. Your organs then use the glucose.

Your body even has a backup plan. Say you've been feeling unwell for a few days and haven't been eating properly. You may not have been eating enough to keep up with your body's demands for glucose, and your liver's stores of glucose (glycogen) may already have been all used up. So where will your body turn for its source of fuel? Well, your clever body will, like a hybrid car, look for alternative fuels and start to break down fat tissue, which releases *fatty acids* into the blood. These fatty acids serve as an alternative source of energy to keep you and your organs going.

Insulin does the following:

- ✔ Allows your muscle cells to extract glucose from your blood (to be used as a source of energy to power your muscles).

- ✔ Allows your fat cells to extract glucose from your blood (to be stored as fat).

- ✔ Stops your liver from releasing excess glucose into your blood.

What Happens When Your Organs Hit the Wrong Notes?

The intricate system we describe above is the way things are *supposed to* work. And if they did, you wouldn't have diabetes. But you do have diabetes, so something has gone wrong. That's not your fault. You didn't want things to go wrong and you sure as heck didn't intentionally make things go wrong. So don't feel guilty.

If you have type 2 diabetes (far and away the most common form, as we discuss further in Chapter 4), your *main* problem is that the insulin your pancreas is making is not working properly. This is called *insulin resistance*. As you eat, your blood glucose level goes up and your pancreas releases more insulin into the blood, but, using the analogy above, your insulin cannot unlock the key on the cell lining and so the glucose cannot enter your cells. Instead, it hangs around in your bloodstream. And that is why your blood glucose level goes up as high as it does. Eventually it gets so high that it spills out into the urine, making both you and your urine the sweet things that you are.

The degree to which you may have insulin resistance is significantly related not just to how much fat tissue you have, but also to where it is located. Visceral fat (the stuff within the abdomen) is the type of fat most likely to cause insulin resistance, followed by fat within the abdominal wall and fat elsewhere on your body.

If you have type 1 diabetes (which we discuss further in Chapter 4), your *main* problem is that your pancreas is unable to make insulin in the first place. As you eat, your blood glucose level goes up, and, try as it might, your pancreas is unable to respond.

A colleague of Ian's recalls the time that a young woman with type 2 diabetes came to the office, two of her friends reluctantly in tow. "Doctor," she said, her voice ringing with frustration, "I know that I'm overweight, and that is part of the reason I have diabetes, but I wanted you to see my two friends here. They're the same weight and height I am, but they don't have diabetes. Why is that?" Ian's colleague looked at the three ladies, and then once again focused his attention on his patient. "Beth, I see your point. There can be *many* reasons why one person gets diabetes and somebody else does not. But at least in terms of body weight, not all pounds are created equal. Take a close look at your friends and you will find that even though they may have the same weight and height, their bodies look different. Your friends have their fat tissue evenly distributed on their bodies, but in your case you have it mostly on your belly. That makes you more 'insulin resistant.' Lose that abdominal fat and I bet you will find that your glucose levels will improve." Beth heeded the words and within a few months she was quite a bit trimmer — as were her glucose readings.

It's worth mentioning that the problems that we just discussed are often relative. In other words, if you have type 2 diabetes, your organs can *partially* respond to the insulin you have. And if you have only recently acquired type 1 diabetes, your body may still have *some* ability to produce insulin.

Regardless of which type of diabetes you have, if you are not able to use glucose properly for fuel, your body starts to use other tissues for this purpose. You break down fat and, eventually, you break down muscles. The excess glucose spills into the urine. And that is why, if you have uncontrolled hyperglycemia (high blood glucose) you may have noticed that you are losing weight and muscle bulk. But of course that either already is — or soon will be — behind you, because from this point on you are going to make sure that your glucose levels are controlled and you are healthy.

In summary, insufficient, or ineffective (as seen with insulin resistance), insulin has the following effects:

- Prevents your muscle cells from extracting glucose from your blood (therefore depriving your muscles of a source of energy and leading to high blood glucose levels).

- Prevents your fat cells from extracting glucose from your blood, therefore leading to high blood glucose levels.

- Allows your liver to release excessive glucose into your blood, therefore leading to high blood glucose levels.

- Causes your fat cells to start releasing fatty acids into your blood stream.

- Leads to loss of fat and muscle tissue.

The discovery of insulin

When you were told you had diabetes, most likely you were anything but happy about it. But as badly as you may have felt, imagine if you were told you had this diagnosis back, say, in 1771, when *The Encyclopedia Britannica* described diabetes this way: "In the beginning, the mouth is dry . . . a heat begins to be perceived . . . the patient falls away, and the mind is anxious and unstable. In time the thirst greatly increases, the urine is plentiful and the body wastes. . . . There is a swelling of the loins . . . and . . . death is at hand."

And as for treatment, how about these commonly prescribed therapies: the oat "cure" (you ate pretty well nothing but oatmeal); overfeeding (sometimes with diets rich in sugar!) and, on the other side of the fence, starvation diets that were sometimes so awful that patients were kept locked in their rooms so they would not have access to food.

Until not too long ago, type 2 diabetes was uncommon. To have diabetes was to have type 1 diabetes. And to have type 1 diabetes before the discovery of insulin, was to have a terminal illness. Imagine therefore the euphoria that greeted the discovery of insulin. It must surely have been equal to what the discovery of a universal cure for cancer would be nowadays. And it happened right here in Canada.

In 1889 a scientist discovered that if a dog's pancreas was removed, the dog became diabetic. This was the first strong clue that the pancreas and diabetes were intimately related. But how they were related remained a mystery.

In 1920, Dr. Frederick Banting, a Canadian surgeon from Alliston, Ontario, was working as a very junior lecturer at the University of Western Ontario in London. Whilst preparing for a class, he read an article on diabetes and the pancreas, and that sparked an interest — soon to be an obsession — in finding out what secretion the pancreas might be making that prevents diabetes.

Dr. Banting, all of 29 years of age at the time, approached Dr. John Macleod, a professor at the University of Toronto, and asked permission to use a laboratory. Dr. Macleod agreed and assigned Charles H. Best, a science student, to assist. How was Best chosen for a role that was soon to make him world famous? Through a rigorous selection process, you might think. Well, it wasn't quite like that. In fact, Best was "picked" by virtue of winning a coin toss!

Dr. Banting and Mr. Best (he wasn't a doctor yet) began their work in May 1921 and in December they were joined by J. B. Collip, a biochemist from the University of Alberta. After some initial setbacks (and what would science be without setbacks?), they eventually purified a pancreatic extract that they felt could be given to people with diabetes.

On January 11, 1922, their extract was administered to Leonard Thompson, a 14-year-old boy in the Toronto General Hospital. The treatment was a dismal failure. Thankfully, the young scientists and Leonard were not deterred and, after some further work in the laboratory, they tried again on January 23. We do not know if they shouted "Eureka!" but they must have wanted to when they saw Leonard's glucose level fall and his well-being suddenly improve. The boy had been rescued from death. Insulin was born.

That is the end of one story and the beginning of another, for the subsequent personal rivalries between Banting and Best on the one side and Collip and Macleod on the other is the stuff of legend. The Nobel Prize in physiology or medicine was awarded to Banting and Macleod in 1923. Banting shared his portion with Best, and Macleod did likewise with Collip. Michael Bliss, a Canadian historian, has written an absolutely wonderful book, *The Discovery of Insulin,* which chronicles the story and is as entertaining and fascinating to read as any detective novel you are likely to come across.

Chapter 4

What Type of Diabetes Do You Have?

In This Chapter
▶ Identifying the symptoms and causes of type 1 diabetes
▶ Identifying the symptoms and causes of type 2 diabetes
▶ Comparing type 1 and type 2 diabetes
▶ Understanding the Metabolic Syndrome
▶ Finding out the importance of pre-diabetes
▶ Looking at gestational diabetes

*Y*ou might think that diabetes is diabetes is diabetes. And, true enough, in many ways the various forms of diabetes have much in common. Everyone with diabetes is combating a tendency to have high blood glucose levels and everyone with diabetes has to make appropriate dietary changes to enhance their health. And whether you are age 5 or 95, it is essential that you have proper eye care, proper foot care, and all the other things that go along with achieving and maintaining good health.

Having said that, there are certain things that are unique to the different forms of diabetes and that require special attention. In this chapter we look at these different forms of diabetes, determining what they have in common and how they differ.

Jim Tucker, a 50-year-old assembly-line worker at a car plant, had always been the picture of health. Indeed, he never saw doctors. He was a hard-working man who enjoyed spending time playing ball in the summer and hockey in the winter. Over the past few months he had noticed that he was going to the bathroom night and day. And he was constantly thirsty. Thinking that he needed better nutrition he had started to drink glass after glass of orange juice. But that didn't make him feel better. One day he got on the scale and realized that, although he was still overweight, during the past six months he had lost fifteen pounds without even trying. Jim was hesitant to see a doctor, but his wife finally convinced him that he had to get checked out. He went to see his family physician, a blood test was done, and a day later Jim got a call at work that he had to come in to see the doctor right away. His blood glucose level was 25. Jim's doctor told him the result and what it meant. Jim had *type 2 diabetes*.

Mary was a 5-year-old girl. She was a beautiful, healthy, and happy child, but had suddenly become irritable and in just a matter of days had started to look increasingly unwell. She was quickly losing weight and had started to wet her bed. Mary's parents became alarmed and took her to the local emergency department, where doctors found that she had a blood glucose level of 15 and that her urine contained a substance called ketones. Mary was diagnosed as having *type 1 diabetes*.

Fatima was pregnant with her third child. She had had no problems during the first two pregnancies, and with this one she also felt fine. As a matter of routine procedure, when Fatima reached her 24th week of pregnancy, her doctor sent her for a glucose tolerance test wherein she had to ingest a sugar-rich drink and her blood glucose level was checked a couple of hours later. Her result was 11.2. Fatima's doctor diagnosed her as having *gestational diabetes*.

What do Jim, Mary, and Fatima have in common? That is easy to answer and takes but one word: *diabetes*. But if we were to write about how they *differ*, that would take a whole chapter. This chapter . . .

You Have Type 1 Diabetes

Until just a few years ago, the way that diabetes was classified was very different (and very confusing!). What we now refer to as type 1 diabetes used to be called "juvenile-onset diabetes" or "insulin dependent diabetes." And what we now call type 2 diabetes used to be called "adult-onset diabetes" or "non-insulin dependent diabetes."

The problem with the old terms is that many people don't fit the descriptive titles. For example, many children who get diabetes actually have type 2 diabetes. And many adults who get diabetes actually have type 1 diabetes. So if we had stuck with the old terms we would be telling tons of kids they have "adult-onset diabetes" and tons of adults they have "juvenile-onset diabetes." Now, in our books, even if you have got a thick head of jet-black hair, a "six-pack" muscled belly, and nary a wrinkle on your perfect skin, it still doesn't seem right to say that you have a "juvenile" disease if you are 40 years old. And telling a 10-year-old that he or she has an "adult" disease doesn't seem sensible either.

Unfortunately, you are still likely to come across the outdated names because many people — including some health care providers — haven't caught up yet with the new terminology.

You can have type 2 diabetes and require insulin, but that does *not* mean you now have type 1 diabetes. You still have type 2 diabetes even though you require insulin therapy.

Identifying the symptoms of type 1 diabetes

Type 1 diabetes almost always gets discovered *before* it has caused any irreversible damage to your body. Why? Because once type 1 diabetes has developed, symptoms tend to come on quite quickly. Symptoms include the following:

- **Frequent urination:** As we explain in Chapter 2, passing lots of urine is a typical symptom of diabetes. You experience frequent urination because once your blood glucose level rises to above 10 or so (people without diabetes seldom have values above 8), glucose passes through the kidneys and spills into the urine, drawing extra fluids along the way.

- **Increase in thirst:** Because you are losing excess fluids in the urine, you are at risk of getting dehydrated. Your clever body tries to prevent this by making you feel thirstier, which, of course, encourages you to drink more.

- **Weight loss and increased hunger:** It is no coincidence that long, long ago, if someone was suspected as having diabetes, their urine was placed near an anthill to see if the little critters would be attracted to it. They knew dinner when they smelled it. If you have (uncontrolled) type 1 diabetes, you are passing urine that is rich in glucose and, thus, is rich in calories. This wasted nutrition is going down the drain in a manner of speaking. The body then starts to break down muscle and fat tissue. Your body doesn't like that one bit, so it makes you hungry, hoping that that will encourage you to eat more to maintain your health.

- **Fatigue:** When type 1 diabetes first strikes, you suddenly start to lose body fluids, muscle mass, and fat tissue, and you quickly become malnourished and are on the verge of being (or actually are) dehydrated. In the face of this onslaught, it is no wonder you feel fatigued. If you have type 1 diabetes, you probably recall how quickly your energy improved once you started insulin therapy.

- **Fruity breath:** When your body cannot use glucose as a fuel, it looks for alternative sources of energy, one of which is fat tissue. As fat tissue breaks down, it releases acids called ketones and these typically make the breath smell fruity, very much like a candy mint. If lots of ketones are present this can be a sign of a dangerous condition called *ketoacidosis,* which we discuss further in Chapter 5.

- **Blurred vision:** When the glucose levels in your body undergo a big change, the fluid content of the lens of your eyes also changes. That, in turn, alters the way that light bends as it passes through your eyes and leads to blurring. Maybe you have noticed the way that a knife in a glass of water looks bent. It is much the same phenomenon.

Investigating the causes of type 1 diabetes

If you or someone you love has type 1 diabetes, after you get over the shock of hearing the news, the next thing you will probably ask is "How could this have happened?" And that is an excellent question. In fact that is the same question scientists have been asking for many, many years, and it still goes unanswered.

We *do* know that type 1 diabetes is not contagious and you can rest assured that you did not get it from someone with diabetes sneezing on you or coughing on you. And you did not get type 1 diabetes from eating the wrong foods or not exercising enough or from being under stress. In fact, you did nothing wrong at all. Type 1 diabetes is *not* something that you brought on; it is something that happened *to* you.

Type 1 diabetes is an *autoimmune disease*, meaning that your body has been unkind enough to react against itself. There are many different types of autoimmune disease, including certain types of thyroid disease and arthritis conditions such as lupus and rheumatoid arthritis.

We all make antibodies to fight off infections, but in the case of type 1 diabetes your body creates antibodies that have decided that your own insulin-producing, islet cells of your pancreas are the enemy and have attacked these cells. This can be demonstrated by checking for certain antibodies in the blood stream, including islet cell antibodies, insulin antibodies, and GAD *(glutamic acid decarboxylase)* antibodies. It is seldom necessary to test for these antibodies outside of research settings (and in Canada the cost for these tests is usually not covered by health insurance plans — another strong disincentive to ordering them).

We don't know why your immune system would turn against your pancreas, but there are a number of theories:

- ✔ At various times in our lives we develop viral infections and our bodies fight these off by producing antibodies. It could be that one of these viruses shared something in its appearance with an islet cell and the body's antibodies couldn't separate out the good guys (your islet cells) from the bad guys (the virus) and attacked both.

- ✔ Non-breastfed babies have a higher risk of developing type 1 diabetes. It could be that a protein in cows' milk causes the same sort of response as a virus and, just as we discussed in the preceding paragraph, leads to an antibody attack on your own pancreas. This possibility is being looked at in the TRIGR study (*T*rial to *R*educe *I*DDM in the *G*enetically at *R*isk; www.trigr.org). This study looks at the risk of developing diabetes in babies who, if they are unable to breastfeed, are given one of 2 types of formula; either a standard, cow's milk based formula or a formula that is made up of smaller, less complex proteins that will possibly be less likely to stimulate an inappropriate immune system response (which, in turn, may reduce the likelihood of diabetes).

✔ A virus may damage the pancreas by directly attacking it. Indeed, there have been small outbreaks of type 1 diabetes that give support to this idea.

✔ As a result of normal chemical reactions in our bodies we produce highly reactive molecules called *oxygen free radicals.* Despite the name, we can assure you that they bear no similarity to hippies from 1960s Berkeley, California. Oxygen free radicals can be produced in excess numbers by exposure to air pollution and smoking. They can also be produced by exposure to high glucose levels and substances called *free fatty acids.* It is possible that oxygen free radicals accumulate in and damage the pancreas.

✔ Certain chemicals are known to cause type 1 diabetes. One such example is a rat poison called Vacor, which, if ingested, can damage the pancreas.

There are other theories as well, but the simple truth of the matter is that we don't know what has caused your type 1 diabetes. We do know, however, that there are certain underlying genetic characteristics that may make you more susceptible to getting type 1 diabetes. Individually they would not cause you to develop diabetes, but when taken together with some other trigger, they might. All of us have our genetic "blueprint" laid out for us in our DNA. And DNA in turn is made up of smaller portions called genes. It is our genes that cause us to be short or tall, blonde or brunette, blue- or brown-eyed, and so forth. People with type 1 diabetes are more likely to have certain types of genes called HLA-DR3 or HLA-DR4. Even though these sound like they should be pals with R2D2 and C3PO, they are not quite so foreign as that; indeed, 95 percent of people with type 1 diabetes have one of these genes.

The best possible illustration of how getting type 1 diabetes must be a combination of a genetic susceptibility *and* an environmental trigger is found in one extraordinarily simple fact. If you have type 1 diabetes and you have an identical twin (who would, therefore, have the same genes as you do), the likelihood of your twin getting type 1 diabetes is somewhere between 25 to 50 percent. If the cause was purely genetic, the odds would be 100 percent. Something else clearly must be at play here. But what? At this time, we simply do not know.

The great British prime minister, Benjamin Disraeli, may have been right when he said there are "lies, damn lies, and statistics," but when it comes to the inheritance of type 1 diabetes, certain statistics do seem to be true. In particular, if you have a parent or a (non-identical) sibling with type 1 diabetes you have approximately a 5-percent risk of developing type 1 diabetes. This risk rises to about 30 percent if *both* your parents have type 1 diabetes.

Preventing type 1 diabetes

It would give us untold pleasure to be able to make this the shortest chapter in this book. How wonderful to be able to write: "Take Vaccine X and you will be guaranteed to avoid type 1 diabetes." Well, we could write it but it would not be truthful. In fact there is no known way to prevent type 1 diabetes. But it is certainly not from lack of trying.

A variety of drugs (even including insulin) have been tried on people at high risk for developing type 1 diabetes, but these people ended up faring no better than those who did not receive the treatment.

Things are not all doom and gloom, however. Researchers are hard at work trying to solve the mystery of type 1 diabetes prevention. And unlike years ago, when scientists often worked in relative isolation, researchers now routinely pool their resources to improve their odds of success. Indeed, a new organization has been formed, TrialNet (www.diabetestrialnet.org) — of which the Hospital for Sick Children in Toronto is a member — that is "solely dedicated to testing new approaches to understanding, preventing and treating type 1 diabetes." This type of intensive, integrated approach by researchers is wonderful news, indeed.

In Chapter 22 we take a look at some innovative strategies that may one day help us to prevent or even cure type 1 diabetes.

You Have Type 2 Diabetes

Type 2 diabetes is much, much more common than type 1 diabetes (10 times more common, in fact). Whereas type 1 diabetes tends to develop in children and young adults, type 2 diabetes typically affects middle-aged or older people. Over the past 10 years, however, there has been an epidemic of type 2 diabetes in children and, remarkably, up to 25 percent (or, in some communities, even more) of kids with newly diagnosed diabetes have the type 2 variety. The reason why this is particularly sad is that type 2 diabetes is often avoidable and these children (some under the age of 10) might have been spared if they had played more hockey and basketball and spent less time watching television. If you have type 2 diabetes and want to help protect your young child or grandchild from also getting type 2 diabetes, perhaps for next year's birthday gift consider giving a YMCA/YWCA membership rather than a video game. Even better, while you're at it, get a membership for yourself, too, and go together!

When Paul, Anne's 10-year-old son, fell off the honour roll for the first time in four years, she thought it was time for him to start to buckle down on his homework. Anne spent extra time reviewing Paul's homework with him, but found it increasingly difficult to get her son to stay focused on his work. He seemed kind of fatigued, but otherwise healthy apart from his being considerably overweight. Anne herself had a weight problem and could readily relate to how tired it sometimes made her to carry her extra bulk around. As the semester went on, both Paul's marks and his energy continued going rapidly south, so Anne decided it was time to take her son to see a doctor. It took the doctor little time to find out what was wrong. "Anne, your son has diabetes; that's why he's not feeling right." Anne remembers how stunned she felt upon hearing the news. Diabetes? How could that be? That's what older people or underweight kids got, she thought. It was a shock to her to find out that overweight children are also prone to diabetes. Fortunately, both Anne and Paul were receptive to the types of changes they had to make to improve their health and they both immediately set about to lose weight and to exercise. What a thrill it was for them when within weeks they both felt newly energized and Paul was once again getting As.

In Chapter 3 we talk about the cause of type 2 diabetes and how, with this condition, the pancreas is able to make insulin but the body's tissues are not able to use it properly. This is called *insulin resistance,* and we look at this in more detail later in this chapter.

It is crucial to know that if you have type 2 diabetes, you do not have a less severe or less important form of diabetes than if you had type 1 diabetes. You do not have a "touch of diabetes"; you have the real thing, meaning you require intensive therapy and equally intensive monitoring to keep you healthy. Don't let anyone try to convince you that if you are being treated with nutrition ("diet") therapy alone, your diabetes is less serious than if you were on insulin. On the other hand, do not let anyone try to convince you that if you are on insulin, your condition "must be worse" than someone with diabetes who does not require insulin. All diabetes is serious. All people with diabetes are at risk of complications, but, equally important, working with their health care team, they have the means to reduce that risk

Type 2 diabetes is written as, well, type 2 diabetes, not type II diabetes. The little in-joke amongst diabetes specialists is that this nomenclature was chosen so that doctors wouldn't think it was to be called type eleven diabetes!

Identifying the symptoms of type 2 diabetes

Nicholas had always been a very healthy man. Indeed, the last time he had seen a doctor was when he had his appendix taken out 10 years ago, when he was 40 years of age. The only reason he was now in the family doctor's office was at his wife's insistence. Starting a year ago, he had noticed some mild numbness in his right big toe. A month or two later, the same thing developed in his left big toe. Nicholas was not a complainer and he figured it was just because of some new, overly tight-fitting shoes he had yet to break in. Nonetheless, as the months passed, things got worse and worse and now the numbness involved all his toes and had started to feel increasingly painful. When his doctor examined Nicholas's feet they looked healthy enough, but when the doctor pressed on the toes with a thin nylon rod, Nicholas hardly noticed. A few tests later and the doctor had made her diagnosis. Nicholas had diabetes. It was a shock for Nicholas. He had no recollection of having been overly thirsty or passing excessive quantities of urine. Indeed, he had felt perfectly fine otherwise. Not in a million years had he imagined that diabetes could show itself in such an unusual way.

Unlike type 1 diabetes, the symptoms of type 2 diabetes tend to come on gradually; often so gradually that people who later discover they have the condition have discounted the symptoms, blaming them on something else. Perhaps before you were diagnosed as having type 2 diabetes, you attributed your weight loss to a new diet you had put yourself on. Or maybe you remember blaming your thirst on a particularly hot summer. Indeed, the symptoms of type 2 diabetes can come on so gradually and so imperceptibly that by the time it is discovered, your blood glucose may be extraordinarily high and, moreover, may have been high for so long that damage has already occurred to your body. In fact, up to 50 percent of people newly diagnosed with type 2 diabetes *already* have some degree of damage to their bodies. (It is for this reason that the Canadian Diabetes Association recommends people be routinely screened for diabetes; the goal is to try to make the diagnosis as early as possible so that treatment can be given before damage to the body occurs. The Cheat Sheet at the front of this book describes when screening should be done.)

Many of the symptoms of (uncontrolled) type 2 diabetes are common to type 1 diabetes, including the following:

- ✔ Frequent urination
- ✔ Increase in thirst
- ✔ Weight loss and increased hunger
- ✔ Fatigue
- ✔ Blurred vision

Weight loss is more common with newly diagnosed type 1 diabetes but also occurs fairly frequently with type 2 diabetes. There are some other differences in symptoms, and the following ones are much more likely to be present with type 2 diabetes:

- **Slow wound healing:** If you have high blood glucose levels, your body's ability to heal itself becomes impaired and you may find that seemingly minor cuts don't heal as quickly as they used to.

- **Yeast infections of the vagina and penis:** High glucose levels make the genital areas of your body prone to yeast infections. In a woman this may manifest as a vaginal discharge and, in a man, as a reddish rash at the end of the penis (balanitis).

- **Numbness of the feet:** This is not so much a symptom of high blood glucose as it is a symptom of nerve damage. If you have had high blood glucose levels for a number of years you may develop an uncomfortable burning or numb feeling in your feet. As Nicholas (in the preceding anecdote) discovered, this can be the first clue alerting you to the fact that you not only have diabetes, but that it has been there for quite some time. We discuss nerve damage further in Chapter 6.

Investigating the causes of type 2 diabetes

Although finding the initial trigger leading to type 1 diabetes has proved very elusive, we know a lot more about why people develop type 2 diabetes.

When you were told you had diabetes you may have thought of relatives of yours who shared the same problem. Indeed, you may have thought of *many* relatives who had diabetes. What you and your extended family have in common is, of course, more than being at risk for diabetes. You share many *genes* in common, including those that make you prone to getting diabetes. Note that the fact that your father or mother or sister or brother may have diabetes does *not* guarantee that you, too, will get it, but it does increase your risk.

If you have a parent with type 2 diabetes you have approximately a 15-percent risk of developing type 2 diabetes. This risk rises to about 50 percent if *both* your parents have type 2 diabetes. If you have a sibling with type 2 diabetes your risk is only 10 percent, but — and this is startling — if your sibling is your identical twin, your risk of developing type 2 diabetes rises to 90 percent. But before you throw your hands up in despair, please note there is a very, very large "but" here.

The "but" is that there is more to getting type 2 diabetes than family background alone. In addition to having relatives with diabetes, most people who acquire type 2 diabetes are overweight and sedentary. And we have recent scientific studies showing overwhelming evidence that your risk of developing type 2 diabetes can be drastically reduced by making appropriate lifestyle changes. Just like Tom Cruise discovers in the movie *Minority Report,* we have control over our destiny. (We discuss this further in the next section, on prevention).

In the early stages of type 2 diabetes your pancreas produces large quantities of insulin. The main problem is that the insulin is not working effectively. As we discuss in more detail in Chapter 3, insulin is like a key that opens up the cells (especially your fat and muscle cells) to allow glucose to enter. In type 2 diabetes this key is malfunctioning. This is called insulin resistance (see "You Have the Metabolic Syndrome" below for a further discussion on this topic).

Although the initial problem with type 2 diabetes is that your insulin is not working properly, as time passes the pancreas also runs into difficulties and eventually cannot make enough insulin. That is one of the main reasons that so many people with type 2 diabetes end up requiring insulin as time goes by. If you have type 2 diabetes and you require insulin to keep your blood glucose levels under control, this does not mean you have failed. It is **not** your fault. It simply means that your pancreas is unable to produce sufficient insulin for your body's needs.

People often think that sugar and stress cause type 2 diabetes, but in fact, they don't. Eating excessive amounts of sugar may bring out the disease to the extent that it makes you overweight, but that is quite different from saying sugar "causes diabetes." Indeed, eating too much protein or fat will do the same thing. As for excess stress, it can make your glucose control worse *if* you already have diabetes, but it does not *cause* diabetes.

Thrifty genes

In countries where people do not get enough food, people whose genetic makeup enables their bodies to use carbohydrates in a very efficient manner have an advantage over the rest of the population because they can survive on the low food and calorie supplies. When these people finally receive ample supplies of food, their bodies are overwhelmed and they are more likely to become fat and develop diabetes. This may explain why people in developing countries are the most at risk to develop type 2 diabetes. The same theory may explain why First Nations have a higher risk of developing diabetes. This proposal is called the *thrifty gene hypothesis*.

Preventing type 2 diabetes

Unlike type 1 diabetes, type 2 diabetes can be prevented, or at the very least delayed, according to recent medical studies.

Type 2 diabetes almost always occurs in people who are overweight and sedentary. Like anything in life, there are exceptions, but over 90 percent of the time this is the case. However, by losing weight and exercising regularly you can reduce your risk of developing type 2 diabetes by over 50 percent. If you already have type 2 diabetes, then do your loved ones a favour and share this information with them so they can start to consider making the necessary lifestyle changes to help them avoid getting (or at least delaying the onset of) type 2 diabetes.

To achieve this huge reduction in risk, all you need to do is lose 5 percent of your body weight and exercise for 150 minutes per week (which is only about 21 minutes a day)!

Research reveals that prevention is most likely to succeed with lifestyle therapy (that is; weight loss and exercise), but we must say that this is often the most difficult prescription of all. Fortunately, these same studies show that you can still achieve nearly similar benefit by using certain medications (such as metformin, or acarbose). We discuss these medicines in Chapter 11.

The medical studies just alluded to looked at people who already had problems with elevated blood glucose levels. They had *pre-diabetes*, meaning their readings were higher than normal but not high enough to classify them as having diabetes. We talk more about this condition later in this chapter.

There are several ways to determine whether or not you are over weight including:

- ✔ **Body Mass Index (BMI):** This is the most commonly used technique to determine if someone is overweight. Basically, BMI is an indicator of whether you are the right weight for your height. It can be calculated — though nobody ever does it this way — by dividing your weight in kilograms by the square of your height in metres. Uh-huh. Realistically, you can just look it up on a graph (see Figure 4-1) or use an online calculator (www.nhlbisupport.com/bmi/bminojs.htm). A normal BMI is 18.5 to 24.9. Note that the normal range for BMI does NOT apply to pregnant or breastfeeding woman, nor does it apply to infants, children, or adolescents (nor to particularly muscular individuals).

- ✔ **Waist circumference:** Another way to establish whether you are overweight is to measure your waist circumference. Your health risk goes up if your waist circumference is equal to or greater than 88 centimetres (35 inches) for women, 102 centimetres (40 inches) for men.

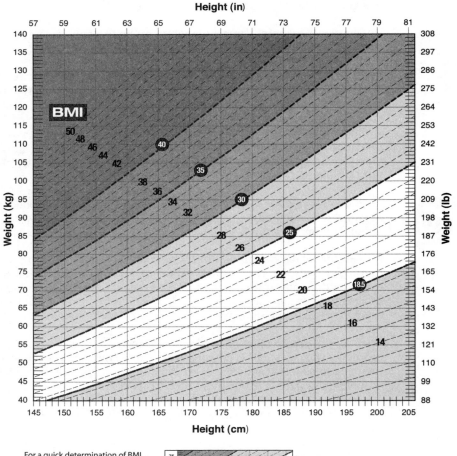

For a quick determination of BMI (kg/m²), use a straight-edge to help locate the point on the chart where height (in or cm) and weight (lb or kg) intersect. Read the number on the dashed line closest to this point. For example, an individual who weighs 69 kg and is 173 cm tall has a BMI of approximately 23.

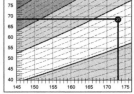

Refer to the table below to identify the level of health risk associated with a particular BMI.

BMI	Risk of developing health problems
< 18.5	Increased
18.5 – 24.9	Least
25.0 – 29.9	Increased
30.0 – 34.9	High
35.0 – 39.9	Very high
≥ 40.0	Extremely high

Figure 4-1:
The Body
Mass Index.

Adapted from: WHO (2000) Obesity: Preventing and Managing the Global Epidemic: Report of a WHO Consultation on Obesity.

When it comes to having too much fat in your body, not all fat is equal. If you have extra fat around your belly but not over other areas of your body, that puts you at much higher risk of getting type 2 diabetes than if you had extra weight distributed over all parts of your body. This is because fat over your midsection is more likely to cause insulin resistance (which we discuss in the preceding section and will discuss further later in this chapter).

Knowledge is power. And now that you know the main risk factors leading to type 2 diabetes, you have the ability to lessen the likelihood of getting it. And if you already have it, reducing your BMI and your extra fat tissue can markedly improve your health anyhow. The point of finding out your BMI is not that you should get angry or frustrated with yourself. Rather, you know what the problem is and can now take steps (both figurative and literal) to improve it.

Key Differences Between Type 1 and Type 2 Diabetes

There are many similarities between type 1 and type 2 diabetes; however, there are also some important differences. The following table highlights some of these differences. (Please note there are *many* exceptions to these):

Table 4-1	Differences Between Type 1 and Type 2 Diabetes	
	Type 1 diabetes	*Type 2 diabetes*
Age at time of diagnosis	Less than 20	More than 40
Length of time present before diagnosis	Months	Years
Weight status at time of diagnosis	Normal or underweight	Overweight
Most common symptoms at time of diagnosis	Thirst, frequent urination, weight loss	Thirst, frequent urination, visual blurring
Insulin defect	Insufficient insulin ("beta cell failure")	Ineffective insulin ("insulin resistance")
Antibodies present to insulin and/or islet cells	Yes	No
Family history of diabetes	Sometimes	Almost always
Initial therapy	Lifestyle & insulin	Lifestyle (with or without medication)

You Have the Metabolic Syndrome

Over the past several years a number of pieces of a puzzle have been found to fit together. Researchers have observed that people who have insulin resistance (we discuss insulin resistance in Chapter 3) are prone to developing not only type 2 diabetes but other health problems as well (including conditions as varied as heart disease and infertility). This problem is called the Metabolic Syndrome.

In your Internet travels you may have come across other names for this condition. One is "Insulin Resistance Syndrome." This term has not yet come into common use. Another name is "Syndrome X." The problem with this term is that there is more than one type of health condition called Syndrome X. You'd think there was a shortage of letters in the alphabet! Anyhow, to avoid confusion, it is best to refer to the metabolic syndrome as, well, the metabolic syndrome.

The definition of the Metabolic Syndrome is in evolution (that is a nice way to say that doctors can't agree on it), but it is usually considered to be present if you have *three or more* of the following:

- Fasting blood glucose of 6.1 mmol/L or higher
- Blood pressure of 130/85 or higher
- Triglycerides of 1.7 mmol/L or higher (triglycerides are one of the fats in the blood)
- HDL cholesterol (the "good" type of cholesterol) less than 1.0 mmol/L (for men) or less than 1.3 mmol/L (for women)
- Abdominal obesity (as defined as a waist circumference of more than 102 cm — about 40 inches — for men; more than 88 cm — about 35 inches — for women)

If you have the Metabolic Syndrome, take that to be a wake-up call: You need to make crucial lifestyle interventions to reduce your risk of the condition deteriorating into diabetes, heart attacks, and other serious health issues. Your destiny is largely in your hands (and brain, in a manner of speaking). We talk more about the various ways to improve your health throughout this book. In particular, we address high blood pressure as well as cholesterol and triglyceride issues in Chapter 6 and weight issues in Chapter 10.

You Have Pre-diabetes

You may be tolerant of your children and you may be tolerant of your neighbours and workmates. Heck, you may be the most tolerant person in the world but, alas, that does not mean you are tolerant of your glucose. With impaired glucose tolerance (IGT), you could say, to paraphrase Hamlet, "Diabetes or not diabetes; that is the question." If you have IGT, your post-meal blood glucose levels are not high enough to say you have diabetes, but not low enough to be normal either. In other words, when you have IGT, your diabetes (or not diabetes) future is being decided.

A physician will diagnose IGT if you have a blood glucose of 7.8 to 11.0 mmol/L two hours after drinking 75 grams of glucose. A related condition (with similar implications and importance) is *impaired fasting glucose* (IFG) which is diagnosed if your blood glucose is 6.1 to 6.9 after not having ingested any calories for the preceding eight hours. *Pre-diabetes* is a very recently coined term and refers to both impaired fasting glucose and impaired glucose tolerance.

Pre-diabetes is important to know about for two main reasons:

- **High risk of developing type 2 diabetes:** Think of pre-diabetes as an early warning system. It is an alert that you are at high risk of getting type 2 diabetes. Indeed, the risk of pre-diabetes developing into type 2 diabetes is as much as 10 percent in any year and about 90 percent over 10 years (hence the reason for calling this condition "pre-diabetes"). Not good odds, eh? But there is a "but": despite the name, pre-diabetes does *not* have to progress to type 2 diabetes. As you read in the preceding section, appropriate lifestyle (and sometimes, medication) intervention can halt (or, at the very least, slow down) this progression.

- **High risking of developing damaged blood vessels:** Having pre-diabetes puts you at very high risk of developing hardening of the arteries (atherosclerosis), which can ultimately lead to heart attacks, strokes, and amputations. However, this does *not* have to happen. Aggressive treatment of pre-diabetes and other risk factors for vascular disease can keep you healthy. This means paying attention to your diet, being physically active, making sure your blood pressure and lipids (cholesterol and triglycerides) are good, and, of course, not smoking.

Although the term "pre-diabetes" is very apt in that it hammers home the message that IFG and IGT are huge risk factors for getting type 2 diabetes, it implies an inevitability about something that we know is not necessarily inevitable. IFG and IGT do *not* have to lead to diabetes.

You Have Gestational Diabetes

If you are pregnant (yes, that excludes you men, but read on, gentlemen — you *do* have something to do with your partner's pregnancy) and you did not have diabetes prior to your pregnancy, during the course of your pregnancy you could acquire a form of diabetes called *gestational diabetes*. If you already have diabetes when you become pregnant, that is called, simply enough, pregnancy with pre-existing diabetes (sometimes also referred to as *pre-gestational diabetes*).

How to define gestational diabetes and the implications of having it have been subjects of controversy for a very long time. Most moms with gestational diabetes have perfectly healthy babies, but others do run into problems, particularly with having large babies. However, the importance of pregnancy with pre-existing diabetes is not controversial. It is a terribly important condition with major implications for both mom and baby, including a much higher rate of miscarriages and birth defects.

We discuss pregnancy issues in detail in Chapter 7.

If You Don't Fit Any of These Categories (and Why LADA Isn't Just a Russian Car)

The great majority of diabetes cases fall within the categories we have just discussed (that is, type 1, type 2, and gestational diabetes). There are, however, other causes of diabetes including the following:

- ✔ **Surgical removal of the pancreas:** If your pancreas has been surgically removed, you will no longer have the ability to produce insulin and, hence, will have diabetes.

- ✔ **Destruction of pancreatic tissue:** Severe inflammation of the pancreas ("pancreatitis") may so badly damage the insulin-producing beta cells of the pancreas that you lose the ability to produce insulin.

- ✔ **Medicines:** Some medicines can cause diabetes. Prednisone (and similar drugs) is a type of steroid that is wonderful at treating some very serious diseases (such as asthma), but unfortunately has the potential — especially if used in high doses for long periods of time — to cause diabetes. Some blood pressure medicine (for example, hydrochlorothiazide) and some newer psychiatric medicines (for example, risperidone and clozapine) can occasionally do this also. That does *not* mean you should never take these medicines. What it does mean, however, is that if you are taking one of these medicines and you have symptoms of diabetes (which we discuss earlier in this chapter) you should see your doctor to have your blood glucose level checked.

- **Alternative and complimentary treatments:** There is evidence that some "natural" therapies, including glucosamine (which many people take to treat arthritis), can cause insulin resistance and, at least in theory, lead to diabetes. Just as with prescription drugs, if you are considering taking alternative or complimentary therapies it is wise to know both the potential pluses *and* minuses.

- **Maturity Onset Diabetes of the Young (MODY):** MODY is a rare genetic disease in which young, non-overweight people develop a condition similar to type 2 diabetes.

- **Other Hormonal Diseases:** See the sidebar below.

A new term has recently come on the scene. *LADA* stands for "*L*atent *A*uto-immune *D*iabetes of *A*dults" and is an unofficial name given to certain non-overweight adults who develop type 1 diabetes. It usually comes on quite gradually and almost always ends up being treated at first as if it were typical type 2 diabetes. Inevitably such treatment fails and people with LADA require insulin therapy. LADA also goes by other, non-official names such as "slowly developing diabetes" and "type 1.5 diabetes."

Mohammed was a 55-year-old man with a long history of severe bronchitis. He came to the emergency department because he was having increasing difficulty catching his breath despite taking a number of different "puffers." The emergency room physician prescribed prednisone and advised Mohammed to follow up with his family doctor in 3 weeks. Within a couple of days, Mohammed's breathing had started to improve and he was feeling very encouraged. A week later, however, he found himself having to get up during the night to go to the bathroom. Initially he blamed this on his prostate, but it kept getting worse and worse and by the time he saw his doctor a week later he had already lost 4.5 kilos (10 pounds) and was feeling miserable. Hearing Mohammed's story, his doctor immediately sent him to the laboratory and the subsequent result confirmed his suspicion: Mohammed's blood glucose level was high — 25 mmol/L, in fact. Fortunately, by that time his breathing had improved and he was able to come off the prednisone. Within 2 weeks his glucose level had returned to normal and his diabetes symptoms resolved.

Conditions and hormones that can lead to diabetes

The following is a partial list of hormonal disorders that can lead to diabetes by causing insulin resistance:

- ✔ **Cushing's Syndrome:** This is a disease in which the body produces excess amounts of steroid hormones (similar to prednisone).

- ✔ **Prolactinoma:** This is a pituitary disorder wherein excess quantities of prolactin hormone are made.

- ✔ **Acromegaly:** This is another pituitary disorder, in this case involving excess levels of growth hormone.

- ✔ **Pheochromocytoma:** This is an adrenal gland disorder in which too much adrenaline (or similar hormones) is made.

- ✔ **Hyperthyroidism:** This is a condition in which the thyroid gland gets overstimulated and produces excess quantities of thyroid hormone.

- ✔ **Glucagonoma:** This is a rare tumour of the pancreas that leads to over-secretion of glucagon hormone.

And now you can consider yourself sufficiently armed to win your next dinner-party game of trivia.

Part II
How Diabetes Affects Your Body

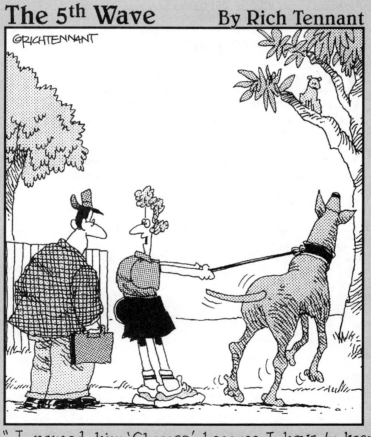

The 5th Wave   By Rich Tennant

"I named him 'Glucose', because I have to keep him under control every day."

In this part . . .

Diabetes can have profound effects on your body. This part explains these effects, how they occur, the kinds of symptoms they produce, and what you and your health care team can do to treat them and, even better, to prevent them.

This part also looks at the special issues surrounding diabetes and pregnancy and discusses those measures that will help you to have a healthy pregnancy and a healthy baby.

Chapter 5

Dealing with Acute Glucose Problems

Glucose control in diabetes involves two separate issues. On the one hand, there is your long-term goal of maintaining good glucose levels to feel well and to avoid damaging the body as time goes by. On the other hand, there are those situations when glucose control suddenly deteriorates and requires urgent attention. We address the long-term issues in Chapter 6. In this chapter we discuss those circumstances that require immediate action.

Hypoglycemia (Low Blood Glucose)

Hypoglycemia is an oft-misunderstood term that gets thrown about with the randomness of a knuckle-ball pitch on a windy day. (You may notice as you read this book that references to hockey keep appearing. But, lest we offend fans of the Toronto Blue Jays, we thought we'd throw in this baseball analogy.) Many people mistakenly believe that hypoglycemia leads to diabetes. So let's set the record straight. It doesn't. Remember, you read it here first.

Hypoglycemia is defined as a blood glucose level below normal. That much is straight-forward. The problem is defining precisely how low a normal blood glucose can be. This is a subject of some controversy in the medical community, with numbers ranging from 2.5 to 4.0 mmol/L having been proposed, however the current guidelines issued by the Canadian Diabetes Association (www.diabetes.ca) consider hypoglycemia to be a blood glucose level of 4.0 mmol/L or less.

Your body doesn't function well when you have too little glucose in your blood. Your brain needs glucose to allow you to think properly, and your muscles need the energy that glucose provides in much the same way that your car needs gasoline to run. So, when your body detects that it has low blood glucose, it sends out a group of hormones that fight to raise your glucose level. But if you're taking medication to reduce your blood glucose (see later in this chapter), those hormones have to fight the strength of the diabetes medication that has been pushing down your glucose levels.

Not every person develops symptoms of hypoglycemia at the same level of blood glucose. Some people notice it at blood glucose levels of 3.8, others only when their blood glucose level is between 2 and 3. Moreover, a person might notice it on one occasion when his or her blood glucose level is below 3.6 and that *same* person might not notice it on another occasion until it is below 3.2. It is crucial also to remember that glucose meters are not perfect. You may have already discovered that you can check your reading seconds apart and find discrepancies of up to 15 percent. That does not mean your blood glucose level changed that much in that brief interval. It simply means the machines are not precision instruments. (Your machine, however, should not give readings — checked moments apart — that differ by *more than* 15 percent. If it does, have your device checked to make sure it is not malfunctioning.)

Symptoms of hypoglycemia

Doctors traditionally divide the symptoms of hypoglycemia into two major categories:

- ✔ **Symptoms that are due to the effects of the hormones (especially epinephrine, also called adrenaline) that your body sends out to counter the glucose-lowering effect of insulin.** These are called *autonomic* symptoms.

- ✔ **Symptoms that are due to your brain not receiving enough fuel with the result that your intellectual function suffers.** These are called *neuroglycopenic symptoms,* derived from *neuro* (referring to the nervous system), *glyco* (glucose), and *penic* (insufficient).

Autonomic symptoms are your best friends. They are your warning system alerting you to a problem of low blood glucose and demanding you attend to it, before it progresses to the more dangerous neuroglycopenic stage (which we discuss shortly).

Autonomic symptoms are:

- ✔ Trembling (shaking of your body; especially of the hands)
- ✔ Palpitations (noticing a rapid or excessively forceful heartbeat)
- ✔ Sweating
- ✔ Anxiety
- ✔ Hunger
- ✔ Nausea
- ✔ Tingling

As you look through the above list, you may recognize having had some or all of these symptoms at various times in your life, even if you have never been on medicine that could cause low blood glucose. The reason: these symptoms can occur in *any* situation where epinephrine levels are high, and that includes so-called fight or flight situations where you are under extreme stress. (Examples are if you are about to write a difficult exam, about to have a job interview, or, let's say you were Ed Belfour and you look up and see Jarome Iginla coming toward you on a breakaway . . .)

Shortly after you begin therapy for high blood glucose you may find that you are experiencing autonomic symptoms, suggesting you have hypoglycemia even though your blood glucose levels may not be low. This is perfectly normal — it will take a few days for your body to become accustomed to having normal blood glucose levels, at which point your symptoms will resolve.

Neuroglycopenic symptoms are much more of a problem. These symptoms are most definitely not your friends. Quite the opposite. Whereas autonomic symptoms alert you to a problem, neuroglycopenic symptoms often interfere with your ability to recognize and deal with hypoglycemia. By the time these symptoms develop, your blood glucose level is usually profoundly low and has become a true emergency. These symptoms include:

- ✔ Difficulty concentrating
- ✔ Confusion
- ✔ Weakness
- ✔ Drowsiness
- ✔ Vision changes (such as double vision or loss of vision)
- ✔ Difficulty speaking
- ✔ Headache
- ✔ Dizziness
- ✔ Tiredness

People lose their ability to think clearly when they become hypoglycemic. They make simple errors, and other people often assume that they are drunk. Suffice to say, if Albert Einstein were having an episode of hypoglycemia, he may have ended up mistakenly deciding E = mc or, in keeping with our hockey analogy, Wayne Gretzky would have been the not-quite-as-Great One. Fortunately, adult brains have an amazing capacity to put up with insults like hypoglycemia, and long-term damage to the brain from low blood glucose almost never occurs. Because the brains of infants and young children are more sensitive to injury, however, it is especially important to avoid severe hypoglycemia in this age group (see the following list for a definition of severe hypoglycemia).

Hypoglycemia can be classified as:

- **Mild:** Autonomic symptoms are present and you are able to treat yourself.

- **Moderate:** Autonomic and neuroglycopenic symptoms are present and you are able to treat yourself.

- **Severe:** Hypoglycemia is bad enough that you require someone else to assist you. Unconsciousness may occur. (With severe hypoglycemia the blood glucose is typically less than 2.8 mmol/L.)

One of Alan's patients was driving on a highway when another driver noticed that she was weaving back and forth in her lane and reported her to the highway patrol. A patrolman stopped her, concluded that she was drunk, and took her to jail. Fortunately, someone noticed that she was wearing a diabetes medical alert bracelet. After promptly receiving the glucose that she needed, she rapidly recovered. No charges were filed, but clearly this is a situation that you want to avoid.

If you take medicines that can cause hypoglycemia, for your own safety it would be very wise to wear a medical alert bracelet or necklace. At the very least (and it is certainly not as good), carry some form of identification in your purse or wallet noting that you have diabetes. You may never need them, but it is a good idea to be prepared just in case.

Most people with diabetes go their entire lives without ever experiencing even a single episode of *severe* hypoglycemia. The vast majority of the time if hypoglycemia is being experienced the early-warning, autonomic symptoms kick in and allow you to quickly rectify the problem.

If you are on medications such as insulin or glyburide (glyburide is a type of oral hypoglycemic agent), it is quite possible that you recall having had at least one episode where your hands started to shake, you became sweaty and hungry, and you recognized that something wasn't quite right. You probably reached for your glucose meter, checked your blood glucose level, and found it be somewhere in the low 3's. You likely took some sugar candies or a glass of juice or pop and felt better within a few minutes. Congratulations: you successfully diagnosed, treated, and cured your first patient. Feel free to write the rest of this chapter. Oh, never mind, we'll do it.

As we discuss earlier in this chapter, symptoms such as sweating or palpitations, which can indicate hypoglycemia, can also occur in situations, such as stress, where your blood glucose level may actually be perfectly normal. For that reason, it is very important to conclude that you have hypoglycemia only if you have demonstrated a low blood glucose level on your glucose meter.

Causes of hypoglycemia

Hypoglycemia does not cause diabetes. Now, in another attempt to dispel popular misconceptions, we wish to hereby announce that diabetes does not cause hypoglycemia. Remember, you read it here first. Certain medicines used to *treat* diabetes can cause hypoglycemia, but it is not caused by diabetes in and of itself. Indeed, if you have diabetes and are being treated purely with lifestyle measures (nutrition and exercise therapy) you will *never* experience hypoglycemia.

Hypoglycemia is always unintended. Ideally, your blood glucose levels would always be normal — never high, never low. Unfortunately, we seldom have that degree of success with our imperfect therapies. Most of the medicines we use to prevent blood glucose levels from being too high have the potential to drop them too low. This is especially likely if you are taking any of the following:

- **Sulfonylurea medicine:** As we discuss further in Chapter 11, medicines from this family (the most commonly prescribed of which is a drug called *glyburide*) have the potential to cause low blood glucose.

- **Insulin:** Unlike insulin made by your pancreas, insulin you inject does not have the ability to turn itself off the instant you no longer need it. An injection of insulin will help to reduce your blood glucose level, but it also has the potential to drop your level excessively. This is called an "insulin reaction." You may have heard the term "insulin shock" used in reference to particularly bad insulin reactions. Insulin shock is not a scientific term, however, and can be misleading. Accordingly, we will not be using it beyond this brief explanation.

- **Meglitinides & D-phenylalanine derivatives:** Never do we, as diabetes specialists, consider ourselves luckier than when we attend conferences where these medicines are discussed. Oh no, not just because they are important drugs to know about. No. We consider ourselves fortunate because it is at these conferences that we learn how to pronounce them! Don't worry; no one uses these names anyhow. Doctors pretty well just use the trade names (Gluconorm, Starlix) for drugs currently available within this group. These drugs, like sulfonylureas, make the pancreas release extra insulin and have the potential to cause hypoglycemia.

Non-diabetes causes of hypoglycemia

Hypoglycemia can occur for many other reasons quite unrelated to diabetes treatment. Fasting hypoglycemia can, for example, occur with certain types of tumours. Hypoglycemia developing a few hours after eating is called reactive hypoglycemia and is generally treated by eating more frequent, smaller meals.

Other commonly used drugs such as metformin (Glucophage) or thiazolidinediones (another impossibly difficult name to pronounce; just call them TZD's and doctors will know what you are referring to) do not cause hypoglycemia unless they are being used in combination with medicines from the list above.

There are many unfair things about having diabetes. It is unfair to get it. It is unfair to develop complications. And it is especially unfair that those people with diabetes who try the hardest to stay healthy are the most prone to getting hypoglycemia. If you have poorly controlled glucose levels with values running between 15 and 20, you may not feel great, but you are highly, highly unlikely ever to run into significant problems with hypoglycemia. But if you look after yourself meticulously and are keeping your blood glucose levels in the 4 to 8 range, you are at much greater risk of having hypoglycemia. Fortunately, it is possible to have excellent control and, at the same time, to minimize the risk of getting hypoglycemia. It ain't easy, but it is doable. We discuss this further later in this chapter.

Treatment of hypoglycemia

The vast majority of episodes of hypoglycemia are mild and you will be able to deal with them easily.

If you find that your blood glucose level is low, then it is imperative that you ingest some sugar to restore your level to normal. The Canadian Diabetes Association (CDA) recommends that if you have mild to moderate hypoglycemia (that is, you are still awake and aware enough to take things by mouth) you should take the following steps:

✔ **Step One:** Eat or drink 15 grams (10 grams for children less than 5 years of age or less than 20 kg; that is, less than 44 pounds) of a fast-acting carbohydrate such as:

- Three 5-gram glucose tablets (for example, BD glucose tablets)
- Five 3-gram glucose tablets (for example, Dextrosol tablets)

- 175 mL (¾ cup) of juice or regular (not diet or sugar-free) pop (but, see the tip below)

- 15 mL (3 tsp) honey

- 15 mL (3 tsp) table sugar dissolved in water

✔ **Step Two:** Wait 10 to 15 minutes, and then retest your blood. If your blood glucose level is still less than 4 mmol/L, ingest another 15 grams (10 grams for small children) of carbohydrate.

✔ **Step Three:** If your next meal is more than 1 hour away, or you are going to be physically active, eat a snack, such as half a sandwich or cheese and crackers. The snack should contain 15 grams of carbohydrate and a source of protein.

Despite what most people think (and do), orange juice is not as effective as products like Dextrosol because it is slower to raise glucose levels and relieve you of symptoms. Nonetheless, if you have some O.J. and it's handier than an alternative, it will work.

If you are being treated with acarbose (Prandase) – see Chapter 11 – and you develop hypoglycemia you should be treated with glucose (such as Dextrosol), not sucrose (such as fruit juice).

If you are hypoglycemic and you're about to eat a meal, you should *still* treat your hypoglycemia with fast-acting carbohydrate as described above. This will ensure that your blood glucose is brought up rapidly.

Because the symptoms of hypoglycemia are so unpleasant and because hypoglycemia is understandably scary, you may find yourself taking candy after candy until you feel better without actually giving time for the first "treatment" to take effect. Then, when all that sugar you have just ingested gets absorbed into your system, you may find that your glucose level is up into the teens. It is best, therefore, to give the first treatment a few minutes to work before you take another.

Because your mental state may be impaired when you have hypoglycemia, you need to make sure that your friends or relatives know in advance what hypoglycemia is and what to do about it. This is especially important if your hypoglycemia is so severe that you are unconscious or nearly so, in which case you will be unable to swallow properly. In this circumstance, people should *not* try to feed you, because you could choke. Instead, your helper should administer glucagon (see below) to you and/or call 9-1-1 to summon an ambulance. If you experience milder hypoglycemia, where you are alert but somewhat confused and unable to obtain an appropriate sugar source, then your helper simply needs to find one for you and help you to ingest it.

Inform people about your diabetes and about how to recognize hypo-glycemia. Let them know where you store your emergency supplies (such as the glucose tablets you use to treat hypoglycemia). Don't keep your diabetes a secret. The people close to you will be glad to know how to help you.

Glucagon is available by prescription from pharmacies in a package called a glucagon kit. This kit includes a syringe and 1 mg of glucagon, one of the major hormones that raises glucose, which your helper should inject into your leg muscle. (Half that dose – that is, 0.5 mg – should be used if you are treating a child five years of age or less.) The injection of glucagon raises the blood glucose and within 15–20 minutes you will likely become fully alert. Be sure to check the expiry date marked on the glucagon kit to make certain that it hasn't become outdated if you haven't used it for a long time.

If you have just experienced a severe episode of hypoglycemia and you required an injection of glucagon, then once you have fully come around and are again able to swallow properly, you should consume some quick-acting hypoglycemia treatment (see the list earlier in this section) followed by food to help prevent your redeveloping hypoglycemia as the glucagon wears off.

Some people are, understandably, just too nervous or too intimidated to take it upon themselves to administer glucagon. In that case, they should just call an ambulance.

Remember that when you pick up the glucagon kit from the pharmacy, the person that is most likely to be giving it should go with you. The pharmacist MUST sit down and explain to both of you how it is to be given.

If you live, work, or play in an area where emergency health care services are more than just minutes away, it is especially important for you to have a glucagon kit. Do you snowmobile? Hunt? Hike? Boat? Do you live in a remote area? Does your job take you into the bush? All of these situations would warrant having a supply of glucagon readily available. Keep in mind the Boy Scouts' motto: 'Be prepared.'

If you have experienced severe hypoglycemia — even if you quickly recovered — it is crucial that you notify your family physician or your diabetes specialist so that they can make appropriate adjustments to your therapy to lessen the likelihood of your having another severe attack. If you are feeling well and have fully recovered from the episode, you do not have to call your health care team right away, but it would be wise to get in touch with them within a day or two.

Preventing hypoglycemia

Not everyone with diabetes experiences hypoglycemia. As we discussed earlier in this chapter, if you are being treated with lifestyle therapy alone, you will not have low blood glucose. However, most people with diabetes at some point will require use of medicines (such as insulin or glyburide) that will put them at risk of hypoglycemia. Although there is no foolproof way to avoid hypoglycemia, there are a few techniques to remember:

- **Do not miss or delay meals:** Because pills and insulin that are used to reduce blood glucose do not have the good sense to know exactly when to stop working, like the famous battery-operated bunny they sometimes tend to keep going and going. (Precisely how long depends on the particular type of pill or insulin that you are using; we discuss this in Chapters 11 and 12). That would be fine if your glucose level is still high, but not so fine if your level has come back to normal, as it most likely will have by the time your next meal rolls around. If your meal is unduly delayed, the medicine may pull your glucose level down too low.

- **Have a bedtime snack:** Eating a bedtime snack is not necessary for most people with diabetes unless you are taking evening doses of insulin and your bedtime blood glucose level is less than 7 mmol/L in which case a bedtime snack containing at least 15 grams of carbohydrate and 15 grams of protein will help you avoid having a low reading overnight. If you find that going to bed with a higher glucose level does not prevent overnight lows then you should take a snack even if your bedtime reading is higher than 7 mmol/L. (As we discuss in Chapter 9, if you are on insulin it is a good idea to periodically test your blood glucose level at about 3 a.m. to make sure it is not going low overnight without your having recognized it.)

- **Plan your exercise:** Exercise is an essential component of your diabetes therapy (particularly if you have type 2 diabetes) as we discuss in Chapter 10. But it is important for you to be aware that exercise accelerates the rate at which glucose moves from the blood into muscle (where it is used as fuel) and, thus, can cause you to have hypoglycemia. By all means *do* exercise; however, if you know from experience that when you perform a certain type or amount of exercise you develop hypoglycemia, speak to your diabetes educator or physician about how to adjust your medicines or diet to reduce the risk of developing low blood glucose. Often the solution is something as simple as having a small snack before you work out. The worst thing is to have hypoglycemia every time you exercise; we can't imagine a stronger disincentive to exercising than that!

✔ **Avoid (or minimize) the use of other drugs that can cause hypoglycemia:** There are several drugs (not specifically being used to treat your diabetes) that you may take from time to time that have the potential to lower your blood glucose levels. These drugs include alcohol and *high* doses of aspirin (ASA). We discuss alcohol further in Chapter 10. If you are experiencing hypoglycemia, make sure you review *all* your medicines (and any alternative and complementary therapies; we discuss these in Chapter 13) with your doctor to see if some changes should be made.

If you are on intensified insulin therapy (see Chapter 12), episodes of hypoglycemia are inevitable. Ian has found that, as a very rough rule of thumb, to achieve excellent overall blood glucose control you can expect to have *mild* hypoglycemia about two times per week. More frequent hypoglycemia may put you at undue risk of severe hypoglycemia. On the other hand, if you are on intensified insulin therapy and you are *never* experiencing episodes of hypoglycemia, your average blood glucose level is probably too high.

We give you other tips for people on insulin therapy in Chapter 12.

Hypoglycemia unawareness

Samantha was a 28-year-old patient of Ian's. She had developed diabetes when she was only 5 years of age. Samantha was a highly motivated patient and was monitoring her blood glucose levels many times per day. With aggressive use of insulin, nutrition therapy, and exercise she was able to keep her glucose readings between 3.8 and 6.6. Recently, while she was at work, her boss had found her staring vacantly into space. He was able to get her to drink some juice and she quickly came around, but the next day the same thing happened again. Two days later, her husband awakened to find Samantha soaking wet in bed beside him. He couldn't awaken her. He tested her blood and found her glucose level to be 1.8. He gave her an injection of glucagon (see above for a discussion about glucagon) and over the next 15 minutes she gradually awakened. Later that day, she went to see Ian in the office, her therapy was adjusted, and soon thereafter she was able to once again recognize when her blood glucose levels were too low.

Samantha's story is quite typical of patients with *hypoglycemia unawareness.* As the name suggests, this is a condition where you lose your ability to recognize when your blood glucose level has fallen below normal. This can occur for several reasons:

- ✓ **Repeated hypoglycemia:** If you have been experiencing frequent hypoglycemia — even if mild — your autonomic warning system (such as sweating and palpitations; see above) may start to fail and the first clue that you have low blood glucose can be when you are confused and unable to look after yourself.

- ✓ **Longstanding diabetes:** Occasionally, if you have had diabetes for a very long time (generally speaking, we are talking decades), your autonomic warning system may fail and, as in the situation above, the first clue there is a problem may be when you become confused.

- ✓ **Other drugs impairing your ability to recognize hypoglycemia:** Several drugs can interfere with your body's ability to produce autonomic symptoms. Such drugs include beta blockers (such as Inderal), which are often used to treat heart disease and high blood pressure. Another drug that some of you may have passing acquaintance with is alcohol, which, if used in sufficient quantities to impair your alertness, can blunt your ability to recognize when you are hypoglycemic.

Fortunately, in *almost* all cases you can restore your ability to recognize hypoglycemia. Sometimes it is simply a matter of avoiding alcohol. Other times it is adjusting your medicines.

Ketoacidosis

If you have type 1 diabetes, you are at risk for developing a temporary condition called *ketoacidosis.* Ketoacidosis (abbreviated DKA) is a condition in which your blood glucose level is high (typically above 14) *and* you have excess quantities of a type of acid called ketones in the blood. High blood glucose *without* the presence of ketones does not indicate DKA. (Though, of course it might indicate your glucose control is pretty crummy, but that is a different story.)

Ketoacidosis requires urgent attention because, if severe, it can be life threatening. Occasionally, the first clue that you have type 1 diabetes is when you become ill with ketoacidosis. More commonly DKA occurs after you already know that you have the disease.

As we say in Chapter 3, the main source of energy for your muscles is glucose. And for glucose to be used properly you must have sufficient insulin in your body. If you have type 1 diabetes you lack the ability to produce insulin and, thus, you need to give it to yourself by injection.

But what happens if your body requires more insulin than you are giving? Several things can happen. Your blood glucose levels will climb (because the glucose cannot get into your cells without sufficient insulin to help it). Your body will start to break down fat (and muscle) because it cannot use glucose as a fuel. And, as fat tissue breaks down, it releases acids ("ketones") into the bloodstream. The result is that you develop ketoacidosis.

Symptoms of ketoacidosis

Depending on the severity of your DKA you will have some combination of the following symptoms:

- **Nausea, vomiting, and abdominal pain:** It is noteworthy that many people with diabetes — and many doctors also, by the way — mistakenly attribute these symptoms to "stomach flu" (*gastroenteritis*) even when it is due to DKA. (Of course you *may* simply have "the flu," but a doctor should come to this conclusion only after DKA has been discounted.)

- **Rapid breathing:** You experience rapid breathing when your blood is so acidic that your body tries to compensate by ridding itself of acids through the lungs.

- **Fruity breath:** The presence of ketones in your system gives your breath a fruity, not unpleasant odour. Most people with DKA do not notice it even though it might be apparent to bystanders.

- **Extreme tiredness and drowsiness:** If your DKA is mild, your tiredness may also be mild, but as your DKA worsens you will feel increasingly drowsy, and if your DKA becomes severe you can lose consciousness.

The Canadian Diabetes Association recommends that people with type 1 diabetes test for ketones:

- During periods of acute illness
- When pre-meal blood glucose readings are above 14 mmol/L
- When symptoms of DKA (see above) are present

Ketoacidosis occurs rarely in type 2 diabetes. Nonetheless, if you have type 2 diabetes and you develop typical symptoms of DKA, it would be a good idea to check for ketones.

Ketones can be tested in either the urine (with Ketostix test strips) or, preferably, in the blood (with use of the Precision Xtra ketone testing meter made by MediSense; www.medisense.com).

If you notice that you have some symptoms of ketoacidosis and you test your blood ketone level and find it to be elevated (0.6 mmol/L or higher), you should contact your health care team. In most cases, the safest and best thing to do is to be seen at the closest emergency department. However, if you are fortunate enough to be working with a diabetes nurse educator who is both trained — and empowered — to deal with DKA and is immediately available, you can first contact him or her for detailed advice (unless you are feeling particularly unwell in which case you should simply proceed directly to hospital).

Causes of ketoacidosis

Ketoacidosis is caused by a *relative* lack of insulin. And no, this does not mean that it is caused by your first cousin Sally not having enough insulin. (Though perhaps she doesn't. We wouldn't know.) When we say *relative* lack of insulin, we mean that the amount of insulin in your body — no matter how much there is — is not enough for your body's needs. It follows, then, that DKA will develop in one of two general circumstances:

- **You are missing insulin doses:** If you have type 1 diabetes, your pancreas is unable to manufacture insulin, so you must give yourself insulin. Because most types of injected insulin don't last all that long in the body, if you miss doses your body quickly detects this and your metabolism will promptly suffer. (See Chapter 12 for a detailed discussion on insulin.) The occasional missed dose will not likely harm you, but if you miss several consecutive doses, you will be at substantial risk for developing DKA.

- **You are not taking high enough doses of insulin:** It is quite possible that day to day you give yourself a fairly similar quantity of insulin and get along quite nicely, thank you very much. That is great. But if you are experiencing some additional stress (emotional or, more commonly, physical) on your body, you will likely require higher doses of insulin to meet your body's increased needs. Examples would be if you develop, say, pneumonia or a kidney infection.

If you have type 1 diabetes, you are dependent on insulin injections not only to preserve your health, but to preserve your life. Even if you are feeling rotten and are eating nothing, you CANNOT forgo taking your insulin. In fact, you may need to give yourself *more* insulin than usual. The sickest patients that diabetes specialists ever see are those people with diabetes who, unfortunately, either weren't given this advice or knew it but didn't follow it.

Treatment of ketoacidosis

Ketoacidosis is a serious condition that requires very careful treatment. If you have mild DKA, you will possibly be treated as an outpatient under the very, very close supervision of your diabetes educator (see the preceding section). The following will probably be part of your treatment:

- **Ensuring proper hydration:** Achieved by making sure you are drinking sufficient quantities of fluids.

- **Giving yourself frequent insulin injections:** You may be asked to give yourself injections of rapid-acting insulin as often as every 2 hours.

- **Testing blood:** You will need to check your blood glucose and blood ketone levels often.

If you have anything more than mild DKA, you should be treated in a hospital. The treatment will consist of the following:

- **Ensuring proper hydration and sodium balance:** Achieved by intravenous administration of sodium-rich fluids.

- **Restoring proper potassium and mineral balance:** This is achieved by intravenous or oral administration of potassium and, at times, calcium, phosphate, magnesium, and bicarbonate.

- **Administering insulin:** This is usually done intravenously.

- **Testing blood:** Oh yes, where would we be without blood testing? You will likely be poked and prodded quite a bit, but fortunately that can usually be done by inserting a small tube into a blood vessel that can, in a sense, be turned on and off at will (sort of like a tap), so you may not have to be jabbed afresh each time.

- **Looking for the cause:** If the reason for your having developed DKA is not apparent (like missing insulin doses, for example) you may require additional blood and urine tests, X-rays, and so on to try to determine what may have triggered the episode (pneumonia, for example).

Prevention of ketoacidosis

How truly wonderful it is that what was once both unavoidable (and fatal!) is now almost always avoidable. It does, however, take a fair bit of effort to accomplish this. The key measures to prevent DKA are:

- **Monitor, monitor, monitor:** Often the earliest signs of developing DKA are rising blood glucose readings. If you are testing your blood frequently you may well detect a problem before it gets out of hand.

✓ **Take your insulin:** Whatever you do, do not fall into the trap of figuring that if you are feeling unwell and not eating or drinking properly, you do not need insulin. Trust us; you *do* require insulin. Sometimes less than usual, sometimes the same as usual, and often, more than usual.

Beth was a 13-year-old girl who had had type 1 diabetes for three years. After visiting a friend at a cottage she came down with terrible diarrhea. She spent the better part of the day on the toilet, but with her mom's encouragement, she was able to drink lots of fluids. Beth usually required three injections of insulin per day and her total daily dose of insulin was generally about 20 units. When she became ill, her blood glucose level rose to 22 and her blood started to test positive for ketones. Beth contacted her diabetes educator, who advised her to test her blood glucose every 2 hours and told her to take extra rapid-acting insulin every 2 hours if her blood glucose level was elevated. Over the next 12 hours she ended up taking an *extra* 30 units. By the next day, Beth was feeling back to normal, her glucose levels were normal, she had no ketones in the blood, her insulin doses were back to usual, and she was out playing with her friends. Beth was thrilled. Her mom was thrilled. Her educator and her doctors were thrilled. Everyone was thrilled, in fact, except for Beth's friend, who felt terribly guilty when they found out their lake water was contaminated with giardiasis ("Beaver Fever"). Ah, but we'll leave that to another book.

Hyperosmolar Hyperglycemic State

The name *hyperosmolar hyperglycemic state* refers to a situation where there are tremendously excessive levels of glucose in the blood. *Hyper* means "larger than normal," *osmolar* has to do with concentrations of substances in the blood, and *glycemic* has to do with blood glucose. In this particular situation, hyperosmolar hyperglycemic means that the blood is simply too concentrated with glucose.

Hyperosmolar hyperglycemic state (fortunately, abbreviated HHS) occurs in people with type 2 diabetes. Like ketoacidosis, HHS is a medical emergency; unlike ketoacidosis, HHS *always* requires treatment in a hospital.

Hyperosmolar hyperglycemic state goes by a variety of other names, including hyperosmolar hyperglycemic nonketotic coma, hyperglycemic hyperosmolar nonketotic coma, and hyperglycemic hyperosmolar nonketotic state. What all these terms share in common is that they are a mouthful to say and impossible to remember!

Symptoms of hyperosmolar hyperglycemic state

The symptoms of HHS arise in part from the effects on the body of very high glucose levels and in part from whatever condition (for example, a heart attack) triggered it. In terms of the high glucose levels — values as high as 100 are not unheard of — symptoms may include:

- ✔ Frequent urination
- ✔ Excessive thirst
- ✔ Dry mouth
- ✔ Leg cramps
- ✔ Weakness and lethargy
- ✔ Unconsciousness

The diagnosis of HHS is actually quite straightforward. If a person with known type 2 diabetes develops extraordinarily elevated blood glucose readings with evidence of dehydration and without the typical blood chemistry picture of ketoacidosis, the diagnosis is readily made.

If you measure your blood glucose on a daily basis, you should never develop HHS because you will notice if your blood glucose is getting high and you will take corrective action before it reaches a critical level.

HHS requires immediate and skilled treatment at a hospital. If you think you may have it, go to the nearest emergency department. The great majority of the time, however, it is not the affected person who recognizes the problem; it is a loved one (or, in the case of nursing home residents, a nurse) who detects something is wrong. The affected person is usually too sick to even know that they are unwell.

Not all elevations of blood glucose indicate HHS. If you are feeling well, not having the symptoms described above, and your blood glucose level is only mildly to moderately elevated (10 to 25 mmol/L or so), that does *not* mean you have HHS. It may mean, however, that you need to speak to your health care team about improving your overall glucose control.

Causes of hyperosmolar hyperglycemic state

HHS is most common among elderly people with diabetes, though it can occur in younger individuals. Whereas ketoacidosis (see the preceding section) most often occurs when people have not been taking sufficient insulin, HHS is most likely to occur if you have some additional serious illness that has triggered it. This may be, for example, a stroke, a heart attack, or a severe infection (such as pneumonia).

Typically, HHS develops in an infirm person whose diabetes is reasonably well controlled until some additional factor (like those just mentioned) develops. Whereas an otherwise healthy person with type 2 diabetes would recognize the presence of the additional problem and seek medical attention, an infirm individual may not know something is amiss or may not be able to deal with it. They then become increasingly unwell from the additional illness, from their worsening blood glucose levels, and from dehydration. Indeed, HHS leads to profound dehydration.

Treatment of hyperosmolar hyperglycemic state

Similar to the treatment of ketoacidosis, HHS treatment includes the following:

- **Ensuring proper hydration and sodium balance:** Achieved by intravenous administration of sodium-rich fluids. This is absolutely essential. Dehydration in HHS is usually very, very severe.

- **Restoring proper potassium and mineral balance:** This is achieved by intravenous or oral administration of potassium and, at times, calcium, phosphate, magnesium, and bicarbonate.

- **Administering insulin:** This is usually done intravenously. (Incidentally, insulin is of lesser importance than restoring proper hydration, and often insulin can be stopped altogether within a few days.)

- **Testing blood:** Monitoring of blood glucose levels as well as electrolytes, calcium, magnesium, phosphate, and other key blood constituents is crucial.

- **Looking for the cause:** HHS is almost always caused by something in addition to diabetes. A physician must make a meticulous search for this other cause and this likely will include blood and urine tests, X-rays, and heart tests amongst other things.

Even with the best possible therapy, the death rate for HHS is high because most people who suffer from it are elderly and often have other serious illnesses that both trigger it and complicate treatment.

Preventing hyperosmolar hyperglycemic state

There are two broad ways of looking at preventing hyperosmolar hyperglycemic state, depending on where you or your loved one live:

- ✔ **In the community:** If you or a loved one has type 2 diabetes and lives in the community, follow the treatment plan detailed in this book. With proper therapy (including nutrition, exercise, medicines, and so forth) you will likely never develop HHS. And, importantly, if despite following proper therapy your blood glucose levels keep climbing, contact your health care team to see if your treatment program needs to be adjusted or if a new health issue has come up that has made things worse.

- ✔ **In nursing homes:** If you or your loved one has diabetes and is resident in a nursing home, speak to the staff (or the physician) to ensure that blood glucose levels are being checked regularly and even more often in situations where you or your loved one is not feeling well. That way, if the blood glucose control is deteriorating, it can be picked up rapidly and dealt with before it spirals out of control.

Chapter 6

Handling Long-Term Problems

You may think that diabetes has made your life more complicated. And of course it has. What with having to alter your diet and your exercise pattern, having to monitor your blood glucose levels, and so on, you may feel that it is just too much hassle. And who could blame you? But the thing is, our long-term objective is not to make your life more difficult but to make it easier. Because looking after your diabetes before you run into complications is immeasurably easier than dealing with complications after they develop.

This chapter discusses the long-term complications that diabetes can cause, the best ways to avoid them, how to recognize them, and how to deal with them if they are already present. (We deal with acute glucose problems in the Chapter 5.)

As you read through this chapter you will come across complications that you will deem, correctly, to be minor, and others that will scare the pants (if that is your chosen attire) off you. Please, please do yourself and us a favour and if you see something that frightens you, keep repeating to yourself the following mantra:

Complications Are Not Inevitable

Long-term complications can take years to develop, so with excellent diabetes care you will be able to avoid the great majority of these problems. It ain't easy, but it is doable. By the way, if anyone who does not have diabetes has the temerity to tell you it is easy, ask them to try it and see how many takers you get!

Before we get into the details of the different long-term complications that can develop, it is worth noting that many of these problems can be lumped into two broad categories:

- **Small blood vessel damage** (called *microvascular disease*): This type of problem leads to disease of the eyes (retinopathy), kidneys (nephropathy), and nerve endings (neuropathy). Microvascular disease is primarily the result of inadequate blood glucose control.

- **Large blood vessel damage** (called *macrovascular disease*): This type of problem leads to disease of the circulation to the brain (cerebrovascular disease), heart (coronary artery disease), and legs (peripheral vascular disease). Macrovascular disease is particularly likely to occur if you smoke or have inadequate control of blood pressure and cholesterol. The bad news: macrovascular disease is the cause of death of 80 percent of people with diabetes. The good news: macrovascular disease is often preventable and always treatable.

If you have been diagnosed recently as having type 2 diabetes, it is quite possible you have already had it for several years without knowing it and, as such, you potentially already could have run into complications that you had no idea were present. For that reason, it is absolutely essential that your physician carefully check to determine if you have any evidence of damage to your body — even if you were diagnosed yesterday. This chapter as well as the Cheat Sheet in the front of this book will detail what you and your doctor should look for.

Eye Disease

A variety of different types of eye problems can occur in people with diabetes. Some eye diseases, such as glaucoma (raised pressure within the fluid of the eye) and cataracts (cloudiness of the lens of the eye), also occur in the nondiabetic population, though you are more likely to get them if you have diabetes. The eye diseases of greatest concern to people with diabetes are *macular edema* (swelling of the small area at the back of the eye where vision is sharpest leading to blurred vision) and *retinopathy* – damage to the back ("retinal") surface of the eye. Retinopathy is the most common cause of new cases of adult-onset blindness in Canada.

Retinopathy

Diabetic retinopathy refers to several different types of injury that occur to the back surface of the eye. It is this surface that allows you to see the world around you. The earliest feature of retinopathy is a tiny ballooning of small blood vessels called *microaneurysms*. One stage later in severity is the development of small areas of bleeding called *dot hemorrhages* or slightly bigger ones called *blot hemorrhages*. These changes usually do not cause loss of vision.

Sometimes retinopathy progresses to a more serious stage, which, if untreated, can threaten your eyesight. Abnormal blood vessels can form (*neovascularization*). These vessels are fragile and have the potential to bleed, which, in turn, can both obscure vision and lead to a potentially catastrophic *retinal detachment*.

If by this point you are not frightened out of your mind — or, for that matter, even if you are — you might wish to see pictures of these different features. Go to Google (www.google.com) and type in any of the terms above, then click Images. For the greatest number of results use "diabetic retinopathy" as your search term and you will come up with thousands of images.

Pregnancy can cause retinopathy to worsen rapidly. If you have pre-existing diabetes (see Chapter 7) and you are considering getting pregnant, it is imperative that you see an eye doctor *before* you try to get pregnant, then regularly during your pregnancy. (This does not apply to gestational diabetes since retinopathy does not develop in this condition.)

If you look in the mirror one day and see that you have "pink eye" or that you have a small area of bleeding in the whites of one of your eyes, you can rest assured that these are not features of diabetes eye damage. Diabetes damages the *inside* of the eyes, not the *outside*.

How you can prevent retinopathy

It is crucial to keep reminding yourself of what we said at the outset of this chapter. Damage to your body from diabetes — including serious eye disease — is not inevitable. By paying careful attention to your diabetes and obtaining appropriate monitoring by health care professionals, you can minimize the likelihood of running into sight-threatening eye damage.

Here are the most important ways to protect your vision:

- Maintain excellent blood glucose control (see Chapter 9).
- Maintain excellent blood pressure (see later in this chapter).
- Maintain excellent lipids (see later in this chapter).
- Don't smoke (reason number 4,362, last time we checked).
- Obtain regular, expert eye care from a highly skilled optometrist or ophthalmologist.

As we discuss in Chapter 4, if your blood glucose levels are in a period of major change (high to normal, or normal to high) you may develop temporary visual blurring. This is *not* a sign of retinopathy.

If you have had chronically poor blood glucose readings and are then placed on aggressive (as it should be!) treatment to improve things, there can be an initial worsening of retinopathy *if* you already have it. Ultimately, better blood glucose control will help protect your eyes, but because of the initial potential for worsening it is crucial that you see an eye doctor shortly after being placed on aggressive blood-glucose-lowering treatment. Most doctors do not know this, so you may have to tell them. Feel free to show them this page. Don't worry about offending your doctor. No doctor in the world knows everything. (Just ask their kids.)

No drugs are of proven value in treating retinopathy, but laser surgery is an excellent treatment option. Sometimes, for particularly severe cases, an operation — called a *vitrectomy* — is done where fluid (and any blood that is present) is removed from the back portion of the eyeball and replaced with a sterile solution.

Contrary to what is commonly thought, aspirin (ASA) does *not* increase the risk of serious bleeding within the eye. If you need to take aspirin (see the next section), having diabetic retinopathy should not prevent you from taking it unless your eye doctor has very specific concerns for your particular situation.

Resources to help you if you are blind or visually impaired

In the event you need them, many devices are available to assist you, including:

- Glucose meters that have speech capability (well, they will talk to you, but don't bother trying to speak to them; not yet anyhow). We discuss glucose meters in Chapter 9.

✔ Insulin pen devices that "click" as you dial them. This makes it easier to keep track of how much insulin you are about to give. For some types of insulin pens you can obtain a miniature magnifying glass that fits over the numerical display to make it easier to see the dose of insulin you are about to give. We discuss insulin pen devices in Chapter 12.

There are many Internet resources also available to assist you. Particularly helpful Web sites are listed in Appendix C.

If you are visually impaired, remember that you can change your Internet browser settings to enlarge the print on a web page (for Internet Explorer, click View, then Text Size, then choose the size you would like to try from the various options displayed). Your computer's operating system also probably has options to make it easier for you to read your screen. For example, in Windows XP, you can click Start, then All Programs, then Accessories, then Accessibility, then Magnifier. Unless you have a prodigious memory, we suspect you will find it easier to do this if you have this page in front of you as you navigate!

If you are using insulin syringes, you may find it helpful to have someone pre-load them with the required amount of insulin. You can then store them in the refrigerator until you need them. In general, however, it is easier to use an insulin pen device if you are sight-impaired.

One of Ian's patients is a 35-year-old man who uses a bar code reader to scan in his grocery store purchases. The device has a speech synthesizer so that whenever he is looking for, say, a can of chicken soup, he will scan the cans on his shelf and, *presto,* his can announces its contents.

Which eye doctor should you see: An optometrist or an ophthalmologist?

As you read this chapter you may be thinking to yourself, "Boy, I'd better make sure I see my eye doctor." You bet. But which one? Should you see an optometrist or an ophthalmologist? An optometrist is trained to detect eye disease and can prescribe glasses, but he or she is not a medical doctor and cannot perform eye surgery. An ophthalmologist is a medical doctor who is trained to detect and treat eye diseases — with medicines and, if necessary, surgery. An optician, by the way, is someone who is trained to fit you with glasses but not to detect or treat diabetes eye disease.

If you do not have diabetes eye disease and simply need to have routine screening to ensure your eyes are in good health, it does not matter whether you see an optometrist or an ophthalmologist. If, however, you have diabetes eye damage – especially if it is severe — you should be referred to an ophthalmologist. The key thing is to see a highly skilled eye specialist.

Current Canadian Diabetes Association recommendations for retinopathy screening are:

If you have type 1 diabetes, you should be assessed by an experienced eye specialist annually 5 years after the onset of diabetes in individuals age 15 or over.

If you have type 2 diabetes, you should be assessed by an experienced eye specialist at the time of diagnosis. The timing of follow-up assessments should be based on the degree of eye damage (if any) that you have. If you have no or minimal retinopathy, you should be seen every 1 to 2 years.

Some provincial health insurance plans will pay for only one optometry visit (but an unlimited number of ophthalmology visits) per year. We think this is foolish, but hey, we don't make the rules. (Sure wish we did, though.)

Heart and Circulatory Disease

Although we (physicians and patients) talk about heart *disease*, in fact what we should be doing is talking about heart *diseases*. Most commonly, the term *heart disease* refers to *coronary artery disease*, but people with diabetes can, on occasion, run into other heart ailments. When you are said to have "problems with your circulation" that usually means poor blood flow to your legs and feet, but it can also refer to impaired blood supply to your brain. The most common cause of death in people with diabetes is related to heart and circulatory disease. This section talks about these crucial issues and, most important, what you can do to help ward them off.

Coronary artery disease and heart attacks

The heart is, essentially, a pump. An amazing, complex, wonderful pump (when was the last time you went to the hardware store and bought a pump that was likely to last for 80-plus years?), but a pump nonetheless.

Coronary artery disease (CAD) is the term for blockage ("plaque") within the arteries (the *coronary* arteries) that supply blood to the heart muscle. Plaque is composed of a mixture of cholesterol, fat, and calcium. The presence of plaque within blood vessels is called *atherosclerosis*. Because the blood vessels become very stiff from all this scarring, atherosclerosis is commonly referred to as *hardening of the arteries*.

The most common symptoms of coronary artery disease are chest discomfort ("angina") and shortness of breath. Other symptoms can include dizziness or fatigue. Symptoms of coronary artery disease are especially likely to occur if you are exerting yourself, such as walking up a hill or a flight of stairs.

If ever you develop symptoms like those just described, it is essential that you arrange to see your doctor promptly. If, however, you experience chest discomfort or shortness of breath that lasts more than a few minutes you must call 9-1-1 and be taken by ambulance to hospital. YOU SHOULD NEVER, EVER DRIVE YOURSELF TO HOSPITAL IF YOU THINK YOU ARE EXPERIENCING A HEART ATTACK. (And don't get your loved one or next-door neighbour to drive you, either. Unless of course they happen to be a paramedic and have an ambulance parked in the driveway!)

These are the most important risk factors for developing CAD:

- ✔ Abnormal lipids (cholesterol and triglycerides)
- ✔ High blood pressure ("hypertension")
- ✔ Smoking
- ✔ Diabetes
- ✔ Family history of coronary artery
- ✔ Obesity (especially in the abdomen)
- ✔ Sedentariness

As you can readily see, many of these factors are reversible. You can lose weight, exercise, bring your blood pressure and cholesterol under control, stop smoking, look after your diabetes, and choose different parents (oops, forget about that last one!).

More than one patient has told us that quitting cigarettes is easy; they've done it hundreds of times! Okay, so quitting *is* easy; but to remain a quitter is difficult. Still, it can be done, *if* you are ready. Quitting "cold turkey" is the best option for some people. For others, using a nicotine patch or a medication called Zyban is helpful. If you have tried quitting but have gone back to smoking, then try again the next day. And if that doesn't work, try again the next day. The key to success is not giving up. Ignore your failures and start your efforts afresh each day. Ultimately you can and will succeed.

You can also help prevent a heart attack by taking aspirin. ASA is a mild blood thinner and helps prevent blood clots. Most people with diabetes *should* be on aspirin unless there is some reason you cannot or should not take it. The usual dose is 81 to 325 milligrams per day. If you are unable to tolerate plain aspirin (for example, if it gives you an upset stomach) try taking a *coated* aspirin. If you cannot tolerate that either, a suitable alternative is another type of blood thinner called clopidogrel (Plavix). (The most common reasons for *not* being able to take aspirin are being under 21 years of age – because of the risk of Reye's syndrome – having a bleeding disorder or having had recent internal bleeding.) Be sure to speak to your doctor about whether you should be taking aspirin.

Also, there is recent evidence that drugs called *ACE inhibitors* can prevent cardiovascular damage – such as heart attacks and strokes — in many people with diabetes who are at high risk for attacks. Most people with diabetes over the age of 55 should be on an ACE inhibitor as should many younger people with diabetes if they are considered at high risk for vascular disease. Be sure to speak to your doctor about whether you should be taking an ACE inhibitor. You (and your doctor) can learn more about the rationale for taking an ACE inhibitor by reading about the HOPE study (www.aventis-pharma.ca/Glo.htm).

There are excellent therapies available to treat coronary artery disease, and more and better ones are coming out all the time. We have medicines, angioplasty (therapy where a blockage is opened with a balloon, then kept open with a tiny device called a "stent"), and bypass surgery. And not to be underestimated is the impact of following a healthy diet and exercising.

If you have a heart attack, your outlook for recovery is much better if your blood glucose levels are excellently controlled while you are in the hospital (and, of course, after you are back home). There is an understandable tendency for health care providers to focus on the most pressing issue — your heart attack — and to not pay sufficient attention to things like glucose control. If you have the misfortune of having a heart attack, it is imperative that your glucose control be treated aggressively — often intravenous insulin is necessary for a few days. If your doctor does not know about this, tell him or her to refer to the DIGAMI study. You can tell them Ian and Alan said so.

Cerebrovascular disease and strokes

The same processes that affect the coronary arteries (the arteries that feed the heart with oxygen) can affect the arteries to the brain. This is called cerebrovascular disease (CVD). CVD can lead to strokes.

Having read the preceding paragraph, you may already have concluded that if cerebrovascular disease and coronary artery disease have a similar underlying process, then the risk factors leading to CVD are probably the same. You are right.

If you want to know what therapies you can use to prevent having a stroke, read the section immediately above, where we talk about ways to prevent heart disease. The same information applies.

Peripheral vascular disease (problems with circulation to the legs and feet)

Diabetes can do many things that are scary. For most people, high up on this intimidating list are perfectly justified fears about "poor circulation" leading to amputations. Poor circulation to the legs is called *peripheral vascular disease* (PVD) and is due to atherosclerosis obstructing the flow of blood. It is caused by the same factors that lead to coronary artery disease and cerebrovascular disease. Similarly, you can avoid it by following the measures that we described earlier in this chapter.

A diabetes educator that Ian works with recalls the time, about 30 years ago, when she was sitting in a room with a 45-year-old man who had been newly diagnosed with diabetes. After they had chatted for a while, the doctor entered the room and nonchalantly said to his patient, "You may as well start preparing for your amputations now. It's just a matter of time, after all." The poor man's face sank. The doctor was clearly heartless and tactless, but even worse, he may have had some reason for saying this. The knowledge and therapy we had back then were vastly inferior to what we have nowadays and this particular doctor had likely had all too much experience at seeing the devastation that could occur. But — drumroll please — we've got news for him (and you). It is most definitely *not* "just a matter of time." Amputations are almost always avoidable. But the time to start your program of healthy foot maintenance is *now*. Think of it the way you would car maintenance: Much better to keep your car in a top state of repair than to run into engine problems halfway between Quebec City and Montreal on a − 30°C Christmas Day (Ian speaks from experience, as you may have suspected).

Far and away the most common symptom of PVD is an aching discomfort in your calves as you walk. This is called *intermittent claudication* (usually abbreviated to "claudication"). Generally speaking, the sooner the discomfort occurs as you walk, the worse are the blockages in the arteries.

If PVD is very severe it can lead to changes in the feet, including the following:

- Pale appearance
- Loss of hair
- Constant pain in the toes
- Small, usually red or black, spots on the tips of the toes
- Open sores or ulcers on the bottom or sides of the feet

If you have developed any of the symptoms above, it is important that you let your family physician or diabetes specialist know. If you have developed either of the last two items on the list, you may have gangrene and/or a foot infection, in which case you need to seek *immediate* medical attention.

Peripheral vascular disease is difficult to treat, but there are helpful therapies available, including medications and, in some cases, surgery to open up or bypass a blocked artery. It is, of course, crucial that you not smoke and it is also important that your cholesterol and blood pressure are well controlled. Your physician can also discuss certain helpful types of exercises that you can perform or alternatively, can refer you to a specialist in this field.

There are, of course, numerous reasons not to smoke, but it is worth making special mention of the influence of smoking on PVD. Smoking will make you much more prone to PVD. Even more important, if you continue to smoke when you *already have* PVD it is a certainty you will develop worsening circulation problems and you will put yourself at enormous risk of developing foot ulcerations and gangrene. Trust us; you will not be a happy camper if this happens.

We will talk more about foot care later in this chapter (see "Foot disease in diabetes").

The lowdown on high blood pressure

High blood pressure is a common health problem regardless of whether or not you have diabetes. It is, however, especially common among people with diabetes. Not that diabetes *causes* high blood pressure; it's just *associated* with it. Yet another unfair thing about having diabetes (as if there were not enough already).

The medical term for high blood pressure is *hypertension*. You may have noticed that your doctor refers to your blood pressure as being *something* over *something* ("140 over 90," for example). The first number represents the *systolic* value and the second number the *diastolic* value. The systolic value is the amount of force exerted by the heart when it contracts to push blood around the body. The diastolic value is the pressure in the large arteries when the heart is at rest.

Keeping your blood pressure *normal* is essential. High blood pressure can lead to all sorts of problems — particularly if you have diabetes — including:

- ✔ Strokes
- ✔ Heart attacks
- ✔ Blindness (hypertension aggravates retinopathy)
- ✔ Kidney failure

Now, a list like this is not designed to depress you. It is to alert you to the importance of the issue, because with proper therapy you can help avoid these problems. Indeed, modern medicine has very, very effective therapy for high blood pressure.

What exactly is "normal" blood pressure? This should be such a simple question to answer, but in fact it is not. Sometimes it seems that each year some new study comes out showing that we should be aiming lower. Ian recalls being at a lecture where a highly respected blood pressure specialist facetiously said: "If your patient can still stand up, then their blood pressure is still too high!" Suffice to say, if you have diabetes your target blood pressure is less than or equal to 130 over 80 (usually written as 130/80 — which, by the way, is not to say you should divide 130 by 80 and walk out of your doctor's office thinking your blood pressure is 1.625. A blood pressure of 1.625 would likely make an earthworm dizzy!).

Never let your doctor or any other health care provider simply report to you that your blood pressure is "good" or "fine" or "okay," or some other equally vague and ultimately meaningless term. If they do not volunteer what your measurement was, ask them and write the number down in your blood glucose logbook (we talk more about logbooks in Chapter 9) or, even better, on the Cheat Sheet at the front of this book. Furthermore, if your blood pressure is above target (remember, target is less than or equal to 130/80), ask your doctor how you and he or she are going to improve it. Do not settle for second-rate blood pressure control. We're talking your health here!

The CDA recommends that you have your blood pressure measured every time you see your doctor for a diabetes-related visit (since diabetes can affect pretty well all your body, that would mean almost every visit).

The following are treatments for high blood pressure:

- Diet (reduce salt, minimize caffeine, limit alcohol)
- Exercise
- Weight control
- Medicines (often a combination of 2, 3 or even 4 different medicines is required)

The ACCORD study

With every passing year it seems that we are aiming for a lower target blood pressure. The ACCORD study (Action to Control Cardiovascular Risk in Diabetes; www.accordtrial.org) is an ongoing research study involving thousands of people with diabetes. The ACCORD study will help us to determine how low we should be trying to get blood pressure. It could be that a systolic value of under 120 is best. This study should help to tell us. The ACCORD study is also looking at whether we should be aiming for even lower blood glucose readings than our current targets. Results of the study will not be available anytime soon; the study's conclusions will not be known until 2010. When it comes to scientific progress, patience is truly a virtue!

Dyslipidemia (Abnormal Cholesterol and Triglyceride Levels)

In much the same way as, with each passing year, some new study comes out telling us that we should be aiming for lower blood pressure values, so too do we keep discovering that we have not been aggressive enough about cholesterol and triglyceride management. In the last section we emphasized the importance of your knowing your blood pressure number and discussing with your doctor how you are going to work *together* at optimizing it. In this section you will learn what cholesterol and triglycerides are all about, so that, once again, you and your health care team can work *together* toward our common goal of keeping you healthy.

There are many types of lipids, but you should be aware of these five important ones:

- **HDL:** This stands for *high density lipoprotein*. You *want* your HDL to be high since it is actually protection for your blood vessels; it removes cholesterol from the walls of your arteries. HDL is thought of as the *good* cholesterol. You can remember this by the phrase: "A **h**igh **H**DL keeps you **h**ealthy." (We haven't taken out a copyright on the phrase, so feel free to share it with your friends.)

- **LDL:** This stands for low density lipoprotein. You want your LDL to be low. LDL is thought of as the *bad* cholesterol. You can remember all of this by the phrase: "**L**DL is **l**ousy and should be **l**ow." (Once again, no copyright.)

- **Triglycerides:** These are the main fats in the blood. Their role in the development of atherosclerosis is not quite as proven as LDL and HDL, however it is wise to keep your triglycerides in the normal range (see below).

- **Total cholesterol:** This is a measure of a combination of various forms of cholesterol.

- **Total cholesterol/HDL ratio:** Just as it sounds, this is a ratio of total cholesterol to HDL cholesterol and is used in helping to decide if you require treatment. The lower the ratio, the better.

The CDA recommends that you have your lipid levels checked at the time of diagnosis of your diabetes and then every 1 to 3 years (more frequently if treatment has been initiated or changed).

You should be fasting when your blood sample is taken to measure your lipids, as this allows for a more precise determination of your levels. When your doctor fills out the requisition for your lipid measurement, make sure he or she writes on the requisition precisely how long they want you to fast. If your doctor does not do this, the lab may tell you that you must be fasting for 14 hours before they will do the test. But that can be dangerous if you are taking certain oral hypoglycemic drugs (we discuss these in Chapter 11) or insulin. If you are on these medicines, *never* fast for anywhere near 14 hours unless you have first checked with your doctor. In most cases an 8-hour fast is sufficient.

Although pretty well everything you read about cholesterol discusses how bad it is, in fact cholesterol is an essential substance required for maintaining healthy cells and manufacturing certain vitamins and hormones. Problems arise when we have too much cholesterol or too much of the wrong type.

If your lipids are abnormal, you are at higher risk for developing hardening of the arteries *(atherosclerosis),* which can, in turn, lead to strokes, heart attacks, and amputations. Keeping your lipids under *great* (don't settle for just "good") control will help you to maintain good health. Here are the current Canadian Diabetes Association (CDA) recommended targets:

- **LDL:** *Less* than 2.5 mmol/L (less than 3.5 if you are not at high risk of vascular disease; this is seldom the case)
- **Total cholesterol/HDL:** *Less* than 4.0 (less than 5.0 if you are not at high risk of vascular disease; this is seldom the case)

Although the CDA does not have a specific treatment target for triglycerides, they note that a triglyceride level of less than 1.5 mmol/L is considered optimal.

For people with diabetes, the most common problem is high LDL, low HDL, and high triglycerides. Fortunately, there is very effective therapy for this.

How to keep your lipids under control

These are the ways to improve your lipids:

- Eat healthfully
- Exercise regularly
- Achieve (and maintain) a healthy weight
- Take medication

We discuss the first three of these therapies in Chapter 10.

The Heart Protection Study

The Heart Protection Study (www.hpsinfo.org) which was recently published may turn our approach to treating lipids on its ear. That study showed that if you have diabetes and you are 40 years of age or older, you can reduce your risk of developing a heart attack or stroke by about twenty-five percent by taking a cholesterol medicine called simvastatin (also known as Zocor) in a dose of 40 mg per day even if your LDL is less than 2.5 (that is, within target) to start with. The study results are compelling, but somewhat controversial and it remains to be seen whether or not this new therapeutic strategy will be widely adopted. Stay tuned.

Some medicines used to improve cholesterol levels work better if taken in the evening. If you are prescribed cholesterol-lowering pills, be sure to ask your doctor or pharmacist when you are to take them.

Most of the cholesterol in your body is actually manufactured *by* your body (your liver to be precise). Although you may be able to limit your cholesterol intake, it is quite a different thing to get your liver to stop making cholesterol. Thus, lifestyle therapy (diet, exercise, weight control) is often not sufficient to bring your lipids into line — and medication (typically a member of the "*statin*" class of drugs; examples include Zocor and Lipitor) becomes necessary. A common mistake is for people to stop their medicine after they have completed their first prescription, mistakenly thinking that they no longer need it. Unless you change livers (which we imagine is not very likely), you will need to continue to take the medicine.

Kidney Disease

You can think of your kidneys as filters. And what amazing filters they are. Not only can they rid your body of toxins that are produced as a normal byproduct of metabolism, but also they can maintain your salt and water balance, keep the level of acids in your body under control, and release hormones that regulate your body's production of blood. Sometimes it seems the only thing these amazing filters can't do is help make coffee.

Unfortunately, diabetes can damage the kidneys. In fact, diabetes is the most common cause of kidney failure in Canada. Fortunately, this damage is largely preventable.

It takes years and years for diabetes to cause kidney damage. That means we have lots of opportunity to prevent damage from occurring. A doctor's earliest clue that there is a problem is that he or she discovers excess levels of *albumin* (a type of protein) in your urine. This is called *microalbuminuria* and can be screened for with a very simple urine test (a urine *microalbumin/creatinine ratio;* abbreviated as *ACR*). Your doctor should be testing you for this routinely (see the Cheat Sheet at the front of this book to find out how often), since it will not cause symptoms to alert you that there is a problem. If damage progresses, it leads to larger quantities of protein in the urine and can cause your feet and legs to swell ("edema"). If things continue to worsen, your kidneys can become unable to purify your blood of toxins. This last stage is called *kidney failure* and typically makes people feel unwell in many ways; it can cause fatigue, weight loss, and, if severe, confused thinking. (Incidentally — and contrary to popular wisdom — kidney damage from diabetes does *not* cause back pain.)

Because the ACR can be temporarily elevated if you are ill with other problems such as heart failure, a kidney infection or even if you have uncontrolled hyperglycemia (that is, very high blood glucose) or you have recently done heavy exercise, your ACR should not be tested until these other conditions have passed.

The new CDA Guidelines recommend that an additional kidney test called the blood creatinine level should be tested annually (and at least every six months if you have excess albumin in your urine). Your creatinine level is used to calculate – with something called the *"Cockroft-Gault equation"* – your *creatinine clearance* which is a measure of how efficiently your kidneys are able to purify your blood. (This equation is available at www.nephron.com/cgi-bin/ CGSIdefault.cgi). Incidentally, most doctors have not likely ever heard of the Cockroft-Gault equation and it will likely take some time before Canadian physicians are routinely using it.

Many other diseases can cause kidney damage, but often not in the same typical series of stages that we just outlined. For example, if your doctor were to find that you had kidney failure but you did not have excess levels of protein in the urine, that would suggest that your kidneys had been damaged by something other than diabetes.

The most important factors in leading to diabetes kidney disease are inadequate blood glucose control and elevated blood pressure. Other, unknown (perhaps genetic) factors must be present too, since most people with diabetes never develop kidney malfunction. Since it is impossible to predict whether you will always have healthy kidneys, it is crucial that you take all possible precautions to protect these important organs.

Now that you've read all about the bad things that can happen to your kidneys, we can tell you the good news. Not only is diabetes kidney disease preventable (by maintaining excellent blood glucose and blood pressure control), but also, in the majority of cases if it is caught early, we can slow down its progression or even halt it in its tracks. We do this through:

- ✔ **Excellent blood glucose control**
- ✔ **Excellent blood pressure control**
- ✔ **Medication** (For type 1 diabetes, drugs called ACE inhibitors should be used; for type 2 diabetes either ACE inhibitors or drugs called ARB's should be used.)
- ✔ **Low protein diet** (This is usually only prescribed if you have quite advanced kidney malfunction and it is of less proven value than the three previous treatments.)

ACE inhibitors and ARB's will occasionally lead to potentially dangerous accumulation of potassium in the body and can, rarely, make kidney function worse, not better. For these reasons, 1 to 2 weeks after you are started on one of these types of drugs your doctor should send you to the laboratory for a blood test to check your potassium and creatinine levels. Although the creatinine typically goes up shortly after starting ACE inhibitor or ARB therapy, it should not rise by more than 30 percent. If it does, it may signify worsening kidney function caused by the drug and your doctor may have to stop the medicine.

If despite our best efforts your kidneys have progressed to the point where they have almost completely stopped working (*end-stage kidney failure*), you will require dialysis (a method of purifying the blood) or a kidney transplant.

Sandra was 13 years old when she found out she had diabetes. Over the next 10 years she didn't look after herself all that well. In fact, she seldom checked her glucose readings, hardly ever saw her doctor, and never met with her diabetes educator. Now, however, she was "getting her act together" as she herself said when she came for her appointment with Ian. She was engaged to be married and had new interest in her health. Ian ran some basic investigations and determined that Sandra had excess albumin in her urine. Sandra was devastated. Now that she was keen to be healthy, she felt guilty about her "past sins" (as she called them). But Sandra was a determined woman and put her full effort into her diabetes. She got her glucose under control, quit smoking, and started ACE inhibitor medicine. Over the next year when we rechecked her urine, her albumin level returned to normal. Ian has rarely seen a happier face than Sandra's the day he told her the good news. We've come a long way from the days, not all that long ago, when once the kidneys showed any evidence of damage things only got worse and worse.

Neuropathy (Nerve Damage)

Nerve damage from diabetes is a very common but *very* preventable problem. There are many different types of nerve damage and this topic alone could fill an entire book. Most forms are uncommon or downright obscure, however, so we will concentrate on the more frequent types of nerve damage that you should be aware of.

You can think of the nervous system as a complex network of electrical circuitry with signals going in every direction as messages are relayed from one part of your body to another. Suffice to say that no computer system yet designed has even 1 percent of the complexity of the human nervous system. Shakespeare sure knew of what he spoke when he said "What a piece of work is man."

Peripheral neuropathy

The peripheral nervous system is made up of the nerves that travel from the spinal cord to the *periphery* of your body, including your arms and legs. Peripheral neuropathy is damage to the nerves that make up the peripheral nervous system.

Although the precise mechanism of injury is not known, there are two main theories as to why people with diabetes develop peripheral neuropathy. One proposal is that elevated blood glucose levels lead to damage to the very small blood vessels that supply oxygen and nutrients to the nerves. The second theory is that various sugars accumulate within the nerves and cause changes in the way nerves function.

Note that peripheral neuropathy can occur with many dozens of different diseases unrelated to diabetes, so clearly elevated blood glucose is but one possible cause of this disorder.

The most common symptoms of peripheral neuropathy are abnormal sensations (*paresthesiae* and *dysesthesiae*) such as a burning or hot feeling in the toes (and, if more advanced, the feet also). Other sensations that can be experienced include throbbing, aching, numbness, prickling, sharp, shooting pains, or even a tickling. Sometimes, people say they feel like they are "walking on marbles." If neuropathy progresses, it can lead to lack of ability to perceive pain. Although lack of pain is wonderful when you are having an operation, it is not a good thing when it comes to your feet, because in the absence of pain you may not recognize when a sore or injury has developed.

Peripheral neuropathy is usually diagnosed on "clinical grounds," which is a fancy way of saying that doctors generally make the diagnosis based on what symptoms you are having and what they find upon examining you. Your doctor may check to see if you can feel a vibrating tuning fork or if you can recognize the feel of a thin nylon rod (*a 10-gram monofilament*) when they are pressed against your foot (in particular, the big toe). We will discuss additional issues in foot care later in this chapter.

The 10-gram monofilament test is very, very easy to do and tells us crucial information. If your test is abnormal it means that you are at much greater risk of developing a foot ulcer, and, as you may recall, foot ulcers can lead to gangrene (and, ultimately, put you at risk for amputation). You can see an online demonstration of how this test is done at `www.bphc.hrsa.gov/leap/default.htm`. This Web site discusses the LEAP (Lower Extremity Amputation Prevention) Program. You can order your own monofilament (free of charge) from them.

Although highly effective therapy is available for the great majority of diabetes complications, regrettably, the treatments available for peripheral neuropathy are not quite as good. They are not bad — just not quite as good. The most commonly used medicines are amitriptyline and gabapentin. These are taken orally. If the area of discomfort is very small, you can try applying a topical medicine called capsaicin. (Since capsaicin is derived from chili peppers, you might think that it could really sting if it got in your eyes. And you would be right. After you apply the capsaicin to your feet, make sure you wash your hands really well before you touch *anything* else.)

We do not have great treatment for peripheral neuropathy, so if you are not responding to the medicines available, you might consider contacting the neurology department of a university-affiliated hospital to see if you are eligible to participate in any ongoing research studies.

Although good blood glucose control will not cure your neuropathy, many people find their symptoms substantially improve as they bring their glucose readings into line. Yet another reason (we must be up to a hundred by now) for making sure your blood glucose control is as good as possible.

Prevention of course is always best. Since peripheral neuropathy is caused by elevated blood glucose levels, the way to prevent it is — no surprise here — making sure your blood glucose level is under control.

Autonomic neuropathy

The autonomic ("automatic") nervous system works behind the scenes, controlling many body functions that you do not directly control, including bowel and bladder function. Autonomic neuropathy is nerve damage to the autonomic nervous system. This occurs quite commonly if you have had diabetes for a long time, but often the symptoms are passed off to something else. Some of the most common problems encountered include the following:

- **Sexual dysfunction:** We discuss this further in Chapter 7.

- **Disorders of the stomach and large intestine:** We discuss this in the next section.

- **Bladder difficulties:** You may not recognize an urge to empty your bladder even when it is full (*neurogenic* bladder). This can lead to distension of the bladder, which in turn can make you more prone to urinary tract infections and, in the most severe cases, kidney malfunction. The most common symptom that may alert you to the development of bladder malfunction is the repeated passage of only tiny quantities of urine (basically a problem with overflow akin to water dripping down the sides of an over-filled glass).

- **Abnormal heart rate:** Your heart has the ability to slow down and speed up to match your body's needs. If you develop damage to the part of the autonomic nervous system that helps regulate your heart, your heart may end up going too fast or, conversely, too slow.

- **Sweating problems:** Excess sweating can occur. One very unusual and intriguing problem is the development of sweating over the forehead as you start to eat your food. This is called *gustatory* sweating.

One last form of neuropathy that we would like to mention is what is called an *extra-ocular muscle palsy*. In this condition one of the muscles that controls eye movement becomes damaged and typically leads to double vision. Fortunately, this spontaneously corrects, but it can take a number of weeks or even months to come around.

Having diabetes and reading about the various neuropathies that can occur may make you feel either discouraged or alarmed, or both. Although that makes perfect sense, it is crucial that you remind yourself that most of these complications are avoidable. Ultimately, we hope the closest you will ever get to a nerve problem will be when you try to get a date with that cute neighbour of yours.

Stomach and Intestinal Function

Your "gut" can be thought of as a long, hollow tube extending from your mouth to your anus. Stretched end to end it would reach over 8 metres (25 feet — once again, please do *not* try this at home!). Diabetes can affect the gut in a variety of ways.

Gastroparesis is a condition in which your stomach becomes less efficient at propelling food into your small intestine. As a consequence, you may find that you get full very quickly as you eat. Additionally, because nutrients do not get absorbed as rapidly (nutrients get absorbed almost exclusively from the small bowel, not the stomach), your blood glucose control may become erratic. We treat gastroparesis with medicines (such as metoclopramide and domperidone) that enhance stomach emptying.

Diarrhea can occur for one of several reasons, including damage to the nerves that control intestinal function and excess numbers of bacteria ("bacterial overgrowth") within the bowel. Depending on the specific nature of the problem, your doctor may prescribe either antibiotics or medicine to slow down bowel function.

Foot Disease in Diabetes

The most serious threat to your foot is an ulcer, because this can lead to worsening infection and, ultimately, the need for amputation. For this reason, it is essential that you keep your feet healthy and happy. You must develop an obsession with your feet. A veritable love affair with your feet. Indeed, you must develop a foot fetish!

In a sense, foot disease is really a combination of many of the different topics we cover in this chapter. Typically, a person with diabetes who runs into foot problems has a combination of peripheral neuropathy and peripheral vascular disease and may have skin problems as well (which we discuss in the next section). In addition to the advice that pertains to those specific topics, there are a number of things you can do to protect your feet:

✔ **Look at your feet:** Inspect your feet carefully at least once a day. Usually this is most convenient after you complete your shower or bath. Check your toes (including between your toes) and check your soles and the sides of your feet. You are looking for cuts, cracks, calluses, flaking skin (which may indicate a fungal infection called athlete's foot), dry skin, sores, blisters, and foreign bodies. (No, this doesn't refer to Brigitte Bardot. It refers to things like tacks, which, if you have significant nerve damage, could be imbedded in your foot without your even knowing it.) Most important, you are looking for openings in the skin, such as ulcerations (which appear as small holes in the skin surface) and areas of redness with heat and pus (which likely indicate an infection; see the 'warning' below).

✔ **Determine if you have lack of sensation:** As we discussed above (see the section on peripheral neuropathy), diabetes can make you less able to feel pain in your feet and this puts you at much higher risk of developing foot ulcers. Touch different parts of your feet to see if there are any areas where the sensation is impaired. If your sensation is impaired (and in fact even if it is not), you should avoid using a heating pad on your feet.

✔ **Put your shoes on your hands before you put them on your feet:** Never put your shoes on before you first look inside them and feel inside them (with your fingers, not your toes) to make sure there are no errant pebbles, tacks, paper clips, or any other object that doesn't belong there and that could damage your feet. And speaking of shoes, make sure you are very careful to buy only very comfortable, well-fitting shoes. (If you have new shoes, break them in by wearing them initially for no more than 1 to 2 hours at a time.) The heels on your shoes should be under 2 inches high. And before you put on those comfortable, low-healed shoes (without over-the-counter insoles we would add – they can cause blisters), make sure the socks you use are not overly tight. Because your feet may swell over the course of the day, be sure to buy your shoes in the late afternoon (that is when your feet will be at their largest).

✔ **Keep your feet well groomed:** Your toenails must be kept short (but not too short). Cut them straight across (use an emery board to smooth the edges). Better yet, have someone else cut them for you, especially if you have impaired feeling in your feet. Keep the *soles* of your feet from getting overly dry (if dryness is a problem for you, apply a good skin lotion in the morning and at bedtime). Keep the *spaces between your toes* from getting overly moist by applying liberal quantities of powder after you bathe. Remember, you want the spaces between your toes to be dry and the soles of your feet to be moist. Check your feet for calluses. These are often a trigger leading to foot ulceration. If you have calluses, corns or warts you should not treat them yourself; they should be dealt with professionally (generally, a podiatrist is the best person to see for these problems)

✔ **Test the waters:** You would never dive into unknown waters, right? Well, you should never *step* into unknown waters either, even in your own bathroom. Before you step into a bath, use your hand (or, even better, your elbow) to make sure the water is not too hot.

✔ **Remember that *Barefoot in the Park* was only a movie:** It may have been okay for Jane Fonda and Robert Redford to go barefoot in the park (assuming they do not have diabetes), but it is not okay for you. Not in the park, or anywhere else for that matter. Your feet are just too valuable to risk injuring them.

✔ **Don't smoke:** 'Nuff said.

If you see an open sore on your foot — in particular if there is pus present and/or surrounding redness — you *must* seek *immediate* medical attention as you likely have an infection. If you have a foot infection, time becomes of the essence. Every day that goes by without proper treatment increases your risk of the infection worsening, potentially leading to amputation. If you have a minor cut or scratch, clean it with soap and water and then cover it with a dry dressing; be sure to change the dressing daily.

If you are unable to lift your feet up close enough to your eyes to inspect them, then you can try using a mirror propped up against a wall (like you see in shoe stores) or you can buy a mirror with an angled handle (available at drugstores). If that is still not effective, then have a loved one check your feet for you. Don't worry about asking. Remember, if they love you, they love *all* of you.

You may be surprised to read this, but soaking your feet is seldom a good idea as it can lead to maceration of the feet and actually increase your risk for getting a foot infection. If you really want to soak your feet, ensure the water is not too hot *and* limit your soaks to no more than 10–20 minutes.

Skin Disease in Diabetes

You may already have discovered that to cope with diabetes it sometimes helps to have a thick skin, in a manner of speaking. Well, we will save for another time our discussion about how to deal with well-meaning but irritating casual acquaintances who insist on instructing you about what you "can and cannot eat." In this section we will focus on the less figurative "thick skin" that people with diabetes can get as well as other skin problems that are of special importance.

There are not many serious skin problems that you have to be concerned about, but there are a few:

- **Lipohypertrophy:** This is a build-up of fatty tissue under the skin in areas of repeated insulin injection (especially if you are reusing your needles). It appears as bumps — sometimes as large as tennis balls (or even cantaloupes!). It is not a danger in and of itself, but it is of major importance in another way. Insulin absorption from areas of lipohypertrophy is erratic and, not surprisingly, causes erratic blood glucose control. Insulin should *never* be injected into areas of lipohypertrophy. By avoiding injecting insulin into these affected areas, the lipohypertrophy will gradually shrink, but it can take years to see much improvement.

- **Sores on the feet:** Take *any* wound, ulcer, sore, or other form of skin breakdown on the feet very seriously. See the detailed discussion on foot care immediately preceding this section.

Some skin problems may raise worries, but in fact they are fairly harmless. These include the following:

- **Bruising:** This may occur at insulin injection sites.

- **Vitiligo:** People with this condition lose normal skin pigmentation and look very pale. Vitiligo is not unique to diabetes, but type 1 (not type 2) diabetes does put you at increased risk of developing it. Vitiligo has cosmetic importance (especially for African Canadians), but is not a threat to your health.

- **Necrobiosis Lipoidica Diabeticorum:** Try saying that quickly three times (assuming you can pronounce it in the first place)! This mouthful of a disease affects the legs and feet (rarely the upper limbs) and presents itself as reddish-brown, shiny patches. The skin is often thinner in these areas. Only rarely does it lead to significant problems apart from its cosmetic importance. There is no particularly effective treatment, but often the areas fade with time.

- **Xanthomata:** These are small, yellow marks that can occur in a variety of parts of the body, especially the eyelids (where they are called xanthelasma). Their importance is confined to the fact that they are often a clue that your lipids may be abnormal (see earlier in this chapter for a discussion about lipids).

- **Nail infections:** The medical term for this is *onychomycoses*. (Unless you are talking to a dermatologist or podiatrist, don't bother using this term because most of us will not have any idea what you are referring to!) People with diabetes commonly develop fungal infections of the toenails. The affected nails appear thickened, yellow-brown. The problem is not serious, but if you have a fungal nail infection you should pay special attention to the health of the skin around the nail to make sure that your nail is not irritating it (and making it red, abraded, or sore). Infected nails can be treated with anti-fungal medicine, but this is seldom necessary. The nails can be quite difficult to cut, in which case we recommend that you have it done professionally (by a podiatrist).

- **Acanthosis nigricans:** This is a dark, velvety increase in pigmentation on the back of the neck and the armpits in some people with type 2 diabetes. (It can also occur without type 2 diabetes if you have insulin resistance.) It is not dangerous and does not require treatment.

- **Thickened skin:** As mentioned in the introduction to this section, people with diabetes can have thickening of the skin. This is felt as, well, thick skin. It is not important and will not make you unwell.

Musculoskeletal Problems (Muscles, Joints, and Such)

The musculoskeletal system in your body is made up of your muscles, bones, joints, and connecting material (such as ligaments and tendons), all of which allow for movement and locomotion. When we think "diabetes," we usually don't think "oh yes, joint problems," but, for unknown reasons, this too (alas) can occur. We will discuss the most important types in this section.

- ✔ **Carpal Tunnel Syndrome:** In this condition the *median nerve* gets compressed as it travels through the wrist. It can cause a feeling of numbness in the hand (particularly the thumb, index, and middle fingers). Carpal tunnel syndrome can occur for many reasons, diabetes among them. Treatment is geared toward avoiding precipitating factors (such as *repetitive strain injury,* as can occur with prolonged typing) and, if necessary, splinting, medication, or even surgery can be used.

- ✔ **Diabetic Hand Syndrome:** In this condition the hands feel stiff and sore. As you might imagine, many people without diabetes can also develop similar symptoms. Treatment is with anti-inflammatory medication and physiotherapy.

- ✔ **Frozen Shoulder:** Even during another muggy, smoggy Toronto summer heat wave, you can run into problems with a frozen shoulder. *Frozen shoulder* is a condition where your shoulder joint becomes stiff (and sometimes a bit painful) as a result of inflammation in the capsule that surrounds the joint. Treatment options include physiotherapy, anti-inflammatory medication, steroid injections into the joint (this procedure is most often done by either a rheumatologist — that is, an "arthritis doctor" — or an orthopedic surgeon), and, in severe cases, surgery.

Gum Disease in Diabetes

If diabetes can affect you from head (hair loss) to toe (peripheral neuropathy), inside (atherosclerosis) and out (necrobiosis), is it any wonder that it can even affect your gums? Regrettably not. But like so much in the world of diabetes, this complication too is one you can avoid with proper attention to your health.

Elevated glucose levels within your mouth can promote the growth of bacteria. These germs can attack the gums, causing *gingivitis* (gum infection), which in turn can lead to problems with your teeth and, of greater concern, blood infections. Conversely, gingivitis, like other infections in your body, can make your blood glucose control worse.

The required treatment is one that your mother (or father, of course) likely prescribed for you when you were 5 years old. Brush your teeth twice a day, floss your teeth once a day, and see your dentist regularly. It's that simple.

Whether you read this chapter beginning to end or simply read those sections of greatest interest to you, most likely there were times when you felt at least a bit overwhelmed at the different problems that diabetes can lead to. But we hope that you will also note that the great majority of complications are avoidable and, even if present, are very treatable. Keeping yourself healthy may not be easy — and don't let anyone tell you otherwise — but it can be done.

We conclude this chapter with one final point.

Despite the fact that diabetes can affect pretty well any part of the body, there is a strong tendency for people (doctors and people with or without diabetes alike) to think of diabetes as being a "sugar problem." But in fact, as you no doubt know by now, diabetes is a "whole body problem." So the next time your doctor (or anyone else, for that matter) asks you how your diabetes is doing, feel free to say, "Thanks for asking, but which part were you referring to?"

Chapter 7

Diabetes, Sexual Function, and Pregnancy

• •

In This Chapter

▶ Treating erectile dysfunction

▶ Dealing with female sexual problems

▶ Handling pregnancy when you have diabetes

• •

As diabetes specialists, for us nothing is quite so thrilling and rewarding as seeing "one of our moms" as she proudly holds her healthy newborn. We look at this beautiful scene and know that until the past few decades, women with diabetes seldom were fortunate enough to enjoy the miracle of creating a new life. It used to be that getting pregnant was difficult, miscarriages were common, and birth defects were all too frequent. But nowadays that has all changed. The great majority of women with diabetes can have successful pregnancies and healthy infants. It is not easy and it is a ton of work for the mom-to-be, but it can be done. Indeed, we see it all the time.

And, of course, sexual intercourse remains the starting point for most babies. People with diabetes — both male and female — can have problems with sexual function, but, once again, very effective therapies are now available for what used to be treated quite ineffectively or ignored (by both doctors and patients) altogether.

This chapter discusses how you can overcome problems with sexual dysfunction as well as the important things you should know about in order to have a healthy pregnancy.

Male Sexual Problems

If carefully questioned, up to 50 percent of all males with diabetes will acknowledge having difficulty with sexual function. This difficulty usually takes the form of *erectile dysfunction,* the inability to have or sustain an erection sufficient for intercourse.

Another form of sexual dysfunction that can occur with longstanding diabetes is called *retrograde ejaculation,* wherein you are able to achieve a normal erection and experience a normal orgasm, but no semen emerges from the penis, having instead been sent the reverse direction into the bladder. This is not a serious problem and only requires treatment should you wish to father a child.

Why the spirit may be willing, but the penis isn't

Erectile dysfunction in a man with diabetes is usually due to poor blood supply and/or nerve damage to the penis. Nonetheless, it is very important that you and your doctor not fall into the all-too-common trap of assuming that if you have diabetes, every conceivable problem you might develop must be diabetes-related. People with diabetes can encounter the same problems as everyone else. Or, as Henry Kissinger (or Golda Meir, some would argue) famously said, "Even paranoids have enemies." Some non-diabetes-related causes of erectile dysfunction include the following:

- **Trauma and other physical abnormalities of the penis.**

- **An adverse effect from medication.** This is particularly common with medicines such as beta blockers, thiazide diuretics and some anti-depressants.

- **Hormonal abnormalities.** Insufficient levels of the male hormone testosterone or excess levels of a pituitary hormone called prolactin can interfere with normal sexual function.

- **Psychological factors.** Problems such as stress and depression can interfere with normal sexual function.

Psychological factors — whether anxiety, stress, depression, etc. — leading to erectile dysfunction are, of course, no less important to address than any other cause, including diabetes. Your family physician can help determine if this is the cause of your sexual difficulties, and effective therapy is available to help you.

Ron, a 30-year-old man, came to see Ian in the office for a routine appointment. He said everything was going well and that he had no complaints. As he regularly does, Ian asked if Ron had had any problems with his erections. Ron denied any difficulties but didn't sound very convincing and, with a bit of prompting, acknowledged that something was amiss. He said he was getting erections but they "weren't straight." Ian arranged for Ron to meet with a urologist (a doctor who specializes in urinary tract and genital problems), who found that Ron had developed some scar tissue on his penis that was making his erections curved ("Peyronie's Disease"). Ron was successfully treated and immeasurably happier at the time of his next office visit. The moral of the story is twofold: first, your doctor is there to help you — *all* of you! — so you should feel free to bring up *any* problems you are experiencing; and second, neither you nor your doctor should automatically assume that every symptom you have is necessarily related to your diabetes.

You can help protect yourself from developing erectile dysfunction by:

- Maintaining good blood glucose, blood pressure and lipid control

- Avoiding the consumption of excess quantities of alcohol

- Not smoking (Smoking leads to blockage of the arteries, including the arteries that supply blood to the penis)

How to improve sexual function

Fortunately, there are many different therapies available to treat erectile dysfunction, with an overall success rate of over 90 percent. Some treatments are geared toward correcting specific reversible causes (such as stopping a medicine if it is causing your problem). Other treatments include:

- **Viagra:** Anyone who has spent any time over the past year or two watching television or reading magazines has seen ads for Viagra (also called sildenafil). The benefits of Viagra are well known. (The drawback of the TV commercials is that they force us to explain to our young children exactly why it is that the men in the commercial are singing "Good Morning" with such fervour). Joining Viagra on the Canadian market are the recently released drugs Cialis (tadalafil) and Levitra (Vardenafil). It remains to be seen if one of these drugs is superior to the other. (Drug companies are responding to a need and they are also responding to a potential profit; since Viagra was released in Canada in 1999, about 20 million pills have been dispensed worth a total – including dispensing fees – of $100 million a year!) For more about how these medications work, see the sidebar "Viagra and you."

- **Injection into the penis:** Several types of medicine can be injected directly into the penis to create an erection. The most commonly used is a medicine going by the trade name Caverject. This may sound pretty nasty, but if you can overcome the understandable fear of giving a needle in the penis, you will find that the amount of discomfort is usually minimal and that this type of therapy is often very effective.

- **Suppository in the penis:** This form of therapy involves inserting a small amount of medicine (MUSE) directly into the urethral opening at the tip of the penis. The success rate is not as good as with the previously two mentioned options.

✔ **Vacuum device:** This is a tube that fits directly over the penis and, with the use of a connected pump, allows for blood to fill the penis, at which point an erection is achieved and a rubber band placed around the base of the penis prevents the blood from escaping. Some men find the device cumbersome to use, but in general it is quite effective, and we feel that this is an under-used therapy.

✔ **Implanted penile prosthesis:** If none of the above measures is helping, another option is to have a prosthesis surgically implanted directly into the penis. There are a variety of types, some of which create a permanent erection and others of which have an implanted pump (placed in the scrotum) that allows for creation of an erection on an "on demand" basis. As with a car, the fancier the equipment, the more expensive the device and the more things that can go wrong, but in general this is a very successful treatment.

Viagra — and other drugs from this family — are almost always the first treatment used. If you do not respond to this type of therapy, we would recommend you be referred to a urologist — they are the experts when it comes to treating erectile dysfunction — to see if you might benefit from one of the other treatment options listed above.

Viagra and you

You take Viagra about 1 hour before sexual intercourse. The dose is usually 50 mg but may be increased to 100 mg if necessary. Viagra is recommended for use no more than once a day. It may accumulate in the body if you have liver or severe kidney disease or you're taking certain drugs, especially erythromycin. In those cases, the starting dose is 25 mg.

Everything in our body is under the control of chemical signals and pathways. As we say above (in the section on how men get erections), certain muscles need to relax for blood to flow into the penis and create an erection. A certain chemical in our body allows this to happen. And our very clever body produces another chemical that gets rid of the first chemical so that we don't have permanent erections. Viagra blocks the action of this second chemical so that the erection can continue. Because Viagra works on the second part of the system, you will require stimulation to get the first chemical flowing.

Viagra is not free of side effects. Some men experience headaches, facial flushing, or indigestion, all of which generally decline with continued use of the drug. Viagra can cause a temporary colour tinge to a man's vision as well as increased sensitivity to light and blurred vision. These side effects too decline with continued use of Viagra.

Drug companies are smart enough to know a good thing when they see one and very soon the Canadian market will be awash in competitors to Viagra. Whether any of the newer drugs within this family are superior to Viagra remains to be determined.

One important group of men must not take Viagra. Men who have chest pain often take nitrate drugs, the most common of which is nitroglycerine. The combination of Viagra and nitrates may cause a significant and possibly fatal drop in blood pressure.

Female Sexual Problems

Sexual problems in women with diabetes have, regrettably, not received nearly the attention that male sexual difficulties have. Some types of female sexual dysfunction, though not unique to people with diabetes, are more common for them. Fortunately, treatment is available that will allow you to have an active and pleasurable sex life. Here are the most frequent issues you are likely to encounter:

- ✔ **Vaginal dryness:** The most common causes are poor glucose control, nerve damage, impaired blood flow, or estrogen deficiency. Vaginal dryness makes intercourse more difficult and less pleasurable (lubrication increases vaginal sensitivity) — sometimes even painful. It can be treated with lubricants that are water-based (such as K-Y Jelly) or oil-based (such as vegetable oil). Water-based lubricants are easier to clean up. Oral stimulation by your partner may also assist in lubricating the vagina. If you are menopausal, lack of estrogen could be the main cause of your vaginal dryness, in which case vaginal estrogen preparations (which are much safer than oral estrogen) may be an option for you. To know if vaginal estrogen therapy is a suitable option for you, your doctor will have to review your specific situation.

- ✔ **Vaginal yeast infections:** Diabetes and, in particular, poor blood glucose control can make you prone to recurrent vaginal infections. Improving your glucose control and taking an anti-fungal medicine would be in order. We discuss this in more detail in Chapter 6.

- ✔ **Vaginal thinning:** Menopause leads to lower levels of estrogen and this, in turn, can not only cause vaginal dryness (see the first item in this list), but can also cause the lining of the vagina to become thin. In this case vaginal estrogen therapy may be an option for you.

- ✔ **Decreased genital sensation:** Nerve damage can lead to reduced sensitivity around the genital area and this, in turn, can reduce sexual enjoyment. Treatment options include gentle stimulation by touch or by use of a hand-held vibrator gently applied to the clitoris.

- ✔ **Bladder problems:** If you have difficulty controlling your bladder (due to *neurogenic* bladder) you may experience leakage during intercourse. Try to empty your bladder before intercourse. Other treatments include both medication and surgery (bladder suspension).

- ✔ **Adverse effects from medications:** Some medicines — particularly antidepressants — can interfere with sexual function. If you have recently started a new medicine only to find your sexual function becomes impaired, speak to your doctor about possibly switching to a different medicine.

✔ **Psychological factors:** Many different psychological factors can influence your ability to enjoy sexual relations, including poor self-image if you are dissatisfied with your appearance *or* if you are concerned that your partner may be dissatisfied with your appearance. As you work with nutrition therapy, weight loss, and exercise to improve your glucose control, you may find you seeing yourself (and your partner seeing you) as more attractive and that, in turn, may be the best therapy of all for your sexual dysfunction. If you are feeling anxious, stressed, or depressed, it would be wise for you to speak to your doctor about this to see what kind of help he or she can offer. In some cases your doctor may wish to refer you to a specialist for therapy.

Although with increasing frequency women with sexual dysfunction are taking Viagra, the drug is not as yet of proven benefit (or safety) in this circumstance.

Pregnancy and Diabetes

If you have diabetes, pregnancy does complicate matters. Nonetheless, it can still be a period of joy, excitement, and anticipation. You will not likely ever have another time where the efforts you apply to your diabetes are so crucial, and you can be assured you will have many people working with you all the way.

When we talk about diabetes and pregnancy it is important that we distinguish temporary, pregnancy-related diabetes (*gestational diabetes*) from diabetes that was present before you got pregnant (*pre-existing diabetes*; also known as *pre-gestational diabetes*). The implications, risks, and treatment are very different for each of these types. The remainder of this chapter looks at these important issues.

Gestational diabetes (diabetes that develops while you are pregnant)

Gestational diabetes (GDM) occurs in women who had normal blood glucose control before pregnancy, but who run into elevations of blood glucose *during* pregnancy. The degree of glucose elevation is so mild that symptoms of hyperglycemia (see Chapter 2) such as increased thirst and visual blurring do not develop. (Of course you may develop a frequent urge to pass urine during your pregnancy, but that is not due to gestational diabetes; it is due to a several-pound, future gymnast having decided to test out their skills by doing flips on your bladder.)

Gestational diabetes is very common, developing in about 4 percent of pregnancies. Most moms with GDM have otherwise uneventful pregnancies and perfectly healthy babies. The reason we look for and treat GDM is to take good odds for a successful pregnancy and make them even better.

The following are risk factors for developing gestational diabetes:

- ✔ Having had GDM during a previous pregnancy
- ✔ Having delivered a large baby with an earlier pregnancy
- ✔ Being a member of a high-risk population (for example, a woman of Aboriginal, Hispanic, South Asian, Asian or African descent)
- ✔ Being 35 years of age or older
- ✔ Having a BMI of 30 or greater (see Chapter 4 to calculate your BMI)
- ✔ Having polycystic ovarian syndrome, excessive facial or body hair growth, or acanthosis nigricans (these conditions are associated with insulin resistance; we discuss insulin resistance in Chapter 4)
- ✔ Taking corticosteroid medication (such as prednisone)

Causes of gestational diabetes

As you might imagine, many hormonal changes taking place during pregnancy, not the least of which is the release of hormones produced by the *placenta*. These placental hormones increase insulin resistance (see Chapter 4 for a discussion of insulin resistance). In a normal pregnancy, the pancreas can respond to this challenge by increasing the amount of insulin it makes so that your blood glucose control would remain normal. If you develop GDM, it means that your pancreas cannot respond sufficiently, so your blood glucose levels rise above normal.

Diagnosis of gestational diabetes

As a result of the fact that we have been able to identify women at higher risk, traditionally doctors have tested only these particular women for GDM. The problem with that strategy was that many women who developed GDM were overlooked. The new Canadian Diabetes Association guidelines therefore have recommended "universal screening"; that is, *every* pregnant woman should be tested for GDM.

The way you should be tested for GDM is as follows:

- ✔ **50-gram challenge:** When you reach 24 to 28 weeks into your pregnancy, your doctor should order this test. It requires you to ingest a sweet drink containing 50 grams of carbohydrate. You do not have to be fasting for this test. One hour after your drink, the laboratory will draw a blood sample from your arm to check your glucose level.

    - If your test result is less than 7.8 mmol/L, it is normal and you do not have GDM

    - If your test result is 7.8 up to (and including) 10.2 then your doctor should send your for a glucose tolerance test (see immediately below)

    - If your test result is 10.3 or higher, you have GDM and no further testing is required to make the diagnosis

- ✔ **75-gram glucose tolerance test (GTT):** An abnormal 50-gram challenge is not sufficient to indicate that you have GDM unless your result is 10.3 mmol/L or higher. All the 50-gram challenge does is determine if you have a strong enough likelihood of having GDM to proceed with the next stage of screening — that is, a GTT. During this test a health care professional will draw blood from you (after 8 hours of fasting) *before,* and then one and two hours *after* drinking a sweet solution containing 75 grams of carbohydrate. You have GDM if you have *two* or more abnormalities on the GTT. These are the *normal* blood glucose levels:

    5.2 mmol/L or less on the fasting sample

    10.5 mmol/L or less on the 1-hour sample

    8.8 mmol/L or less on the 2-hour sample

If you have multiple risk factors (see the list of risk factors earlier in this section), your risk of redeveloping GDM is high enough that you should be tested during your first trimester (that is, the first one-third of your pregnancy), and if your test result is normal, you should be re-tested periodically throughout your pregnancy.

Treatment of gestational diabetes

The most important element in treating GDM is dietary therapy (more appropriately called *nutrition therapy*). Your physician should refer you to a diabetes education center, where you will meet with a highly skilled diabetes educator and a registered dietician who will teach you the best ways for you to look after your gestational diabetes including the following two important things:

✔ **The best nutrition plan for you to follow during your pregnancy**. This will be geared toward assisting with blood glucose control while allowing for appropriate weight gain and ensuring adequate nutrition. Your carbohydrate intake will be distributed over 3 meals and at least 3 snacks (1 of which will be at bedtime). Think of this as a therapeutic indulgence! Your target weight gain will be based, at least in part on your pre-pregnant weight.

✔ **How to test your blood for glucose**. Most diabetes education centres (DECs) will be able to lend you a glucose meter for the duration of your pregnancy. The Canadian Diabetes Association recommends the following targets:

Target blood glucose (mmol/L)

Fasting and pre-meals	Less than 5.3
1 hour after meals	Less than 7.8
2 hours after meals	Less than 6.7

We mention above that gestational diabetes is associated with insulin resistance. You may recall that insulin resistance is improved (though not eliminated) by exercise. This holds true during pregnancy as well. A bit of exercise — even a daily walk — can help.

If, despite 2 weeks of appropriate nutrition therapy, your blood glucose readings are exceeding target (see above), you will require insulin and will typically need to give this to yourself four times per day. We discuss principles of insulin therapy in Chapter 12. The idea of having to give yourself insulin may not sound particularly pleasant, but bear in mind two things:

✔ Unlike taxes and Canadian winters, insulin won't be forever. The moment you deliver your baby, you will discontinue your insulin.

✔ Your efforts during your pregnancy will help you have a healthy baby. What could possibly be a better reward than that?

Recent studies suggest that a drug called glyburide (a type of *oral hypoglycemic agent* that reduces blood glucose — we talk more about these in Chapter 11) may be safe and effective if given *after* the first few months of pregnancy. This remains controversial and most diabetes specialists still prefer to use insulin when nutrition therapy is not sufficient to achieve target blood glucose levels.

If you take insulin, you will find that your insulin requirements progressively increase as your pregnancy goes along. This is perfectly normal.

What are the potential complications for Mom?

Most moms with gestational diabetes sail through their pregnancy with no complications and deliver perfectly healthy babies. Serious complications seldom occur. There is an increased likelihood that you will end up delivering by Caesarian section since you will be at risk of having a big baby (see the next section), and your obstetrician may determine that it would be unsafe for you to deliver vaginally. As well, your blood pressure, which could rise, will require extra monitoring.

What are the potential complications for baby?

Your baby will likely be completely fine. Your baby will *not* be born with diabetes and your baby will *not* be at greater risk of birth defects. There are two important possible complications:

- **Macrosomia:** This is the medical term for a large baby. Elevated blood glucose levels put your infant at higher risk of being large (which can complicate delivery). We typically assume the baby to be at risk of being large because if the mom's glucose levels are high, that glucose travels through the placenta into the baby's circulation and it is akin to overfeeding the baby in the uterus. Things may indeed be that simple; but in medicine whenever things seem really simple one can't help but be reminded of a famous quote from H. L. Mencken: "For every complex question there's a simple answer . . . *and it's wrong.*" The reason for a baby having macrosomia is likely far more complex and related to other maternal metabolic factors, genetics, and other, undetermined issues.

- **Hypoglycemia:** This is low blood glucose, and your baby may develop this shortly after it is born. It is usually easily treated by giving your baby sugar water to drink.

Other complications (such as the baby having low calcium or magnesium) occur far less frequently.

When Dominique first found out that she had gestational diabetes, she was certain that meant that her baby was going to be "huge." She had heard that "it's always like that." She had also heard from well-meaning but uninformed friends that her baby would probably have diabetes. When Ian met her for the first time, he spent almost the entire interview reassuring Dominique, not warning her. By the time the appointment was over, newly aware that with proper attention her pregnancy would almost certainly be smooth and her baby would be the picture of health, she was smiling ear to ear. As she passed through the waiting room, Ian smiled equally broadly as he overheard Dominique say to a seated, anxious-appearing pregnant woman, "Hey, don't worry, everything's going to be just fine!"

Controversies in gestational diabetes

It is highly unlikely that a doctor in Canada will tell you that you can ignore your gestational diabetes. The great majority of physicians (including us) treat GDM aggressively. You may be surprised, therefore, to find out that the whole issue of GDM is actually quite controversial and that there are a number of excellent physicians who feel that we are making a mountain out of a molehill. (This feeling is especially prevalent in the U.K.) They argue that very few women with GDM ever develop complications that can be attributed to their GDM unless their blood glucose readings are very high (in which case *every* doctor agrees that aggressive treatment is mandatory). They also say that when a woman is told she has GDM it creates stress and worry that is, for the great majority of women, unjustified based on their low risk of actually developing complications from their GDM.

Women with GDM are more likely to have a Caesarian section. Some doctors argue that this is because once a woman is diagnosed as having GDM, the doctor adopts a lower threshold for recommending the procedure. All told, some doctors feel that we are doing more harm than good for many women. Often times, we feel that way ourselves. Nonetheless, the so-called "standard of practice" in Canada is to treat GDM aggressively, so it would potentially be medico-legally unwise to do otherwise.

The Hyperglycemia and Adverse Pregnancy Outcome (HAPO) study (www.preventativemedicine.northwestern.edu/hapo.htm) is a very large (25,000 pregnant women will be enrolled) study addressing important issues in GDM and should, when published, clarify some of the key areas of uncertainty and controversy.

Although there are some controversies with regard to gestational diabetes, there is one issue about which there is no controversy whatsoever, and this is the most important point of all. If you have (or have previously had) GDM, you are at very, very high risk of developing type 2 diabetes. You can, however, substantially reduce this risk by following a very healthy lifestyle after you have your baby. Do your utmost to achieve and maintain a good weight. Eat healthfully. Exercise. After all, you've got a family to stay healthy for!

You should be monitored over time so that if you do develop type 2 diabetes it will be detected sooner rather than later. The Canadian Diabetes Association recommends that within 6 months of delivery you should have either a 75 gram glucose tolerance test (the preferred test) or a fasting blood glucose level. Additionally, your glucose status should be assessed prior to any future pregnancies.

It would be wise for you to be keep an eye out for the development of symptoms of hyperglycemia (see Chapter 2) and, should they develop, you should have your blood glucose level checked promptly.

Pre-existing diabetes (diabetes before you are pregnant)

As the name indicates, *pre-existing diabetes* refers to diabetes that you had *before* you became pregnant (and will still have after you deliver), whereas *gestational* diabetes is diabetes that is acquired during pregnancy and that resolves once you have had your baby. If you have type 1 (or type 2) diabetes and you get pregnant, then you have pre-existing diabetes.

If *only* the father has diabetes, none of this discussion applies to you. Only when diabetes affects the mom do these issues apply.

If you have diabetes and get pregnant, there is an excellent chance that everything will go well for you and nine months down the road you can have your dream fulfilled and hold a beautiful, bouncing, healthy baby. You are, perhaps, waiting for a "but." If so, then you are right. You *can* have everything go well for you, *but* to achieve your dream you must follow many precautions. We hate to be dogmatic, but we feel so strongly about the issue of pre-existing diabetes that in this section we are going to sound far more "black and white" about things than pretty well anywhere else in this book.

Although the odds are good that you will not run into serious problems during your pregnancy, you will be at increased risk for some complications including:

- **High blood pressure and toxemia**. Toxemia is a condition of raised blood pressure and fluid retention leading to swelling and, at other times, more serious complications. High blood pressure can be treated with medications. Toxemia generally requires hospitalization and early delivery.

- **Deterioration in eyesight**. This rarely occurs unless you have at least some retinal damage before you get pregnant. If severe, you may require retinal laser surgery. We discuss diabetes eye disease in more detail in Chapter 6.

- **Deterioration in kidney function**. This rarely occurs unless you have kidney malfunction *before* you get pregnant. We discuss diabetes and kidney function in Chapter 6.

- **Severe insulin reactions due to hypoglycemia unawareness**. This occurs because during pregnancy your blood glucose control will be kept exceptionally tightly controlled. We discuss hypoglycemia unawareness in more detail in Chapter 5.

- **Miscarriages**. Miscarriages are more common if your blood glucose control is poor in the early stages of pregnancy. If your control is excellent in early pregnancy, your risk of a miscarriage is less.

✓ **Having a baby with a birth defect**. The medical term for "birth defect" is *congenital anomaly*. This is the most dreaded complication of all, but fortunately it is largely preventable. If your blood glucose control at the time you get pregnant and for the first 12 weeks or so thereafter (when your baby's organs are forming) is excellent, your risk of having a baby with a congenital anomaly is about the same as if you never had diabetes (about 2 to 3 percent). On the other hand, if your blood glucose control is poor during this critical period of time, your risk is as high as 30 percent. An astounding difference, indeed. And one that you can directly influence.

✓ **Having a baby with other problems**. These include difficulty breathing, prematurity, small or large size, and disorders of body chemistry such as we listed in the previous section on gestational diabetes. Your baby will *not* be born with diabetes.

We hope that as you read through this rather intimidating list you noticed the recurring theme that these complications are usually avoidable. Most women with pre-gestational diabetes do *not* experience these complications!

Things to do before you get pregnant

To maximize your likelihood of having a healthy pregnancy and a healthy baby, here's what you should do *before* you get pregnant:

✓ **Be in regular touch with your health care team.** We discuss the members of the health care team and their respective roles in Chapter 8. It is essential that you and your diabetes specialist have reviewed whether it is safe for you to proceed. This will be determined based largely on the other factors in this list.

✓ **Maintain excellent blood glucose control.** This will be reflected by your blood glucose test results and your A1C (a blood test that provides an overview of your preceding three months' glucose control; we discuss A1C in detail in Chapter 9). This is terribly important. The better your glucose control, the more likely it is that your baby will be born free of birth defects. Working closely with your health care team, you should strive for an A1C of 7 or less (if you can achieve it, it is even better if your A1C is 6 or less).

✓ **See your eye specialist.** Since retinopathy (we discuss retinopathy in Chapter 6) can rapidly progress during pregnancy, it is crucial that your eye doctor assess the health of your eyes *before* you get pregnant.

✓ **Have your kidneys tested.** If your kidneys are healthy before you get pregnant, they will almost certainly remain healthy during your pregnancy. If your kidneys are damaged to begin with, they can significantly worsen during pregnancy. Your doctor can assess your kidneys through very simple blood and urine tests (as we discuss in Chapter 6).

✔ **Have your blood pressure tested.** If your blood pressure is high before you get pregnant, it puts you at much higher risk of running into more severe blood pressure problems during your pregnancy.

✔ **Have your medicines reviewed.** Your doctor will need to review any medicines you are taking, and if they would be unsafe (as is true, for example, of ACE inhibitors and ARBs) to take during pregnancy, you will need to stop them. If you have type 2 diabetes treated with oral hypoglycemic agents (see Chapter 11) you will need to stop these and initiate insulin well before you try to get pregnant.

✔ **Ask questions.** Nothing in your life will ever be so important as your quest to have a healthy baby. If you have questions about the impact of your diabetes on your pregnancy, *ask*. Ask your family doctor, ask your diabetes specialist, ask your diabetes educators, ask your obstetrician; ask *anyone* who is going to be a part of your health care team. As well, don't forget to make sure your partner is fully involved. Your partner needs to know what you are going to be contending with.

✔ **Take folic acid supplements.** The Canadian Diabetes Association recommends taking a folic acid supplement starting before you try to get pregnant and continued until you are about 13 weeks pregnant. The "best" dose is not known, however, our preference is to take 5 mg per day — and to continue it until breast feeding is completed. (See the following sidebar for more information.)

Folic acid supplements during pregnancy

Folic acid supplements taken during pregnancy will help reduce the risk of your baby developing "neural tube defects." These are serious disorders where a part of the central nervous system fails to develop normally and can result in the fetus having a form of impaired brain growth ("anencephaly") or a spinal disorder ("spina bifida"). Neural tube defects occur in the very earliest stages of pregnancy; indeed, usually before you would even be aware that you are pregnant. Women with diabetes are at higher risk of having a baby with neural tube defects. You should start taking folic acid supplements as soon as you stop using birth control. The amount of folic acid you should take and how long you should take it for are not known for certain. The CDA recommends taking 1 to 4 mg per day until you are 10 to 12 weeks pregnant. The Motherisk Clinic of the Hospital for Sick Children in Toronto (www.motherisk.org/folic/index.php3) however, advises the use of 5 mg of folic acid per day and continuing until breast feeding is completed (because the body requires greater amounts of this vitamin throughout pregnancy and breastfeeding; even after the risk of neural tube defects has passed). Since it is perfectly safe to take this higher dose, we recommend that our pregnant patients with pre-existing diabetes follow this advice.

Things to do while you are pregnant

Congratulations. You have done everything you had to, and you are now a proud, though perhaps apprehensive, mother-to-be. So what next, then? These are the things that you will need to do during your pregnancy:

- **Get a rewards card for your favourite gas station.** You will be spending a lot of time in your car, what with visits to the diabetes educator, the dietitian, your doctors, and so on. So when you fill up, look at the bright side; you're earning points toward that holiday you will so richly deserve (even if you have to delay taking it!).

- **Have your diet adjusted.** Your registered dietician will work with you to devise an appropriate meal plan designed to ensure adequate nutrition whilst assisting with blood glucose control and appropriate weight gain. Your carbohydrate intake will be restricted and you will be advised to eat 3 meals and 3 snacks per day (one of which will be a bedtime snack).

- **Monitor your blood glucose levels frequently.** Our preference is for a minimum of six tests per day (before and after every meal). Testing either 1 or 2 hours after meals is alright so long as the appropriate target value is taken into account as the following table of CDA-recommended goals illustrates:

Target blood glucose (mmol/L)

Fasting and pre-meals	3.8–5.2
1 hour after meals	5.5–7.7
2 hours after meals	5.0–6.6
Pre-bedtime snack	4.0–5.9

- Your A1C should be checked monthly. Target A1C is 6 or less (that is; in the normal range). Keeping your blood glucose under excellent control will help your baby develop normally. It is important to bear in mind, however, that obtaining uniformly normal values for blood glucose or A1C may simply not be possible (for instance, if it is leading to excessively frequent or severe episodes of hypoglycemia). Though we strive for perfect control, the truth of the matter is that it is rarely possible to achieve it. Fortunately, occasional, mild hyperglycemia is not likely to lead to any harm to your baby. Equally fortunately, if you experience hypoglycemia that will *not* hurt your baby.

✔ **Adjust your insulin.** Because the placenta releases hormones that increase insulin resistance (see Chapter 4) your insulin requirement will rise substantially during your pregnancy. By the time you deliver you may be on three (or more) times the amount of insulin you were taking before you got pregnant. This is normal. You should review your blood glucose profile at the time of every visit to your diabetes specialist and your diabetes educator. They will assist you with insulin adjustment however most day-to-day changes in dose you will almost certainly be able to make yourself. (If you have type 2 diabetes and did not require insulin *prior* to your pregnancy, you will, nonetheless, almost certainly require insulin *during* your pregnancy).

✔ **Test for urine (and/or blood) for ketones.** Do this daily before breakfast. If you have ketones present it may signify or indicate that you are not consuming an adequate diet (in which case a call to the dietician is in order). We discuss ketone testing in Chapter 5.

✔ **See your eye doctor regularly.** In addition to seeing your eye doctor before you get pregnant, you should be seen again during your first few months of pregnancy and, depending on the health of your eyes, periodically during the remainder of your pregnancy. Because eye damage can develop or progress even after childbirth, you should also be seen within 1 year of having your baby.

If you are pregnant and have type 1 diabetes, and the idea of participating in research appeals to you, you might wish to look into the TRIGR study on the Web (www.trigr.org) or by phone (888-STOP-T1D). This very important study is trying to determine the cause of type 1 diabetes. We discuss this study further in Chapter 4.

What to expect during labour and delivery

Congratulations once again. You've made it through nine months of pregnancy and you are now ready to have your baby.

When you are brought into hospital, you will likely be given short-acting insulin intravenously (rather than by injection) as this allows for minute-to-minute fine tuning of the dose. Your blood glucose level should be checked often — as often as hourly — and your insulin dose constantly adjusted to keep your blood glucose levels between about 3.8 and 6.6.

During labour and for the first day or two after you deliver, your insulin requirements will be markedly reduced. A day or two after you deliver you will be switched from intravenous insulin back to insulin injections. You will still need to carefully monitor your glucose readings, seeing as your insulin requirements will be changing daily as your body goes through major changes (in case you hadn't noticed!). If you have type 2 diabetes, and if your blood glucose levels necessitate it, your doctor may advise you to resume your oral hypoglycemic agents. This will depend in part on whether you will be breastfeeding (see the next section).

Shortly after you deliver, your doctor will check your baby's blood glucose level and, if it's low, he or she will be given some sugar water to drink. A pediatrician will thoroughly examine your baby to make sure everything is all right.

When Leanne, a newly married woman with type 1 diabetes, asked Ian what would be involved if she were to get pregnant, she was expecting a simple answer. The answer she got, however, was complicated. Leanne was surprised to hear about all the things she would have to do leading up to and then during pregnancy, but she was sure she was up to the challenge and was willing to do "whatever it takes" to have a healthy baby. During her subsequent pregnancy, there were times when, what with visits to doctors, the educator, the dietitian, and so on, she felt as if she was "doing nothing but going to appointments," but she persevered. Although her nine months of pregnancy seemed to Leanne to "take forever," all recollection of the hassles she had gone through instantly disappeared the moment she first cradled her newborn infant lovingly in her arms, her only thought "how lucky" she was to have experienced this joy.

We have looked after hundreds and hundreds of pregnant women with pre-existing diabetes. And while it is absolutely critical that you be aware of the important issues that we discuss during this chapter, it is equally important to recognize that if you look after yourself properly, your likelihood of having as successful a pregnancy as Leanne (in the preceding anecdote) is excellent. It may not be easy, but it can be done. As we said at the outset of this chapter, we see it all the time.

Handling your diabetes for the first few months after having your baby

Unless you are unable to do so, breastfeeding is far and away the preferred way for you to supply your newborn with nutrition. Because you will be providing your baby's nutritional requirements, you will need to ingest an additional 300 calories per day.

Oral hypoglycemic agents can pass from your system into your breast milk and then into your baby's system. For this reason, you should *not* take these types of medicines if you are breastfeeding unless you have first consulted with your diabetes specialist and/or your baby's pediatrician.

By now, you are likely very familiar with all the reasons why excellent blood glucose control is so crucial to maintaining your good health. And in almost all cases you should be striving for optimal glucose control. It is important, however, to recall that the (terribly unfair) price to be paid for so-called "tight" blood glucose control is a much higher risk of severe hypoglycemia (which we discuss in Chapter 5). This is a bad enough problem to begin with, but it is even more of a concern if you are going to be home alone with your newborn. For this reason, if you are prone to severe hypoglycemia, you should speak to your diabetes specialist to determine if it would be best for you to have somewhat looser blood glucose control for the first few months after you are home with your baby.

Part III
Rule Your Diabetes:
Don't Let It Rule You

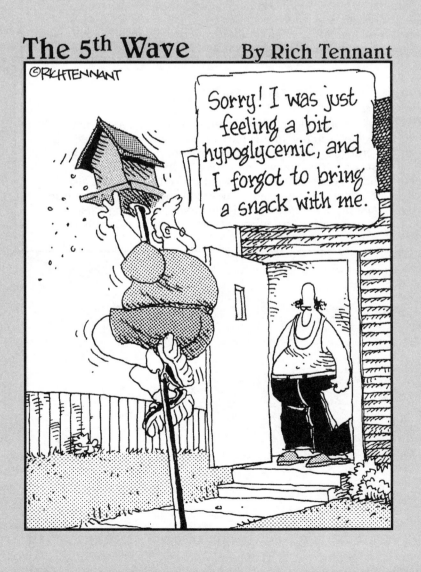

In this part . . .

Is it possible to have diabetes without it dominating your life? You bet! In this part we look at the most effective strategies you can use to control your diabetes and to stay healthy. You will find out who the members of your health care team are and what roles they play. We also examine the important issues of proper nutrition, exercise, and other therapies available to you, including pills, insulin, and alternative and complementary treatments.

Chapter 8

Meet Your Diabetes Team

*T*o the best of our knowledge, no hockey team has ever won a gold medal at the Olympics by sending only one player onto the ice. Nor do we know of any team that ever won gold without having a coach, a general manager, and a slew of fans rooting along the way. And if an Olympic hockey team ever played without a trainer and an equipment manager, it surely must have been way back before Don Cherry put on his first red-checkered sport jacket (with matching lime-green tie, of course!). Heck, it must have been before Howie Morenz notched his first hat trick.

Now it may not be easy to make it onto an Olympic hockey team, but *you* can be the star of *your own* team. Indeed, you should be the star of your own diabetes health care team, because for you to succeed with your diabetes, you must not only be the captain of the team, you must have all the other players working with you. There is nothing second rate about coming home from the Olympics with a silver or bronze, but when it comes to your health, we should always be after the top prize.

In this chapter we will look at the different players on your health care team, starting with the first, second, and third star of each and every game. That would be — you guessed it — you.

The only hockey player we can recall that came close to matching your selection as first, second, and third star of the game is Maurice "the Rocket" Richard who was awarded all three stars back in 1944 after scoring all five Habs' goals in a 5–1 Montreal Canadiens playoff victory. Clearly, you are in rarefied company.

You Are the Captain of the Team

You may not have wanted to be captain of the team; heck, you didn't want to be on a diabetes team to start with, but here you are, the star of the team, and as you might imagine, with stardom come certain responsibilities. Leadership, for example. This is where diabetes differs from almost any other illness. If you have appendicitis, it is not very likely that you will be the one to order the X-ray, deliver the anesthetic, hold the scalpel, and put in the stitches. No, your role would be relatively passive as the experts around you tend to your needs. Diabetes is not like that.

When you have diabetes, *you* have to take charge. *You*, after all, live with you. Day and night. Night and day, too, we suspect. *You* are the one that ultimately decides what you will eat, when you will exercise, when you will test your blood glucose levels, when you will take your medicines, and so forth. Other people can offer advice, other people can prompt or even cajole you, but in the end, the decisions are yours. And with your keen and ongoing involvement in your health care, you will be helping yourself to receive the best possible therapy to achieve and maintain good health. Like we said, you are the star.

It may seem rather daunting for you to have so much responsibility placed upon your shoulders. And there may be times when you simply want people to tell you to "do this" and "do that." But with time and support you will grow into your role and become comfortable with it.

Before we move on to a discussion about your teammates' functions, let's summarize what *your* responsibilities are as captain of your health care team. This list may seem intimidating, but you will be surprised at how quickly these responsibilities can all become part of your normal day-to-day existence:

- ✔ **Follow your lifestyle treatment plan:** This means knowing what foods you should eat, how much, and how often. What exercises you should do and how often you should do them. How much weight — if any — you should lose and the best strategy to achieve this. How much alcohol you can safely drink. If you smoke and want to quit, what cessation strategies are available to you. (We discuss this further in Chapter 6.)

- ✔ **Monitor your blood glucose:** You should become familiar with how to test your blood, how often you should test, what your target blood glucose levels are, and, importantly, what you should be doing to achieve these targets. You should also make sure that you have your A1C checked every 3 months *and* that you find out the result. (We discuss blood glucose and A1C testing in Chapter 9.)

✔ **Keep track of your blood pressure:** Anytime someone checks your blood pressure, ask what it is and write it down. Become familiar with what your target blood pressure is, and if your readings are too high, ask your doctor how he or she is going to help you reduce it. (We talk more about high blood pressure in Chapter 6.)

✔ **Keep track of your lipid levels:** As with your blood pressure, anytime someone tests your lipid levels (see Chapter 6 for a discussion on lipids), you should write them down. Also, you should speak to your doctor to know what your target levels are, and if you are not within those targets, ask your doctor how he or she is going to help you meet those goals.

✔ **Schedule visits to each member of your health care team:** How often you see each member of the team will depend on many circumstances, including your state of health. Anytime you meet with your health care providers (be it your family doctor, diabetes specialist, diabetes educator or other member of your health care team), be sure to ask them when they want you to return. It is best to book the return appointment *before* you leave the office *and* write down the details on your calendar as soon as you get home (or, for the technologically savvy, in your PDA before you leave the office).

✔ **Know about your medicines:** Every time you see a physician or diabetes educator, be sure to bring all your medicines with you. At the very least, bring a list of your medicines, making note of your drugs' names, dosages, and how many times per day you are taking them. Telling your doctor that you are "on a small blue pill once a day" and a "red capsule twice a day" tells your physician more about the state of your colour vision than the nature of your drugs.

✔ **Ask questions:** For you to function as an effective captain of your health care team, you must know how you are performing. And you can't know this without your teammates giving you feedback. So, before you leave an appointment, make sure you have a good understanding of what your health care provider has concluded. Don't accept vague phrases like "your blood pressure is okay" or "your cholesterol isn't bad" or "your sugars are reasonable." As diabetes specialists we can tell you that these terms are meaningless. Meaning*ful* would be to hear that your blood pressure is 125/85, your LDL is 2.4, and your A1C is 7.4.

Dress for success

You might normally think that "power-dressing" is something that is done on Bay Street, not in your doctor's office. Well, you may be amazed at how much more "power" you can have in making sure you get the attention you need by dressing for the occasion. We're not talking business suits here; we're talking "easy access." On the day of a doctor's appointment, you would be well served to dress in such a way that you can easily expose your arm (for a blood pressure measurement) and your feet (for assessment of skin health, circulation, sensation, and so on. We discuss foot health in Chapter 6). Even better, take off your shoes and socks while you are waiting for your doctor to come into the examining room; this will ensure that your feet will get looked at. (Of course, you will not want to do this if the doctor you are seeing is your eye doctor!) You may reasonably conclude that none of this dressing (and undressing) strategy should be necessary and we would agree completely. But in truth, if this technique makes it more likely your blood pressure or feet get checked, it may be a life- and limb-saving measure.

Your physician is dealing with many patients each day and even the most conscientious, well-meaning doctor can easily forget some of the specific issues that surround your particular situation. Therefore, be sure to bring up any concerns or questions you have about your health. Tell your doctor if you are having a problem such as chest pain, numbness in your feet, sexual dysfunction, and so forth. Otherwise, a potentially serious problem may end up being overlooked.

When it comes to your health care, never accept the old adage that "no news is good news." Sometimes, no news means the lab lost your blood sample! If you have had tests done, follow up with your doctor (in person, by phone, by fax, by e-mail, or some other means) to obtain and discuss the results.

The remainder of this chapter looks at the responsibilities of the other members of your health care team. As you see what their roles are, you will further understand the ways that you can help *them* help *you*. After all, as the old expression says, knowledge is power.

The Family Physician (Your Coach)

Your family physician has a major role to play on your diabetes team; indeed, even if you have a diabetes specialist whom you see from time to time, your family doctor will still provide the great majority of your diabetes medical care. For this reason, if you are fortunate enough to live in one of the few communities remaining in Canada where you can actually choose your doctor, it is best to find a family physician that has a particular interest and expertise with diabetes. If you are unsure about this, simply ask them. If they do not feel that diabetes management is their forté, they may be able to recommend another doctor to help you.

Your family physician's responsibilities are far too numerous to list in their entirety (it would take many pages to itemize all the many tasks that these hard-working, dedicated doctors must do), but if we speak specifically in terms of your diabetes, here are just some of the things your family doctor will do:

- **Review any symptoms you may have developed:** In most cases, your family doctor should be your first point of contact if you have developed symptoms (for example, such things as mood problems, vaginal discharge, diarrhea, or numbness in your feet).

- **Review your blood glucose control:** We strongly recommend that you record your blood glucose readings in a logbook (see Chapter 9 for a detailed discussion of blood glucose record keeping) and that you review your numbers with your family doctor on a regular basis.

- **Examine you:** Routine components of your physical examination should include checking your blood pressure and pulse, feeling your thyroid, listening to your heart and lungs, and examining your feet for problems with your skin, circulation, or nerve function (see Chapter 6 for a more detailed discussion on testing for nerve problems).

- **Order screening studies:** There are a number of tests that your doctor should do from time to time, including checking your A1C, cholesterol, urine albumin/creatinine ratio, and so on. See the Cheat Sheet at the beginning of this book for a detailed list of what tests should be done and how often.

- **Help organize your visits to other team members:** This includes things such as reviewing with you when you are due to see other team members — for example, your diabetes educators and your eye doctor — and, if necessary, arranging for visits to other providers, including your diabetes specialist and podiatrist.

Please note again that this list is not meant to be exhaustive and does not include the numerous things your family doctor helps you with, independent of your diabetes.

The Diabetes Specialist (Your General Manager)

Family physicians provide the great majority of diabetes care in Canada. Nonetheless, seeing a diabetes specialist from time to time is usually a good idea — especially if you have known complications from diabetes or if you have type 1 diabetes.

It is surprisingly difficult to define the term *diabetes specialist*. Sure, we can say it is "a doctor who specializes in diabetes," and although that would be accurate, it would still be incomplete. We can arbitrarily classify diabetes specialists into three groups:

- **Endocrinologists** (such as Alan): These are doctors who, after medical school, trained in internal medicine and then did additional training in endocrine ("hormone") disorders such as those affecting the pancreas (diabetes, for example), thyroid, and adrenal glands.

- **Internists** (such as Ian): These are doctors who, after medical school, trained in internal medicine and then usually tailored their practice to a particular area. In Ian's case this was diabetes. For other internal medicine specialists it is, for example, heart disease or high blood pressure.

- **Family Physicians:** This one may surprise you. Not many family physicians are diabetes specialists, but some are. These are doctors who, after medical school, trained in family medicine and then, because diabetes was a particular interest of theirs or because their community may not have had ready access to a diabetes specialist, or both, focused their practice on diabetes. We have given lectures to such family physicians and must admit we have felt that it just as well could have been *them* giving the talk.

The main reason to see a diabetes specialist is the greater likelihood that they will be — by virtue of the time they devote to this one topic — "on top of the literature," that they will know about new research findings and new and innovative forms of therapy.

Your diabetes specialist can assess your diabetes-related issues and develop a treatment plan that they can then share with other members of your health care team.

It is *essential* that your specialist send any reports to *all* relevant parties. Otherwise, using our previous hockey analogy, you and your specialist will be the only players on your team that are handling the puck. And that will make your other teammates less effective. Whenever you see your diabetes specialist, make a point of asking him or her to be sure to send a report to your family physician (*and* your diabetes educator). You shouldn't have to ask, but you do.

Your family physician, your diabetes, and you

As diabetes specialists we are indebted to family doctors. They provide the overwhelming majority of diabetes care in this country. Regrettably, the number of physicians choosing to make a career of family medicine is rapidly dwindling, making it harder and harder for Canadians to obtain basic medical care. Fewer family doctors means that those in this field have to look after more and more patients, which makes it that much harder for them to spend additional time with each individual in their practice. There is also a shortage of diabetes specialists, which puts additional work and responsibility on the shoulders of family physicians. The result is that numerous Canadians with diabetes (and people without diabetes too, of course) are not receiving all the

care they require. All the more reason, therefore, that it is crucial for you to be an "informed consumer" and take on the responsibility of knowing what your health care requires.

Dr. Stewart Harris of London, Ontario, is a family physician. He is also the Chair of the Canadian Diabetes Association's Clinical and Scientific Section. Dr. Harris is a perfect example of why the label (be it "family physician," "internist," "endocrinologist," or whatever) does not necessarily tell the whole story. Indeed, given the realities of diabetes care in Canada, Dr. Harris says, "All family doctors are going to have to be diabetes specialists."

The Diabetes Educator (Your Trainer)

It is for good reason that a recent president of the American Diabetes Association once said, "Diabetes education is the single greatest advance ever made in diabetes care."

Although every member of your diabetes team is, in some way, shape, or form an educator, a diabetes *nurse* educator is typically the health care team member that provides the bulk of your initial and ongoing teaching. In Canada, diabetes educators generally have the initials *C.D.E.* ("certified *d*iabetes *e*ducator") after their names, however there are many excellent educators that do not have such certification. Diabetes educators are typically registered nurses that, after completing nursing school, have worked in hospitals or clinics and then went on to do further training to learn how to teach people about their diabetes.

Many dieticians are also certified diabetes educators (as are some pharmacists and, on occasion, some other type of health care provider) and, in addition to their role in teaching about proper nutrition, they can provide expert guidance about many other aspects of diabetes management; indeed, Claire Lightfoot, a dietician in Campbell River, British Columbia, was the recipient of the Canadian Diabetes Association's Diabetes Educator of the Year award for 2004.

A diabetes educator teaches you how to take your insulin or pills, how to test your blood glucose, and how to acquire many of the other skills you need. And that is just the beginning. They are invaluable resources, and if you have not met with a diabetes educator, you are truly missing out.

Diabetes educators' roles are progressively expanding. Not only do they continue to fulfill their traditional teaching role, they can also keep you up-to-date on new developments in diabetes therapy. Additionally, many educators now have the authority — as well they should — to test your A1C level (see Chapter 9), to help you adjust your insulin dosages, to adjust the dose of your oral hypoglycemic agents, to test your urine for evidence of kidney damage, and to measure your cholesterol levels. There are even some extraordinary (and extraordinarily *rare*) educators that carry pagers so that they can be contacted 24 hours a day if you are having problems.

If you have not met up with a diabetes educator, ask your doctor to refer you to one. If you have not seen your educator for some time, call to arrange a follow-up visit. What health professionals know about diabetes keeps changing, so why should you be left behind? Stay current; see your educator regularly. (If this sounds like a sales pitch, we offer no apologies. We think diabetes educators are wonderful — in case you hadn't noticed.)

The majority of doctors are fully aware of the essential role that diabetes educators and dietitians play and make a routine practice of referring their patients to them. (Trust us; it makes life a lot easier for the doctor to have other members of the health care team sharing the work!) Regrettably, there are some doctors who feel that diabetes educators and dietitians are super-fluous and who will not send their patients to them. If you are placed in this unfortunate situation, ask your doctor to refer you anyhow. If he or she still refuses, call your local hospital diabetes clinic and ask if you can make an appointment without a doctor's referral.

The Dietitian (Your Energizer)

Remember the movie *Ghostbusters*? Well, when it comes to your nutrition plan (also called a "meal plan"), *who you gonna call?* Your dietitian.

Registered dieticians are the pros when it comes to assisting you with your nutrition. To be called a "registered dietitian" in Canada, a person must have official certification establishing that he or she has the appropriate credentials. In Canada, the initials *R.D.* appear after the name of certified dietitians.

What you eat (and drink) is central to your success with your diabetes. Eat poorly, and you will render many of the pills you are taking less effective. Your oral hypoglycemic agents will be less useful. Your blood pressure pills will not work as well. Your cholesterol medicine will be fighting an uphill battle. And so on.

Your dietitian is the most knowledgeable person when it comes to advising you about what you should eat. It would be a terrible disservice to them — and, more important, to you — to think of the dietitian's role as simply "putting you on a diet to lose weight." A dietitian can help you determine the best choice and quantity of foods, and he or she can help you determine the number of calories that your body requires.

If you have type 1 diabetes and are on an "intensified insulin" program (see Chapter 12), your dietitian can teach you how to keep track of your carbohydrates (called "carbohydrate counting"), which is often a highly effective means of achieving excellent blood glucose control. We discuss carbohydrate counting in Chapter 10.

A good dietitian will help you to create a nutrition plan that does the following:

- ✔ Stays flexible
- ✔ Takes into account your particular ethnic and cultural background, and meets your particular religious requirements (if any)
- ✔ Fits with your lifestyle

The importance of tailoring a diet to fit the individual can no be no better demonstrated than by the tale of two brothers that Ian had occasion to meet a couple of years ago. They were both teenagers and both also had type 1 diabetes. Bob was athletic and was captain of his hockey team. David, a year younger than his brother, couldn't have been more different. David could dismantle (and reassemble!) a car or a computer, but the only red line he knew about was the one on the tachometer. For the sake of convenience, the first time they were to meet with their dietitian they went together. The advice they received and the meal plans they took home were as different from one another as night and day. But the plans worked. To each his own (diet, that is!).

If you feel that the treatment plan your dietitian gives you is too rigid, that it is too out of keeping with your tastes, or that it is in some other way simply not realistic or practical, *do not* give up on the idea of proper nutrition therapy. Let your dietitian know of your concerns and he or she will likely be happy to work with you at creating a more appropriate meal plan.

The Eye Specialist (Your Cameraperson)

An eye doctor has special expertise in the detection and treatment of eye disease. There are two types of eye doctors — ophthalmologists and optometrists. In Chapter 6 we look at the differences between them and how often you should be seen by one of them. We also look at the various types of eye disease for which you are at risk.

Eye damage from diabetes seldom causes symptoms until it is very advanced, so it *absolutely essential* that you see an eye doctor routinely — even if you have no problems with your sight!

Although your family doctor and your diabetes specialist may examine your eyes, an eye doctor has additional skills that you should avail yourself of.

Although spending inordinate time in doctors' waiting rooms is the stuff of legend, eye doctors' offices are particularly famous for this. Make sure you bring something to read when you go. Hmm . . . how about *Diabetes For Canadians For Dummies*? And you had best plan on doing your day's reading prior to going into the examining room, because when you see your eye specialist, he or she will dilate your pupils using eye drops. This can affect your vision for a few hours and may make it difficult for you to read, and, more important, may make it impossible for you to drive yourself home from your appointment. It would be wise, therefore, for you to bring someone with you to drive you home.

Sometimes the good deed of restoring vision leads to unexpected, negative consequences. One ophthalmologist told Alan that he restored the vision of a patient with diabetes, only to have the patient buy a gun and nearly shoot someone with whom he had a grievance!

The Pharmacist (Your Equipment Manager)

If you have diabetes, you are invariably going to be on medications to assist with our ultimate goal of keeping you healthy. Now, it may be that when you go to the pharmacy, your first thought is "oh heck, another errand." Okay, so going to a pharmacy isn't the highlight of your day (thankfully!). But what a great resource you have at your disposal in the form of your pharmacist.

Pharmacists have expertise in medicines, so when you pick up your prescriptions, you have a golden opportunity to become an informed consumer. Here are some of the things that your pharmacist should review with you:

- The names of your medicines
- The dosages of your medicines
- How often you are to take your medicines
- What time you should take your medicines (for example, many cholesterol medicines work best if taken in the evening)
- What route you are to take your medicines (oral, vaginal, topical, and so on)
- Whether you should take your medicines with food or on an empty stomach
- Whether it is safe for you to consume alcohol (Some people have bad reactions if they ingest alcohol while on sulfonylurea oral hypoglycemic agents.) We discuss oral agents further in Chapter 11.
- Whether there are any possible interactions between your different medicines (For example, thyroid pills don't get absorbed as effectively if you take them at the same time as calcium pills.)
- What adverse effects ("side effects") the medicines can cause.

A good pharmacist will not simply hand your pills to you with a piece of paper (listing 50 side effects) stapled to your bag and say goodbye. A good pharmacist will sit down with you and not only explain the items listed above, but also review with you *how likely* it is that you will experience the different side effects. Without a pharmacist's help, as you read through the lengthy list of all the bad things that the medicines can do you will not be truly informed. You will simply be scared. And *that* is not effective counselling.

If you are on several (or more) different medicines, ask your pharmacist to prepare a list of your medications that you can keep in your wallet or purse. This list should include the names, doses, and frequency of your drugs. Keeping track of when to take medicines can be very difficult. Your pharmacist may be able to help you out by packaging your medicines in a container where they are laid out by day of week and time of day.

The Foot Doctor (Your Sole Mate)

The foot doctor *(podiatrist)* is your best source of help with the minor and some of the major foot problems that you may encounter. He or she can assist you with such problems as toenails that are hard to cut, bothersome corns and calluses, and difficulties with excessively dry or cracked skin. If you have areas of your feet that undergo excessive pressure as you walk, a foot doctor can also help fit you with special insoles called orthotics, which more evenly distribute the forces upon your feet.

The longer we are in practice as diabetes specialists, the more we have come to rely on and use the expertise that podiatrists have to offer. They truly are the experts when it comes to helping you keep your feet healthy.

Not all podiatry services are covered by provincial health care plans. Before you meet with your podiatrist, you might want to call ahead to find out what charges you may expect.

Your Family and Friends (Your Fans and Cheerleaders)

Okay, so the 1985 Oilers likely would have done just fine, thank you very much, even if they didn't have a single fan in the stands. But they were the exceptions. For the rest of us, it is essential to have people rooting for us as we deal with the trials and tribulations of life. And this is especially true if you are living with a health issue such as diabetes.

Your fans and cheerleaders are the people you live with, eat with, and play with. Your family and friends can be a tremendous source of support, but for them to help you, they will need your guidance. For example, you can teach them what to look for if you become hypoglycemic (see Chapter 5). And you can ask them to avoid eating indiscriminately in your presence. Following your diet is challenging enough; you certainly don't need your family exposing you to constant temptation. Your family or friends can also become your exercise partners. Sticking to a program is a lot easier when a partner is counting on you to show up to work out.

It is often a good idea to have someone accompany you when you see a member of your health care team. (This is especially true if you are meeting the dietitian and you are not the main food preparer at home.) A lot of information is going to be communicated, and an extra set of ears is helpful.

If you do plan to bring an extra set of ears with you to your doctor's appointment, be sure to ask your physician ahead of time if it is okay to bring this person in. There may, on occasion, be some issues that should be discussed in private before your friend or relative joins you. (Important conversations about, say, sexual dysfunction, likely would not take place if you have your daughter or son in the room as you are speaking to your doctor.)

Let people who are important to you know about your diabetes. Showing them this chapter might be a good way to introduce them to their important supporting role.

In this chapter we look at the central players on your diabetes team, but it is important to recognize that there are many other teammates who may be asked to take a face-off from time to time. These include, among others, hospital emergency room staff, heart specialists, neurologists, gastroenterologists ("stomach doctors"), social workers, dentists, psychologists, and psychiatrists.

Chapter 9

Monitoring Your Blood Glucose Control

*I*f you read Part II prior to getting here, you are now familiar with the problems that this part of the book is going to help you avoid. In Chapter 8 we introduce you to the members of your team (including you) that are working diligently to keep you healthy. The remainder of Part III focuses on all the amazing tools we have to help your team. And boy, do we have tools! We have nutrition therapy, we have exercise techniques, we have prescription medicines, and we have non-prescription products. And to make sure that we are reaching our goals, we have the benefit of testing equipment to help us monitor our progress. Sure, it's a bit of a bother and will cost some money, but, hey, you're worth it.

Not only that, but you're among the most fortunate people with diabetes who have ever lived. Most of the products and treatments we cover in this part were not available even 20 years ago. And the new products coming along will knock your socks off (but put them back on because you should not go barefoot).

How can we get you to make use of these great advances? Let's listen in on an excerpt from the *2,000 Year Old Man* album, in which Carl Reiner and Mel Brooks are speaking:

> *Reiner:* "Tell me, sir, what was the means of locomotion 2,000 years ago?"
>
> *Brooks:* "What d'ya mean, locomotion?"
>
> *Reiner:* "What was it that got you to move quickly from one place to another?"
>
> *Brooks:* "Fear."

We did not write Part II with the intention of frightening you. Well, maybe we did a bit when we wrote about the foot stuff, but hey, whatever works.

Testing with a Glucose Meter

In earlier chapters we discuss the bad things that can happen if you are exposed to elevated blood glucose. In this chapter, you discover all you need to know about how to monitor your blood glucose levels.

"Why monitor?" you might ask. "After all, my doctor can just send me to the lab for a blood test when I need it."

True enough. Your doctor *can* just send you to the lab for a blood test when you need it. But that would mean visiting the lab *every* day. Surely, you have better things to do with your time.

Why you should test

Have you even gotten dressed in the dark only to find out as you were heading out the door that your socks were mismatched or the blue pants you put on were actually black or your red purse was actually brown? You probably either made a mad dash back inside to re-dress, or you just headed out, hoping that your gaffe would not be noticed. Well, not monitoring your blood glucose levels is like getting dressed in the dark every day.

If you are not testing your blood, you will never know:

- If your nutrition ("diet") plan (see Chapter 10) is helping your glucose control
- If your exercise program (see Chapter 10) is improving your glucose levels

✔ If your oral hypoglycemic agents (see Chapter 11) or insulin doses (see Chapter 12) need to be changed

✔ If your recent illness, such as a chest infection, is making your glucose readings dangerously high

Basically, you will be in the dark, without guidance, and equally important, without feedback.

But what if your readings are poor? "Why do I want to be frustrated by always seeing crummy readings?" you might ask. And you would be perfectly justified in asking this. At least, you would be perfectly justified if there were no way to improve things. But there are *always* ways to improve things. So if your readings are not good, it is time for you to meet with your diabetes educator and dietitian to see if your lifestyle plan needs adjusting. And to call your family doctor (or diabetes specialist if you are in regular contact with one) to have your oral hypoglycemic agents or insulin therapy reviewed.

There is a tendency for people with diabetes to look at a record of their glucose readings as a report card, keeping constant score and noting whether they have passed or failed. That is understandable, but terribly inappropriate. Your glucose readings are not meant to judge you or your efforts. Your readings are being done to serve as an aid — a tool — to help you and your team know when changes to your therapy are in order. And if your readings are good, they serve as a nice source of positive feedback.

How often should you test?

How often you test is determined by three factors: the kind of diabetes you have, the kind of treatment you are using, and the level of stability of your blood glucose. As you can tell, this is not a "one size fits all" issue. The Canadian Diabetes Association (CDA) recommends the following:

✔ **If you have type 1 diabetes:** Test at least three times daily (and, periodically, overnight). Many situations require more frequent testing to achieve desired blood glucose levels.

✔ **If you have type 2 diabetes:** Test at least once daily if you are being treated with oral hypoglycemic agents or insulin. Many situations require more frequent testing to achieve desired blood glucose levels.

✔ **Tests should include both before-meal and two-hour post-meal readings.** (Tricky indeed if you are testing only once — or even three times — daily! Well, what the CDA means is that you should vary the timing of your tests from one day to the next, not that you need to test before and 2 hours after meals *every* day. We will look at some possible testing schedules in a moment).

In our experience, the more you test, the more information and feedback you have, and, ultimately, the better you do. For this reason we would encourage you to focus on the "at least" wording of the CDA guidelines and aim to test considerably more often than the minimum recommendations. We have found the following schedule to work very well (note that this schedule assumes your overall control is both very good and very stable; if it is not, you should be testing *even more*):

- **If your treatment consists of lifestyle measures alone** (see Chapter 10), test *once* daily, varying the timing of your reading so that over the span of a week or two you will have values from before and after each of your meals.

- **If you are taking oral hypoglycemic agents** (see Chapter 11), test *twice* daily:

  - Before breakfast, *and*

  - Vary the time of the other test (sometimes do it before your other meals and sometimes 2 hours after your meals).

- **If you are an adult taking insulin once or twice a day** (see Chapter 12), test *twice* daily:

  - Before breakfast, *and*

  - Vary the time of the other test (sometimes do it before your other meals, sometimes 2 hours after your meals, and *sometimes at bedtime*).

- **If you are an adult taking insulin three or four times a day (or a child or adolescent taking insulin any number of times a day)** (see Chapter 12), test *four to seven* times daily:

  - Before each meal, *and*

  - 2 hours after some meals (you may wish to rotate so that one day you test after breakfast, the next day after lunch, and the next day after dinner), *and*

  - *Every* night at bedtime, *and*

  - *Occasionally at about 3 am* (to make sure you are not having low overnight readings that have not been awakening you).

- **If you have gestational diabetes** (see Chapter 7) treated with lifestyle measures alone, test before and 2 hours after your breakfast.

- **If you are pregnant and have pre-existing diabetes *or* if you have gestational diabetes treated with insulin,** test *six to seven* times per day (before and 2 hours after each meal and again at bedtime if your bedtime is 4 or more hours after your dinner).

Never fall into the trap of assuming that if you feel well, your blood glucose levels *must* be good and therefore you do not need to test. The truth is, your blood glucose level can be twice (or more) normal and you may not have a single symptom, while all the while your body is being irreversibly damaged.

As you can tell from this list, the frequency of testing is directly related to how often you need the information to make decisions about your care. If you are being treated with lifestyle measures alone, getting feedback once per day is usually enough to let you know how effective your treatment plan is, whereas if you are on an intensified insulin program (see Chapter 12), you should test much more often to know what insulin dose to administer.

Most everyone has periods of time where they get fed up with testing, testing, testing. Don't feel guilty if you feel this way; it is perfectly normal. And if you do happen to go through periods of time where you are not testing nearly as much as you should, there's no need to berate yourself about it. Just grab hold of your meter and get back into the routine.

Mr. Pereira was a middle-aged man with type 2 diabetes who had come to Ian's office for a consultation. Ian asked him how his blood glucose control was, and Mr. Pereira replied, "It was 7.4 today." Ian asked him if he had any other readings to share. "Sure; it was 9.3 last month so it's getting better." Ian explained to his patient that glucose control varies not only month to month, but day to day and even meal to meal, so knowing two readings taken a month apart tells us virtually nothing about how control is or what trend it is following. Hearing this explanation, Mr. Pereira, a math teacher, asked if he could borrow Ian's calculator, and, a moment later, announced, "Gee, Doctor, now I get it. I've told you what my readings were for a total of 2 minutes out of the past 43,200 minutes. That's not even five one-thousandths of 1 percent of my readings. *No wonder* that doesn't tell you much." Couldn't have said it better ourselves.

How do you perform a test?

Just like any test, a blood glucose test requires some basic supplies:

- ✔ **Lancet:** If you happen to be like us, the notion of intentionally wounding yourself is most definitely not your idea of a good time. Well, you need not despair because obtaining a blood sample is a nearly painless procedure. In order to prick yourself you use a small, sharp, disposable *lancet*.

- ✔ **Lancet holder:** Your lancet fits into this spring-loaded holder, and when you push the release button, the lancet springs out and pokes your finger.

- ✔ **Test strip:** This is the small disposable strip onto which you place your drop of blood.

✔ **Blood glucose meter:** This is the device that figures out how much glucose is in your blood sample. We'll talk more about these neat gadgets in a moment.

✔ **"Sharps" container:** This is a small box into which you place your used lancets. You can pick up a sharps container from your drugstore. When the container is full, seal it and bring it back to the drugstore for proper disposal.

Though you may be apprehensive about pricking yourself to obtain a drop of blood, rest assured that you will be far more relaxed than a man in his 20s that Ian knew of. This man was converting to a religion that required a ritual drop of blood to be obtained from the end part of his penis. The man lay down and the appropriate part of his anatomy was exposed. A physician was called into the room to obtain the drop of blood. The physician, a twinkle in his eye, looked down at the anxious man and said he need not worry, the procedure would be over in a minute. "I've got a new medical instrument I just obtained when I was travelling overseas," the doctor said. "It will work perfectly," he added as he reached behind him and brought into full view a Samurai sword! (P.S. The procedure actually did go ahead — the mischievous doctor using a tiny needle in lieu of the sword.)

Now, let's look at the, ahem, more conventional steps in obtaining a blood sample:

1. **Wash your hands (or at least your finger):** Although you do not need to prepare your site — or your psyche — with alcohol, you need to make sure your finger (or arm if you are using an "alternate-site meter," which we discuss in the next section) is clean.

2. **Obtain a blood sample:** Insert a lancet into the lancet holder, press it against the *side* of your fingertip, and activate the trigger. In an instant, you will see a tiny drop of blood appear. It does not hurt much at all, but to make it hurt even less you can:

   • Use a lancet holder that allows you to adjust the depth of penetration. An example is the Softclix Lancing Device.

   • Avoid re-using your lancets since they dull quickly. (It's okay to use the same one a few times, but not more than that.)

   • Change fingers often or, quite the opposite, stick to the side of the same finger and you will find that once you have built up a small callus it hurts less to draw blood from that site.

   • Take blood from an "alternate site" such as your forearm. (To do this you will need an "alternate-site meter.")

3. **Apply the end of the glucose-measuring strip to the blood:** Only a tiny drop of blood is required, but it still has to be sufficient to cover the marked area on the strip. Most strips are designed to draw up the blood in the same way that a strip of paper towel, when dipped into water, draws up the water (a process called "capillary action," in case you were wondering).

4. **Presto, you're done:** Most modern meters will then quickly display your result.

If you have difficulty obtaining a sufficient quantity of blood, try one or more of the following:

- ✔ Warm your finger with warm water.

- ✔ Let your arm hang down at your side for a minute before you test.

- ✔ Hold your finger about 1.5 centimetres (about half an inch) from the tip and squeeze — but only once, as repeated squeezing can interfere with the test's accuracy.

If ever you find that your test result is far lower than you expect, this may be because you had insufficient blood on the strip (this can give falsely low readings). If your blood glucose meter tells you that your reading is, for example, 2.8 mmol/L and you had expected a 12.8 mmol/L, re-test yourself. On the other hand, you can obtain falsely elevated readings if the test strips have been exposed to high humidity or high temperature. Be sure to read the package insert that came with your strips to familiarize yourself with the instructions (and precautions) made by the manufacturer.

Incidentally, when it comes to used lancets, remember the old adage: Neither a borrower nor a lender be. The only time you should share your blood is when you are donating to Canadian Blood Services (which, incidentally, we discuss further in Chapter 12). Similarly, because a meter invariably gets a little blood on it (and hence, can be a source of infection), you should not share your meter.

How a blood glucose meter works

Earlier glucose meters relied on a colour change that appeared on the test strips and that was proportional to your blood glucose level. The new meters use a different process to analyze your blood. They measure an electrical potential that is created when the glucose in your blood sample reacts with reagents (glucose oxidase and potassium ferricyanide) on the electrode of the test strip. This reaction generates electrons that produce an electrical current. The higher your glucose level, the greater the current.

How Do You Choose a Meter?

So many meters are on the market that you may be confused about which one to use. One consideration that should play little or no part in your choice of a meter is the cost, since with rebates, promotions, trade-ins (and, most of all, because the companies are happy to sell their machines at a loss in order to get you to buy their strips), you will find *almost* every meter you look at to be quite inexpensive and competitively priced. Because the meters are so cheap and because the manufacturers replace them with better ones so frequently, it is a good idea to get a new meter every year or two, to make sure that you have the "latest and greatest" device.

Another non-consideration is the accuracy of the various machines. All are accurate to a degree acceptable for managing your diabetes. Keep in mind, though, that they do not have the accuracy of laboratory equipment. (If ever you are experimenting with your machine and test your blood twice within a minute or two, you may find your readings vary by 10 to 15 percent. This is not because your blood glucose level has changed that amount in a matter of seconds; it is simply that the machines are not perfect.)

Although the meters are cheap, the test strips are anything but. Typically they are about a dollar per strip (ouch!), regardless of which meter you are using. If you shop around, however, you will find that some drugstores sell them for significantly less than others.

 Some provinces and territories will subsidize the cost of your blood glucose strips. For more information you can contact your provincial or territorial government or the CDA. (Excellent information is available on the CDA Web site, www.diabetes.ca. Click Advocacy, then click the link entitled Financial Coverage Charts for Diabetes Supplies and Medication.

Capillary versus venous glucose levels

When you test with a finger-prick sample, you are obtaining what is termed a "capillary" blood sample, whereas when a lab takes blood from your arm they are obtaining a "venous" blood sample. The glucose level in a venous sample is typically about 15 percent higher than a capillary sample. This would make your meter's results misleadingly low, so the testing equipment has been designed to correct for this.

Since the machines are similar in price, similar in accuracy, and similar in terms of the costs for their strips, your purchase decision should be based on other factors:

✔ Whether you like products with "bells and whistles" or prefer those that are "plain and simple."

✔ If your eyesight is poor, you will want to make sure the display is easily readable or, if that is not sufficient, you may wish to purchase a meter that can connect with a voice synthesizer. (The SureStep and OneTouch meters can connect to a "voice box" sold by Auto Control Medical — 800-461-0991 — for approximately $400. This synthesizer is truly amazing, but you will have to put up with — how can we say this kindly — the voice of a particularly assertive gentleman.)

✔ If you are likely to be testing in the dark you will want to select a meter that has backlighting. There is even a meter that is itself glow-in-the-dark (the Precision Xtra).

✔ If you want to test from "alternate sites" such as your forearm, there are now meters designed to allow this (such as the OneTouch Ultra and the Freestyle).

✔ You will want to make sure the meter is not too bulky (seldom an issue with current meters), or, conversely, too small to fit comfortably in your hand. For example, the brand new "FreeStyle mini" is an amazingly compact meter which will make it a great choice for some people and not a good choice for others.

✔ Some strips are larger than others. If you have a hard time holding onto very small objects, you may wish to choose a meter (such as the AccuSoft Advantage) that uses larger strips.

✔ You will have to decide how much memory you need in a machine. They can vary considerably in terms of how many readings they store. If you are keeping a written logbook — which we recommend — this is not a particularly important feature, but if you are not keeping a logbook, a memory is a good thing to have (in a meter, not to mention in our heads!). The OneTouch UltraSmart has an excellent, though not perfect, way of presenting records stored in its memory.

✔ If you have type 1 diabetes, it would be a good idea to use a meter that also tests for ketones, such as the Precision Xtra. (See Chapter 5 for more on ketones.)

✔ You may find it more convenient to have a device that can hold multiple test strips. Examples include the DEX2 and the Accu-Chek Compact.

✔ If you like the idea of being able to download your readings onto your computer so you can graph (and print) them, you will want to buy a meter that has this capacity. Bear in mind that you will likely encounter an additional charge for the connecting cable.

✔ If you are using insulin, NovoNordisk and Lifescan have teamed up to make a nice product called the InDuo. It has two components — a meter and an insulin pen device — that fit together into a fairly small package.

✔ If time is of the essence, you will want to have a lightning-fast machine. Depending on the machine, it can take from 5 to 30 seconds to process a sample and display the result.

Alternate-site glucose readings are not reliable if they are obtained when your blood glucose level is rapidly rising or falling. For this reason, you should not rely on alternate-site tests if you are doing a blood glucose test within 2 hours of eating, nor should you use an alternate site test if you suspect you are hypoglycemic.

You will save much time, energy, and aggravation by speaking to your diabetes educator before you buy a meter. Not only can he or she show you the latest meters and point out their pros and cons, but also, more important, *they know you* and will able to help you select a meter that meets your particular needs.

If you would like to do some of your own research, you can find (far from impartial) information regarding meters by going to the different manufacturers' Web sites or by calling them. Here are the main manufacturers in the Canadian market, their current products, Web site, and phone numbers:

Table 9-1	Manufacturers and Meters	
Manufacturer	*Product*	*Contact information*
Abbott Diabetes Care	FreeStyle FreeStyle Mini Precision Xtra	www.abbottdiabetescare.ca 888-519-6890
Bayer	Ascensia Breeze Ascensia Contour Ascensia DEX2 Ascensia Elite Ascensia Elite XL	www.bayer.ca 800-268-1432
Becton-Dickson	BD Logic Latitude Diabetes Management System The Link	www.bddiabetes.com 800-268-5430

Manufacturer	Product	Contact information
Lifescan	OneTouch Ultra OneTouch UltraSmart OneTouch SureStep	www.lifescancanada.com 800-663-5521
Lifescan/ NovoNordisk	InDuo	www.novonordisk.ca 800-465-4334
Roche	AccuSoft Advantage Accu-Chek Aviva Accu-Chek Compact	www.rochecanada.com 800-363-7949

How Should You Record Your Results?

Ian recalls going for a haircut a few years back (when he used to have to go more often) only to find his barber profoundly upset. "What's the matter?" Ian asked, to which his barber replied that he could not find his scissors. "Why not just use somebody else's?" Ian innocently asked. His barber immediately stopped his searching and looked at Ian with disbelief. "Use somebody else's? Would you use somebody else's wife?" And that just about sums up most diabetes specialists' opinions about how glucose readings should be recorded. We are very particular and we each have our own preferences.

So then, we *could* show you many different ways of recording your results, or we could just show you the best way, which, ahem, just happens to be Ian's way!

The first thing you need to do is to obtain a logbook. You can find these at your pharmacy, at your diabetes education centre, and at your diabetes specialist's office. Your family doctor may also have them. Each page in your logbook should be laid out like this:

	Blood Glucose Levels							Insulin Injections					
Date	Breakfast		Lunch		Dinner		Bedtime	Other	Insulin Type	Units Taken				Notes
	Before	After	Before	After	Before	After				Breakfast	Lunch	Dinner	Bedtime	

Figure 9-1:
Logbook
format.

Of course, if you are not on insulin the right hand side of the page will go unused.

Most logbooks, alas, do not have this particular format. If you are unable to find a book with this layout, you can download similar pages from Ian's Web site (www.ianblumer.com).

The one shortcoming with this layout is, potentially, insufficient space for you to write in the Notes column (where you might want to write things such as "birthday party" or "missed snack" to remind you later on of some event that had occurred that might explain a high or low reading). If you need more space, you can always create your own sheet on a piece of paper (which you could photocopy) or with a spreadsheet program such as Excel.

Using this layout allows you to quickly assess your overall blood glucose *patterns, trends,* and *averages* for a given time of day. To illustrate what we mean, let's have a look at two different ways of recording your readings.

The following table is the typical way that a log is kept or that a machine's memory displays results (although a machine would display the time of day, not the meal of the day). The following readings are pre-meal values:

Table 9-2	Blood Glucose Readings Listed Chronologically
Time of Reading	*Blood Glucose Level*
Breakfast	12.6
Lunch	4.1
Dinner	14.7
Bedtime	5.6
Breakfast	11.7
Lunch	5.2
Dinner	12.1
Bedtime	7.0
Breakfast	10.0
Lunch	5.9
Dinner	11.9
Bedtime	4.0
Breakfast	9.9
Time of Reading	*Blood Glucose Level*

Time of Reading	Blood Glucose Level
Lunch	4.2
Dinner	14.4
Bedtime	4.4
Breakfast	11.1
Lunch	6.3
Dinner	12.2
Bedtime	5.1

If you were to record your readings like this, you would likely feel that your glucose values were "all over the place" (or, as Ian often hears, "my sugars are up and down like a toilet seat") and you would likely be feeling frustrated by what you concluded were very inconsistent values. Although your conclusion would be perfectly understandable, you might be surprised to see that if we look at your readings from a different perspective, they could be thought of as being remarkably consistent. Let's take those same readings and chart them differently.

Table 9-3	Blood Glucose Reading Listed by Time of Day		
Breakfast	**Lunch**	**Dinner**	**Bedtime**
12.6	4.1	14.7	5.6
11.7	5.2	12.1	7.0
10.0	5.9	11.9	4.0
9.9	4.2	14.4	4.4
11.1	6.3	12.2	5.1

Now, scan the columns from top to bottom. Aha! You will see that your readings at any given time of day are remarkably similar. You are consistently too high at breakfast, consistently normal at lunch, consistently too high at dinner, and consistently normal at bedtime.

The memory on a blood glucose meter does not allow for this type of instant overview, and hence is almost always inferior to using a logbook. (The only meter that comes close is the OneTouch UltraSmart, but even that one does not give as complete a picture as those old and trusted tools: pen and paper.)

This is of great importance because now that we have identified your blood glucose patterns, we can adjust your therapy accordingly. For example, if you were on insulin therapy, we would know that you need more bedtime insulin to bring down your breakfast blood glucose and more lunchtime insulin to reduce your suppertime readings (see Chapter 12 for a detailed discussion of insulin adjustment). We could have figured this out from the first table, but it would have been much more difficult and time consuming.

If you are using an insulin pump (see Chapter 12) you will need an even more detailed log book; a good one can be found at Rick Mendosa's Web site (www.mendosa.com/logsheet.pdf).

What Is Your Glucose Target?

The Canadian Diabetes Association (CDA) guidelines recommend that *most* adults with type 1 or type 2 diabetes (we look at children's targets in Chapter 14) aim for the following readings:

	Before meals	***2 hours after meals***
Target	4.0-7.0 mmol/L	5.0-10.0 mmol/L
Normal level	4.0-6.0 mmol/L	5.0-8.0 mmol/L

If you can do so safely, target the normal level. Here are some of the things that might make it unsafe for you to aim for normal levels:

- ✔ You have other health problems that make it too dangerous to risk *any* hypoglycemia.

- ✔ You have *irreversible* problems with hypoglycemia unawareness (see Chapter 5).

- ✔ When you try to have readings in this range, you experience excessively *frequent* hypoglycemia.

- ✔ Your life expectancy is such that you are at low risk of developing diabetes-related long-term complications.

No one with diabetes has glucose readings that are always within target. Indeed, having two-thirds of your readings within target is a wonderful accomplishment. And remember that to achieve (or to even come close to achieving) your targets will require a concerted and ongoing effort on behalf of your diabetes team. (And remember, *you* are the first star on this team.)

It can be very difficult to consistently achieve target blood glucose values and, for some people, it may simply not be possible. If you and your health care team have worked hard at reaching these goals but have not been able to achieve them it is essential that you not feel that all is lost. The reason for this is simple; although fantastic blood glucose readings are our goal, any improvement in your blood glucose control will help keep you free of complications from your diabetes. (See the following discussion on A1C testing.)

Testing for Longer-Term Control with an A1C

As Ian's mathematician discovered (in an anecdote earlier in this chapter), individual blood glucose tests are great for telling us how you're doing at a specific moment in time, but they do not give us the big picture. Frequent blood glucose measurements help, but even then, they only provide a series of snapshots of your glucose levels. So what we need is a test that gives an estimate of your *overall* control over a longer period of time. And that is precisely what we can determine from a test called an A1C. As the sidebar in this section discusses, your A1C level is a measure of how much glucose has become attached to your red blood cells over the preceding three to four months.

Knowing your A1C is crucial because the likelihood of your developing microvascular complications (that is, eye, kidney, and nerve damage, as we discuss in Chapter 6) is directly related to your A1C. A normal A1C is 6 or less. An A1C of 7 is good and puts you at quite low risk for microvascular damage. An A1C of 9 or higher is poor and puts you at much greater risk. An A1C that is too high is an alarm to you and your health care team that your control needs to be improved. If you can drop your A1C by even 1 percent you will substantially decrease your risk of microvascular complications. In one landmark study — the "DCCT" — it was found that reducing the A1C from 8 down to about 7 (equivalent to a reduction in average blood glucose of only 2 mmol/L) resulted in an astounding 40 to 50 percent lower risk of retinopathy progression.

You may come across other terms for A1C, including "hemoglobin A1C," "glycosylated hemoglobin," or "glycohemoglobin." You may also come across it abbreviated as HbA1C or HgbA1C. These all mean the same thing. Also you may find an A1C level written as a number ("9," for example) or as a percentage ("9 %," for example); both of these are correct and mean the same thing.

After you have had your A1C tested, be sure you contact your doctor (or educator, if he or she is the one that requested the test) to find out the result!

The A1C does not replace blood glucose meter testing; it is *complementary* to it. Since the A1C represents an overall estimate of your blood glucose control, it does not tell us how many highs and lows you may be having. Your average glucose level may be good even though half your readings are too low and the other half too high. It's sort of like having one foot in ice water and the other in boiling water and saying "on average, I feel fine."

The following table shows what the average blood glucose levels are (over the preceding three to four months) for a given A1C:

Table 9-4	A1C with Corresponding Average Blood Glucose Level
A1C	**Average blood glucose level (in mmol/L)**
5	5.5
6	7.5
7	9.5
8	11.5
9	13.5
10	15.5
11	17.5
12	19.5

As the table demonstrates, the higher your A1C, the higher your blood glucose levels have been running. The lower your A1C, the lower your recent blood glucose levels. The Canadian Diabetes Association recommends that your A1C level be tested every three months. (If you are pregnant it will need to be checked more often, as we discuss in Chapter 7.)

As you can see, your A1C reading is *not* the same as your average blood glucose. This is commonly misunderstood. (For example, an A1C of 8.0 does *not* mean that your average blood glucose level is 8.0 mmol/L; it actually corresponds to average readings of 11.5 mmol/L.)

The Canadian Diabetes Association (CDA) guidelines recommend that *most* people with type 1 or type 2 diabetes aim for an A1C of 7 percent or less (normal is 6 percent or less for most laboratories). If it can be safely achieved (see the earlier discussion about why it might be unsafe), your goal is to have an A1C in the normal range.

As long as you use your glucose meter frequently, your A1C result will likely be as anticipated. When it isn't (for example, if your meter's average was 7.0 mmol/L yet your A1C was 10), you and your health care team will need to figure out why. The most common reason for this is that your readings are up when you are not testing and therefore you would not be aware of the elevations. If your readings have this sort of discrepancy, try testing more often and at times you haven't been testing (including overnight). On occasion an A1C level is affected by other substances in the blood or by anemia. If your physician suspects this, he or she can contact the laboratory to discuss this possibility.

How A1C works

Within red blood cells there is a protein called hemoglobin. Hemoglobin carries oxygen around the body, delivering it to where it is needed to assist with various chemical reactions that are taking place. Hemoglobin is constantly exposed to the glucose within the blood and becomes permanently attached to it. It attaches in several different ways, and the total of all the hemoglobin attached to glucose is called *glycohemoglobin*. The largest fraction, two-thirds of the glycohemoglobin, is in a form called hemoglobin A1C. This is the easiest form to measure. The rest of the hemoglobin is made up of hemoglobins A1a and A1b. The more glucose in the blood, the more glycohemoglobin forms. Hemoglobin is destroyed when the red blood cell that contains it dies. This occurs after the red blood cell has been in existence for about 120 days or so. Because glycohemoglobin remains in the blood for that length of time, it is a reflection of the glucose control over that entire time period and not just the second that a single glucose test reflects.

Apart from going to the lab to have them take blood from your arm, there are two other ways to check an A1C. Some diabetes centres have a desktop machine that can process a fingerprick sample in 6 minutes so that you (and they) will know your result while you are there for your visit. The cost is usually about $10 per test. There is also a disposable test kit for home use called A1C Now. It is expensive, though, at about $50 per test.

Bloodless ("Non-Invasive") Meters

Although pricking yourself to draw blood may not be a terrible experience, it is anything but pleasurable. For now, we do not have an alternative to routine blood testing, but there are some *complementary*, non-blood-requiring devices available.

One such device is the Medtronic Continuous Glucose Monitoring System (CGMS). This is an expensive ($3,000) pager-size device that you wear on your belt. It is connected to a sensor that is inserted just under your skin surface and that stays in place for 3 days. Every few minutes, it automatically measures the glucose level in the *interstitial* fluid (the fluid just under your skin). Because interstitial glucose levels are similar to blood, these readings are essentially the same as glucose meter results. After 3 days, the device is removed and the readings stored in its memory are downloaded into a computer and printed. Your diabetes specialist or diabetes educator may ask you to do a 3 day CGMS test to determine if you are having high or low blood glucose readings that are not being detected with routine blood glucose monitoring.

Because the device (and the electrode that is worn) are so expensive — and because provincial health plans do not cover the cost — you may be asked to pay a fee (usually somewhere between fifty and one hundred dollars) to cover the cost of the test.

Because the CGMS device does not display the results, it does not provide you with moment-to-moment information and, hence, cannot replace blood glucose testing. There are, however, ongoing attempts to improve the device so that it provides real-time results and there are also competing devices under development that will hopefully provide this information. The ultimate goal, of course, is to have a sensor that can be hooked up to an insulin delivery device (such as an insulin pump). The sensor would measure your glucose level and send a message to a pump, which would then figure out how much insulin to give. This would, in essence, be an artificial pancreas. You can see a picture of the CGMS at the manufacturer's Web site (www.minimed.com).

Another device that records your glucose without requiring you to prick yourself is the Glucowatch. This looks like an oversize wristwatch and you wear it on your forearm. It displays your glucose level after a 20-minute delay, and you can set alarms to notify you if your reading is too low or high. It is not yet available in Canada and, in any event, it does have some shortcomings, including the delay between when the sample is obtained and when the result is displayed. Additionally, the skin under the device often becomes a bit swollen and red. As well, the Glucowatch and the supplies are very pricey (the device and 1 year's supplies will run you about US$4,000). At this time, the FDA (the U.S. regulatory body in charge of such issues) advises that Glucowatch wearers must also test their blood. This, of course, largely defeats the purpose of the device. You can see a picture of the Glucowatch at the manufacturer's Web site (www.glucowatch.com).

There are some truly amazing non-invasive sensors under development including ones that give a reading by shining a light through your skin and even one that measures the glucose level in your tears. Developers are well aware of the phenomenal profits that await them if they are successful in their efforts at replacing blood glucose testing. In Chapter 22, we look at some promising technologies under development.

Chapter 10

Lifestyles That Will Help You Become Richly and Famously Healthy

*L*anguage specialists claim that the five sweetest phrases in the English language are:

✔ I love you.

✔ Dinner is served.

✔ All is forgiven.

✔ Sleep until noon.

✔ Keep the change.

To that, most people would certainly add, "You've lost weight."

If you have diabetes and you are overweight and sedentary — and that is true of the great majority of people with type 2 diabetes — appropriate nutrition, weight loss, and exercise are your tickets to success. You have more power at your disposal than any drug that any doctor can dispense to you.

It may well be that you look back at your high school grad photos and point out to your children or grandchildren how slim and trim you were way back when exercise was not a chore, but a matter of routine. Perhaps it was not long thereafter that family and work commitments appeared, followed in short order by some excess weight around your middle. And once your lifestyle had changed, maybe you were like millions of your fellow Canadians and simply could never find the time or enthusiasm to get on track with exercise and shedding the extra kilograms you had acquired.

But the wonderful thing is, you are not too late. You are *never* too late. Whether you are 25 or 85, you can still make changes in your lifestyle to enhance your health. And you do not have to feel intimidated by this. The changes do not have to occur overnight. And the changes do not have to be "all or none," because any change is a change for the better.

And we can promise you that the changes you have to make are not quite so intimidating as those recommended by Hippocrates, the renowned physician of ancient times, who said "obese people should perform hard work, eat only once a day, take no baths, and walk naked as much as possible."

This chapter will provide you with the key information you need to follow a healthy lifestyle. We will review the role of "diet" therapy — we prefer to call it nutrition therapy — and how exercise can become a part of your life. And as for walking naked as much as possible, well, if you choose to, remember to at least wear shoes and socks!

Diabetes and Nutrition — A Recipe for Success

Wanda B. Thinner (okay, we admit it; we changed the name), age 46, was recently diagnosed with type 2 diabetes. When the diagnosis was made, her doctor put her on some pills to reduce her blood glucose, but they were not helping and she continued to be bothered by excessive thirst and urination. When she was referred to Alan, she had a blood glucose of 13 mmol/L. She was 165 centimetres (5 feet 5 inches) tall and weighed 75 kilograms (165lb).

Although she had been told by her doctor that she had to lose weight, no further instructions had been given. Alan immediately arranged for her to meet with a registered dietitian — and diabetes educator — and Mrs. Thinner started a lifestyle treatment program that included a meal plan based on the principles in this chapter. She worked hard over the next few months and successfully lost 9 kilograms (20 lb), which she subsequently kept off. Her blood glucose levels came down to the range of 6 to 7 mmol/L and her readings stayed there even after she stopped taking pills. She felt the best she had in years. Mrs. Thinner was yet another prime example of how pills are second-rate diabetes therapy compared to the impact of lifestyle treatment.

One of the single greatest obstacles to effective lifestyle therapy is expecting too much too soon. If you need to lose 23 kilograms (50 lb) and after a month you have lost only 2 kilograms (4 lb) you may start to feel frustrated, as if you are "never going to get there." But we wouldn't suggest for a second that you have not had success. You would have had *great success!* Diabetes is a long-term disease. Achieving your target weight does not have to occur overnight, or even over weeks or months. Slow and steady surely does win the weight-loss race. In fact, if you lose weight too quickly (see later in this chapter) you will be more likely to regain it. Before we talk further about techniques to help you lose weight, it would be a good idea to first look at the fundamental elements that make for a healthy nutrition plan.

Nothing is so likely to frustrate your efforts at following proper nutrition therapy as trying to figure it out without professional help. We would strongly recommend that in addition to reading this chapter, you see a professional dietitian that has expertise in helping people with diabetes. If your doctor has not referred you to one, as soon as you finish reading this chapter, pick up the phone, call your doctor's office, and ask them to book you an appointment. You'll be glad you did.

The key ingredients

Our diets are made up primarily of carbohydrates, proteins, and fats. These basic groups are rounded out by the other things we need to consume to survive, including minerals, vitamins, and, of course, water. And, for most of us, our diets also include some degree of alcohol and, often, non-nutritive sweeteners. Despite what Ian's boys insist, cookie-dough ice cream *does not* constitute a separate and indispensable food group.

The Canadian Diabetes Association (CDA) recommends that people with diabetes follow Canada's Guidelines for Healthy Eating (you can find it online at www.hc-sc.gc.ca):

- ✔ Enjoy a variety of foods.
- ✔ Emphasize cereals, breads and other whole grain products, fruits and vegetables.
- ✔ Choose lower-fat dairy products, leaner meats and food prepared with little or no fat.
- ✔ Achieve and maintain a healthy body weight by enjoying regular physical activity and healthy eating.
- ✔ Limit salt, alcohol and caffeine.

The CDA guidelines also recommend that your diet be divided (based on energy, or calories) as follows:

- ✔ Carbohydrate: 50–55 %
- ✔ Protein: 15–20%
- ✔ Fat: less than 30%

The number of calories contained in 1 gram is

- ✔ Carbohydrate: 4 calories
- ✔ Protein: 4 calories
- ✔ Fat: 9 calories

Of course, you and your dietitian will have to determine the best diet for you based on your particular needs. Your diet will include not only the best food choices for you, but also, the appropriate number of calories you should consume. With unrestricted calories you could limit your carbohydrates to 50 percent of your diet and still have enough energy to power a Boeing 747.

Technically speaking, there is a "calorie" and there is a "Calorie" and there is a kilocalorie (1000 *calories* equals 1 *Calorie* equals 1 *kilo*calorie). However, almost no one speaks of kilocalories in normal, day-to-day discourse, and it's a chore to capitalize the "c" every time, so we use the conventional "calorie" whenever we are talking about nutrition issues. Sure, it is not perfectly scientific to do so, but we won't tell if you won't. (Also, you may come across the term *kilojoules*. One Calorie is equal to about 4.2 kilojoules. Once again, few people use this unit of measure so we will forgo it also.)

Carbohydrates

Carbohydrates do much more than just fuel our bodies. They also fuel debate. Indeed, there is probably no other area of diabetes management that offers quite the same degree of controversy. In this section we will look at the important issues for you to be aware of, including the pros and cons of low versus higher carbohydrate diets.

Although glucose — a carbohydrate made up of one molecule — gets most of the attention, within our bodies we also have other carbohydrates made up of many molecules, including starches, cellulose, and gums (not the chewing type; although, come to think of it, we can think of more than one occasion when chewing gum has made its way into someone's stomach, but we'll chew on that one some other time).

Carbohydrates are found primarily in things grown in the ground and in dairy foods. Some of the common dietary sources of carbohydrate are bread, potatoes, grains, cereals, rice, dairy products, fruits, and sweet vegetables (such as carrots and squash).

A lot is known about the roles that carbohydrates play in the body:

- Carbohydrates are the primary source of energy for muscles.
- Carbohydrates cause the triglyceride (fat) level to rise in the blood.
- Glucose is the carbohydrate that causes the pancreas to release insulin.
- When insulin is not present in sufficient amounts or is ineffective, ingesting carbohydrate raises the blood glucose above normal.
- Simple sugars (as present in sweets) are not directly harmful (except, perhaps to your teeth) as long as your total number of calories ingested is not excessive.

Consuming "sugar" does *not* cause diabetes. Furthermore, do not let any well-meaning friend or relative tell you that because you have diabetes you cannot eat sugar. You can. Tell them Ian and Alan said so. (We'll leave it up to you if you also want to tell them that you recognize that you have to eat appropriate amounts and types of "sugar.")

A few years ago an 85-year-old man was referred to Ian after having been diagnosed a few months earlier with type 2 diabetes. He was a charming gentleman and clearly was working diligently to maintain his traditionally good health. As they spoke, Ian couldn't help but get the impression that something was bothering his new patient. Finally, because the gentleman was not volunteering anything in this way, Ian asked him point-blank if there might be something on his mind. "Well, Doctor," he said, "I guess I'm just feeling kind of sad that I had my birthday yesterday and everyone got to eat my birthday cake except for me. And it was my favourite, too. Chocolate." Whatever reply this gentleman was expecting, it was clearly not the one that Ian supplied. "Well, sir," Ian said, "I have a prescription I want you to fill. Right after you leave this office I want you to go *not* to the drugstore, but to the *bakery*. Buy the biggest chocolate cake they sell and cut yourself as big a slice as you want. And if anyone tells you that you 'can't eat it because you have diabetes,' you tell them that your diabetes specialist *ordered* you to." The patient left the room literally singing.

Cake is not a four-letter word! If you have diabetes you can eat not only cake, but other sweets too. The point is, nothing is "forbidden," it just has to be consumed in moderation and, most importantly, not at the expense of other, healthier foods that you need. So long as your total number of carbohydrates and calories is appropriate, there is nothing wrong with having occasional treats. Happy birthday!

A greater percentage of Canadians are overweight now than at any other time in our history. This is due primarily to two things. We are not as physically active as we once were. And we are consuming, on average, about 200 calories more per day than we did a generation ago. These extra calories are derived almost exclusively from unneeded carbohydrates in "super-size" soft drinks, "extra-large" candy bars, and excessive consumption of breads, pastries, and the like. Within our bodies, these extra carbohydrates are turned into fat and stored in our fat cells. This ability to store extra calories as fat was great when everyone lived in caves and got little food for prolonged periods of time, but it doesn't fit today's lifestyle, consisting as it does of abundant food (and minimal foraging for it — unless you count hunting through the supermarket aisles).

Because carbohydrate is the food that raises the blood glucose — and high glucose is responsible for many of the complications of diabetes — it is important to consume the proper amount of carbohydrates.

If you are on a 2,000-calorie diet and are consuming 50 percent of your calories as carbohydrate, that would work out to 1,000 calories of carbohydrate per day. Each gram of carbohydrate is 4 calories, so you would be consuming 250 grams of carbohydrate per day. Translating this into foods you know and love, this would work out to about 16 slices of bread (15 grams per slice), 9 cups of cereal (28 grams per cup), or 6 cups of rice (42 grams per cup).

Most people with diabetes do very well on this amount of carbohydrate, but for others a lower percentage works best.

Glycemic index

All carbohydrates are not alike in the degree to which they raise the blood glucose. This fact was recognized some years ago, and a measurement called the *glycemic index* was created to quantify it. The glycemic index (GI) uses white bread as the indicator food and assigns it a value of 100. Another carbohydrate of equal calories is rated according to its ability to raise the blood glucose and assigned a value in comparison to white bread. A food that raises glucose half as much as white bread has a GI of 50, while a food that raises glucose $1^1/_2$ times as much has a GI of 150. The point of the index is to select carbohydrates with low GI levels to try to keep the glucose response as low as possible.

Like most things in life, the GI has its supporters and its detractors. Its supporters point out that relying on foods with a low glycemic index has these advantages:

- ✔ May help improve blood glucose control.
- ✔ May help improve lipids. (There is often a reduction in levels of triglycerides and LDL cholesterol.)

On the other side of the food fence, GI detractors point out these problems:

- ✔ The GI of a carbohydrate may be different when it is eaten alone than when it is part of a mixed meal.
- ✔ The GI of a food may differ depending on how it's processed and prepared.
- ✔ Some low-GI foods contain a lot of fat.
- ✔ Figuring out the GI can be difficult and can lead to confusion.
- ✔ Research has not yet proven long-term health benefits of a low-GI diet.

We can think of no better illustration of the controversy regarding the glycemic index than the point that Alan is a supporter and Ian is not yet convinced. Alan would note that he has observed improved glucose control in his patients that follow a low-GI and Ian would point out that a Snickers candy bar rates better on the GI than does a bowl of cornflakes. (We are not making this up!) Is it possible that some people might mistakenly believe this means that candy bars are a healthy food choice? What a disastrous error that would be!

The Canadian Diabetes Association, quite appropriately, feels that the decision to implement a low-glycemic-index diet should be individualized based on a person's particular interest and ability.

Seeing as we do not yet have proof that a low-glycemic-index diet is the way to go, the most prudent course would be to initiate your nutrition therapy with the standard Canadian Diabetes Association guidelines, as you will learn from your dietitian. If you have been working with this meal plan and not succeeding the way you should, speak to your dietitian and your family doctor (and diabetes specialist if you are seeing one) to see if they feel you would benefit by switching to a low-GI diet.

Should you elect to proceed with a low-glycemic-index diet, you can easily make some simple substitutions in your diet, as shown in Table 10-1.

Table 10-1	Simple Diet Substitutions for a Low-GI Diet
High-GI Food	*Low-GI Food*
Whole meal or white bread	Whole grain bread
Processed breakfast cereal	Unrefined cereals like oats or processed low-GI cereals
Plain cookies and crackers	Cookies made with dried fruits or whole grains like oats
Cakes and muffins	Cakes and muffins made with fruit, oats, and whole grains
Tropical fruits like bananas	Temperate climate fruits like apples and plums
Potatoes	Pasta or legumes
Rice	Basmati or other low-GI rice

Bread and breakfast cereal are major daily sources of carbohydrates, so these simple changes can make a major difference in lowering your glycemic index. Foods that are excellent sources of carbohydrate but have a low GI include legumes such as peas or beans, pasta, grains like barley, parboiled rice, and whole grain breads.

The CDA Web site (www.diabetes.ca) lists additional foods based on their GI in a document entitled Glycemic Index Resource.

Carbohydrate Counting

Glucose levels rise after you eat mainly because of the carbohydrates in your meal (or snack). Also, in general, the greater the number of grams of carbohydrate, the more your blood glucose level will rise. People who are on an intensified insulin program consisting of frequent injections of short-acting insulin can gauge the amount of insulin to inject based on the number of grams of carbohydrate they are about to ingest. (We discuss this further in Chapter 12.)

Fibre

Fibre is the part of the carbohydrate that is not digestable and therefore adds no calories. It is found in most fruits, grains, and vegetables. Fibre comes in two forms:

- ✔ **Soluble fibre:** This form of fibre can dissolve in water and has a lowering effect on blood glucose and fat levels, particularly cholesterol. Soluble fibre gets gooey and sticky when mixed with water. An example is oatmeal.

- ✔ **Insoluble fibre:** This form of fibre cannot dissolve in water and remains in the intestine. It absorbs water and stimulates movement in the intestine. Insoluble fibre also helps prevent constipation and possibly colon cancer. This is the fibre called bulk or roughage. Insoluble fibre does not change much when mixed with water. An example is the skin of an apple.

Before the current trend to refine foods, people ate many sources of carbohydrate that were high in fibre. These were all in plant foods, such as fruits, vegetables, and grains. Animal foods contain no fibre.

The Canadian Diabetes Association recommends you ingest 25 to 35 grams of fibre daily. Because too much fibre causes diarrhea and gas, you need to increase the fibre level in your diet fairly slowly.

Protein

Unless you are a vegetarian, most of the protein in your diet is derived from the muscle of other animals, such as chicken, turkey, beef, or lamb. The main role that protein has in your diet is to maintain the health of tissues such as your muscles. As it turns out, you do not need to consume much protein in your diet to maintain your current level of muscle. Unlike carbohydrates, proteins do not raise blood glucose levels significantly.

Why proteins do not raise blood glucose

When the protein you ingest passes through the stomach and enters the small intestine, it is broken down into smaller molecules called amino acids. The amino acids are absorbed into the bloodstream and head for the liver, where *some* are converted into glucose (others are used to build new protein). So, although dietary protein can raise glucose, this takes place slowly and is not a major contributor to blood glucose.

Your choice of protein is very important because some protein sources also contain very high quantities of fat while others are relatively fat free. The following lists give you an idea of the fat content of various sources of protein.

About 30 grams (1 oz) of **very lean** meat, fish, or substitutes has 7 grams of protein and 1 gram of fat. Examples are:

- Skinless white-meat chicken or turkey
- Flounder, halibut, or tuna canned in water
- Lobster, shrimp, or clams
- Fat-free cheese

About 30 grams (1 oz) of **lean** meat, fish, or substitutes has 7 grams of protein and 3 grams of fat. Examples are:

- Lean beef, lean pork, lamb, or veal
- Dark-meat chicken without skin or white-meat chicken with skin
- Sardines, salmon, or tuna canned in oil
- Other meats or cheeses with 3 grams of fat per 30 grams (1 oz)

About 30 grams (1 oz) of **medium-fat** meat, fish, or substitutes has 7 grams of protein and 5 grams of fat. Examples are:

- Most beef products
- Regular fat pork, lamb, or veal
- Dark-meat chicken with skin or fried chicken
- Fried fish
- Cheeses with 5 grams of fat per 30 grams (1 oz) such as feta and mozzarella

About 30 grams (1 oz) of **high-fat** meat, fish, or substitutes contains 7 grams of protein and 8 grams of fat. Examples are:

- Pork spareribs or pork sausage
- Bacon
- Regular cheeses such as cheddar and Monterey Jack
- Processed sandwich meats

Depending on whether you choose a high- or low-fat-containing protein source there can be a huge difference in the number of calories. For instance, 30 grams (1 oz) of skinless white meat chicken contains about 40 calories whereas 30 grams (1 oz) of pork spareribs has 100 calories. Because most people eat a minimum of about 120 grams (about 4 ozs) of meat at a meal, they're eating from 160 to 400 calories depending upon the source. That is why it is so important to look carefully at the food you are about to eat; the company your protein source keeps can make the difference between you successfully losing weight or not.

If you are on a 2,000-calorie diet with 20 percent being protein, that would call for 400 calories from protein sources. Because a gram of protein is 4 calories, you could eat 100 grams of protein.

Fat

When we think of fat, we tend to think of the fat we see on a steak or in hamburger meat. But there are actually quite a variety of fats and fat-like substances. Although many of these are unhealthy and to be avoided, some, in fact, help to protect our health. This section looks at these different issues.

Cholesterol is the fat-like substance everyone knows. It has been shown to be a major contributor leading to atherosclerosis (such as coronary artery disease, as we discuss in Chapter 6). It is recommended that no more than 300 milligrams a day of fat come from cholesterol. (One large egg has about 210 mg of cholesterol.) Other sources of cholesterol include whole milk and hard cheeses such as Monterey Jack and cheddar.

Most people do not realize the extent to which our bodies (our livers in particular) contribute to our cholesterol levels. In fact, the majority of our body's cholesterol is made by our livers. It is for that reason that so many people with diabetes, even if faithfully following a low-fat diet, end up requiring medication anyhow in order to achieve optimal blood cholesterol levels.

The other kind of fat is triglyceride, which we classify into two groups:

- **Saturated fat** is the kind of fat that comes from animal sources. The streaks of fat in a steak are saturated fat. Butter, bacon, cream, and cream cheese are other examples of foods rich in saturated fat. Eating a lot of saturated fat can make your bad (LDL) cholesterol level go up. And that is not a good thing.

- **Unsaturated fat** comes from vegetable sources such as olive oil, canola oil, and margarine. It comes in several forms:

  - **Monounsaturated fat** does not raise cholesterol. Avocado, olive oil, and canola oil are examples. The oil in nuts such as almonds and peanuts is also monounsaturated.

  - **Polyunsaturated fat** does not raise cholesterol but can lead to a reduction in HDL cholesterol (this is the "good" cholesterol that we discuss in Chapter 6). Examples of polyunsaturated fats are soft fats and oils such as corn oil, mayonnaise, and margarine. Polyunsaturated fats should be less than 10 percent of your total calorie intake.

You may have read recently about "trans" fatty acids. Trans fatty acids also raise LDL levels. They are formed when vegetable oil goes through a process of hydrogenation during the manufacture of many commercially baked goods such as cookies, cakes, potato chips, and some types of margarines.

Saturated and trans fatty acids combined should be restricted to less than 10 percent of your calorie intake.

Lest you think that everything with the word *fat* in it is bad, here is some good news about fat. Some fats are actually good for you. There is mounting evidence that a fat called *omega-3 fatty acids* can help protect you from atherosclerosis. These acids are found in certain fish such as salmon, tuna, mackerel, and trout. Omega-3 fatty acids also help reduce blood pressure and protect against the formation of blood clots in the coronary arteries (thus reducing the likelihood of your getting a heart attack). It is recommended that you eat fish rich in omega-3 fatty acids at least once (better still, two or three times) per week. If you don't like fish, we can't help but think that it must mean you have never tasted salmon cooked on a barbecue or in a dishwasher. (True story: Ian's mom makes marvellous "dishwasher salmon," and no, the fish does not swim around in the water; it is wrapped in tinfoil and put through the entire wash and dry cycle—without soap! Readers can find a variety of dishwasher salmon recipes on the Internet.)

If we go back to your hypothetical 2,000-calorie diet — lest you slowly starve while waiting for us to figure out how much fat to feed you so that you get your final 600 calories — fat has 9 calories per gram, so you can eat about 67 grams of fat daily. Seeing as you may have consumed much of this with your protein source, you may not have much fat left to add.

Vitamins, minerals, and water

Your nutrition plan must contain sufficient vitamins and minerals, but the amount you need may be less than you think. If you eat a balanced diet that comes from the various food groups, you will generally get enough vitamins for your daily needs. Table 10-2 lists the vitamins and their food sources.

Table 10-2	Vitamins You Need	
Vitamin	*Function*	*Food Source*
Vitamin A	Needed for healthy skin and bones	Milk and green vegetables
Vitamin B1 (thiamine)	Converts carbohydrates into energy	Meat and whole grain cereals

Vitamin	Function	Food Source
Vitamin B2 (riboflavin)	Needed to use food properly	Milk, cheese, fish, and green vegetables
Vitamin B6 (pyridoxine)	Needed for growth	Liver, yeast, and many other foods
Vitamin B12	Keeps the red blood cells and the nervous system healthy	Animal foods (for example, meat)
Folic acid (also called folate)	Keeps the red blood cells healthy	Green vegetables
Niacin	Helps maintain healthy metabolism	Lean meat, fish, nuts, and legumes
Vitamin C	Helps maintain supportive tissues	Fruit and potatoes
Vitamin D	Helps with absorption of calcium	Dairy products and is made in the skin when exposed to sunlight
Vitamin E	Helps maintain cells	Vegetable oils and whole grain cereals
Vitamin K	Needed for proper clotting of the blood	Green, leafy vegetables

As you look through the vitamins in Table 10-2, you can see that most of them are readily available in the foods you eat every day. In certain situations, such as if you are pregnant or breastfeeding, elderly, a strict vegetarian, or on a very low calorie diet, you should take a multivitamin daily. (In pregnancy you should also take a folic acid supplement. We discuss vitamin therapy and pregnancy in Chapter 7.)

Although Canadians spend millions upon millions of dollars each year on vitamin supplements, these supplements are seldom helpful (except for the people selling them!). Our clever bodies are quite adept at knowing when we have enough vitamins in our system, and when you take in extra quantities you either store them in your fat or you have very expensive urine. By way of example, recent medical studies showed that taking extra vitamin E provided no additional health value. Yet until those studies were published, tens of millions of dollars (perhaps hundreds of millions) was being spent each year in North America on vitamin E supplements. We would strongly recommend that if you have good nutrition (and thereby will get all the vitamins you need), you take the money you might be spending on vitamin supplements and donate it to your favourite charity.

Not only are routine vitamin supplements not necessary, but a recent study found that Vitamin E supplements may actually be harmful (the study found a higher risk of heart failure in people taking Vitamin E supplements). "Megadoses" of certain vitamins are a particular concern. For example, high doses of vitamin A can lead to liver damage and too much Vitamin D can cause vomiting and muscle weakness.

Minerals are also key ingredients of a healthy diet. Most are needed in tiny amounts, easily consumed from a balanced diet. These are the main minerals you should know:

- ✔ **Calcium:** We need calcium primarily to maintain strong bones. Insufficient calcium intake can be a factor in developing osteoporosis. Milk and other dairy products provide plenty of calcium. It is important to ingest between 1,000 and 1,500 milligrams of calcium per day. If you are not consuming enough calcium in your diet, you should take calcium supplements. If you are growing up (adolescents) or out (pregnant women) this also applies.

  Before you start taking calcium supplements it is important to check with your physician to make sure you are not taking any other medicine or do not have any other health problem that could lead to abnormally high blood calcium levels.

- ✔ **Chromium:** We require chromium for certain internal chemical reactions to take place normally. In areas of the world where there is a severe deficiency of chromium in the diet, people are more likely to develop diabetes. Regrettably, people in areas of the world where we get perfectly adequate quantities of chromium in our diets (this includes Canada) have been inundated with pseudo-scientific and misleading claims that taking chromium supplements will either reduce your blood glucose levels or cure your diabetes. We have no convincing evidence of the former and as for the latter, it is simply false. Once again, the only people benefitting from this promotion are the people selling the products.

- ✔ **Iodine:** Iodine is necessary for our thyroid glands to work normally. You may have noticed that boxes of salt in Canada are labelled "Iodized." Because of this iodine supplementation, Canadians do not develop iodine deficiency (even if you never add salt to your food).

- ✔ **Iron:** We require iron to make red blood cells. A lack of iron leads to anemia. Most of our iron intake comes from consumption of red meat. Menstruating women are prone to iron deficiency (menstrual blood is rich in iron) and often will require iron supplementation. Vegetarians also often require iron supplements.

- ✔ **Magnesium:** Our bodies use magnesium to allow a number of different chemical reactions to occur. Magnesium deficiency can lead to problems with the heart's electrical system. Magnesium deficiency is very seldom a problem and routine supplements are unnecessary.

✓ **Phosphorous:** Phosphorous in our bodies contributes to the maintenance of strong bones. We get ample phosphorous in our diets and routine supplements are not required.

✓ **Sodium:** Getting sufficient quantities of sodium ("salt") in Canadian diets is not a problem. Quite the opposite. We uniformly consume excess quantities. Sodium is present in many of the foods we eat — particularly in processed foods such as prepared meats and some cheeses, as well as packaged snack foods such as pretzels and potato chips. You may be surprised to know that Canadians consume an astounding 20 times more sodium per day than we need. This may be a factor leading to high blood pressure. You would be wise to avoid adding salt to your food, and if you have high blood pressure, make a point of buying foods that are low in salt to begin with.

✓ **Cobalt, Tin, and Zinc:** These minerals are rarely lacking in the human diet and supplements are unnecessary.

Although we have saved our discussion about water to last, it is by no means the least important. Your body is made up of 60 percent or more water. All the nutrients in the body are dissolved in water. You can live without food for some time, but you will not last long without water. Water can help to give a feeling of fullness that reduces appetite. You should make a point of drinking at least 1¹/₂ litres (50 oz) of water per day.

A whole industry has developed based on the assumption that tap water is not as healthy for you as bottled water. There is, in fact, a *huge* difference between tap water and bottled water. Last time we checked, this difference was a penny or two compared to about a dollar. If you want to drink bottled water because you prefer the taste, go for it. If you are drinking bottled water because you think it is healthier, we would suggest that you take the dollar a day you plan on spending and put it toward purchasing some new running shoes that you will be using after you read the section on exercise later in this chapter.

Artificial and sugar alcohol sweeteners

Unrestricted consumption of sugars does not fit with good diabetes management (or, of course, with good health in general). And since there are limits on how much sugar we should consume, artificial sweeteners have a role to play. Of the artificial sweeteners in common use, aspartame (NutraSweet) is the best known. In the amounts commonly used, aspartame provides virtually no calories, yet provides abundant sweetness. In fact, aspartame is 200 times sweeter than sucrose (table sugar). Aspartame has been the subject of many Internet rumours detailing its dangers. These are false. The truth of the matter is that aspartame is completely safe unless you have a rare genetic disease called PKU. The equal truth is that despite common use of aspartame in our society, we as a population are getting larger and larger, not smaller and smaller.

Other approved artificial sweeteners in Canada are saccharin (Sweet'n Low), cyclamate (sucaryl; this is the sweetener used in Sugar Twin), sucralose (Splenda), and acesuflame potassium (Sunett). These are safe for use if you have diabetes — unless you are pregnant or breastfeeding, in which case you should not consume saccharin or cyclamate.

Sugar alcohols (maltitol, mannitol, sorbitol, isomalt, and xylitol) are another type of sweetener. They are not artificial. They do provide calories and can affect your blood glucose levels to a degree. Examples of products that may contain sugar alcohols are chewing gum, hard candies, some jams, and syrups. Consumption of more than 10 grams per day of sugar alcohols can cause abdominal cramping and diarrhea.

Alcohol

Alcohol is a substance that has calories but no particular nutritional value. It has, however, been shown that a moderate amount (a drink or two per day) may reduce your risk of a heart attack.

If you like to have a drink, it is reasonable that you continue so long as you limit yourself to no more than two drinks per day if you are a man, and one drink per day if you are a woman. If you do not normally drink, do not start just because you are at possible risk of developing heart disease down the road. And, of course, if you are pregnant, you should not drink any alcohol at all.

Having two drinks per day is *not* the same as quaffing 14 cold ones on a Saturday evening while you watch *Hockey Night in Canada*. Even if the game goes into overtime.

Because alcohol has calories, you must account for the alcohol you drink in your diet. Depending on the strength of the individual product, 350 millilitres (12 oz) of beer, 150 millilitres (5 oz) of wine, and 45 millilitres (1$\frac{1}{2}$ oz) of hard liquor all have similar quantities of alcohol.

Despite what many people think, drinking beer or wine is not "better for you" than drinking hard liquor. To your liver they all taste the same.

Apart from the consequences of the calories it provides, there are several other important points about alcohol to keep in mind:

  ✔ Alcohol — especially if taken without food — can cause low blood glucose if you are on insulin or some forms of oral hypoglycemic agent therapy (see Chapter 11). It does this by reducing your liver's ability to produce glucose. You can lessen this risk by making sure you eat some food when you are drinking alcohol.

✔ Alcohol reduces your awareness of symptoms of low blood glucose (see Chapter 5) and as a result, makes you less likely to take appropriate corrective action.

✔ Alcohol can interact with some medicines called sulfonylurea oral hypoglycemic agents (see Chapter 11) and cause a variety of unpleasant symptoms including nausea and flushing (even if you are not inebriated).

✔ If you are on insulin (see Chapter 12) or certain medicines that stimulate insulin production (see Chapter 11), drinking alcohol 2 or 3 hours after your supper can result in hypoglycemia occurring the next morning after breakfast.

The Atkins Diet

There is seldom a shortage of controversy over diets, especially when it comes to the diet recommended by the late Dr. Robert Atkins.

The Atkins diet recommends the consumption of very small amounts of carbohydrate and substantial quantities of protein and fat.

The main potential advantages of this diet:

✔ Many people find it allows them to lose weight when other diets have not.

✔ Blood glucose control often improves.

The main potential disadvantages of this diet:

✔ The weight that is lost is often regained.

✔ People commonly develop hair loss.

✔ Most people do not adhere to this diet for very long (as is the case with all diets that are very restrictive, people tire of them).

✔ Many healthy foods are potentially eliminated from the diet.

✔ There is some evidence that a high-protein diet can lead to worrisome problems including calcium loss from the bones (which could potentially lead to osteoporosis), kidney stones, an increase in LDL ("bad") cholesterol, dizziness, and, though not dangerous, problematic constipation and fatigue.

Research has also found that the weight loss that occurs with the Atkins diet is due primarily to lower calorie intake; the fact that fewer carbohydrates are ingested is of less importance.

Suffice to say, there are advocates, fans, and even zealots on both sides of the Atkins fence. Although the jury is out, history shows that diets that advocate an extreme diet management approach have invariably failed because people get tired of the severe restrictions they contain and eventually abandon them. How else to explain the fact that many (perhaps most by now) homes in Canada have so many different diet books, each book having its own particular bent and often saying things opposite to the book sitting next to it on the bookshelf?

Weighty Issues

In Chapter 4 we discuss the various ways you can determine whether you are overweight. If you are, then you are in good company. Millions of Canadians are also overweight, as are the great majority of people with type 2 diabetes. But (we love being able to add a "but" here) we are now going to work our hardest at improving your health, and one of the most important steps is to, well, take steps.

As it turns out, you will soon see the benefits of weight loss, even when you have lost relatively little weight. Blood glucose falls rapidly. Blood pressure declines. Bad (LDL) cholesterol falls as do fats (triglycerides), and good cholesterol (HDL) rises. How neat is that! We suspect that if we were to market a drug that had all these attributes it would be considered a "wonder drug."

You should aim to lose 1 to 2 kilograms (2 to 4 lbs) per month, 5 to 10 percent of your initial body weight over 6 months. Losing weight faster than that increases the likelihood that you will regain it. You should try to burn off 500 calories more per day than you ingest. (To calculate what this requires, have a look at the calorie content of carbohydrates, proteins, and fats earlier in this chapter.) Although you will need to reduce your intake of carbohydrate, you should make sure you consume at least 100 grams of carbohydrate per day. Ingesting less than that will lead to loss of muscle tissue and can affect your fluid balance. Also, if you eat lots of high-fibre foods you will find that you won't feel as hungry.

At the risk of sounding like a late-night TV commercial, when it comes to the benefits of weight loss, "you get all this and more." More? Yes, more. Weight loss will also accomplish the following:

✔ Allow blood pressure and oral hypoglycemic agent medications (see Chapter 11) to work more effectively

✔ Improve your sense of well-being

✔ Make you feel more energetic and more inclined to exercise

✔ Increase your life expectancy

Weight reduction is difficult for many reasons, but perhaps foremost among these is the immense challenge of trying to change lifestyle patterns and habits that you may have lived with for decades. No one should ever tell you that the changes you are being asked to make are easy. They are not easy. In fact, for most people they are downright difficult. But they can be done. And if you have initial success only to then revert back to old habits, that does not mean all is lost. Just pick up where you left off and try again.

Half a kilogram (about a pound) of fat contains 3,500 calories. Therefore, in order to lose this much fat, you must eat 3,500 calories less than you need or you must burn off these calories by exercising. Often the best strategy is to combine reduced calorie intake with increased calorie expenditure. So grab your walking shoes and bypass the fridge as you head for the door for your new, daily walk.

Medication therapy for losing weight

In the event that your best efforts at lifestyle change have not produced a significant fall in your weight, you may be a candidate for medication therapy. Two drugs are available in Canada to assist with weight loss, neither of which tend to be all that successful, but some people do benefit.

- ✔ **Xenical** (orlistat) is taken three times daily with your meals. It works by blocking ingested fat from being absorbed into your blood stream from the small intestine. Unfortunately, most people lose only small amounts of weight while taking this medicine and, significantly, many people run into problems with oily deposits escaping from their rectum and soiling their underclothes. Ugh! We don't want to sound overly negative, however, since some people do benefit nicely and recent evidence also suggests that Xenical can help reduce blood glucose levels.

- ✔ **Meridia** (Sibutramine) assists with weight loss by acting directly on the hunger centre in the brain. Like Xenical, its benefits are generally fairly marginal and it can have significant side effects, including making your blood pressure go up.

Medicines to assist with weight loss do not, of course, replace or substitute for ongoing dietary change and exercise.

Surgery for weight loss

Surgery is sometimes used in the most severe and resistant cases of obesity (BMI 35 or greater; see the chart in Chapter 4). For select individuals it can be a very effective form of therapy, with multiple health benefits including improved glucose control.

The most effective surgical treatment for obesity is the Roux-en-Y gastric bypass operation, where the stomach is stapled to create a small pouch. A section of the small intestine is attached to the pouch so that food passes through very little of the small intestine, reducing calorie and nutrient absorption. Because the pouch is small, you tend to eat less.

As you might imagine, surgery — any surgery — is not to be undertaken lightly. (There is an old expression that "minor surgery" is surgery that someone else has.) Potential drawbacks include direct complications from the procedure (wound breakdown, infection, and so on) and more remote complications (including deficiency of certain vitamins and minerals due to inadequate absorption, anemia, diarrhea, and hypoglycemia).

Behaviour modification

We've already talked about the importance of lifestyle change to help reduce your weight and enhance your health. And we've also already mentioned just how difficult changing longstanding eaten patterns can be. Here are some tips you may find helpful in your quest to adjust your eating habits:

- Eat at set times.
- Eat your food in a single place.
- Slow down your eating.
- Put your cutlery down between mouthfuls.
- Don't put more food in your mouth before you have finished your last bite.
- Concentrate on the taste of each mouthful before you swallow.
- Every few minutes, pause and ask yourself if you are still hungry.
- Don't finish every morsel on your plate. There is nothing wrong with leaving some behind.
- After the food has been served, remove the serving dishes and bread basket from the table.
- Don't keep high-calorie snacks visible in the kitchen or elsewhere in the house. Better yet, don't keep them in the house at all.
- Remember that seemingly innocent things like salad dressings can be very rich in calories.
- Add bulk to your food (adding vegetable to pasta for example). Hunger is often satisfied by increasing the volume of food even if the number of calories is reduced.
- Avoid "impulse buying" when doing your groceries. Bring a shopping list and walk the aisles specifically looking for the items you have written down rather than just wandering from aisle to aisle.
- Get a 5-kilogram weight and carry it around for a while to appreciate the importance of a loss of even that little.
- Incorporate regular exercise into your weight-loss strategy.
- Most important of all, remember that there is no rush. As we say earlier, trying to lose weight too rapidly will make it more likely that you will regain the weight later.

As you go about the difficult task of losing weight and keeping it off, remember to seek the help of those around you. A loving partner provides great help through the roughest days.

Diabetes and Exercise

Decades ago it was thought there were three main components to diabetes therapy:

- ✔ Proper diet
- ✔ Sufficient exercise
- ✔ Appropriate medication

Now, in the next century, guess what? There are three main components to diabetes therapy. (Bet you know what they are). *Plus ça change* . . .

Oh, do I really have to?

We are tempted to make this the shortest section in the book and simply write "yes." But we won't because we know that you are — appropriately, we might add — more likely to follow our advice if you understand the reasoning behind it.

Exercise benefits you in the following ways (whether or not you have diabetes):

- ✔ Improves blood pressure
- ✔ Improves lipids
- ✔ Helps with weight control
- ✔ Reduces risk of death due to heart attacks
- ✔ Improves your energy level and creates a better sense of well-being

If you have type 2 diabetes, exercise supplies additional benefits, including:

- ✔ Improved glucose control because exercise reduces insulin resistance. (This effect can last as long as 18 hours or more after you have completed a single bout of exercising. See the Tip following this list.) We discuss insulin resistance in Chapter 3.

- ✔ Reduced need for medicines to lower your blood glucose. (If you need them anyhow, exercise will allow them to work much more effectively.)

If we haven't convinced you yet, how about this: Studies have shown that if you have diabetes and you exercise regularly, you can reduce your risk of dying in the next 10 years or so by over 50 percent! So, do you need to exercise? Well, only as much as you need to breathe. Literally.

 Because exercise can reduce insulin resistance for many hours after the exercise has been completed – and hence, cause delayed hypoglycemia – it would be a good idea to do more frequent blood glucose testing for the first week or so after you've taken up a new exercise program. See the sections on exercising while taking OHA and insulin toward the end of this chapter.

 Of course, the social benefits of exercise are very important too. You can spend time with people who are also concerned with health. These people usually share many of your interests. The person who likes to jog often likes to hike and climb. And more than one lifetime partnership began on a tennis court.

Precautions to take before you start exercising

 Prior to beginning a new exercise program, check with your family doctor (who may recommend — depending on the nature of the exercise you are about to do and other factors listed below — that you visit with other members of your team, including your diabetes specialist, educator, dietitian, and eye doctor). Although exercise is essential, you must initiate it with caution.

 If you have type 1 diabetes and your fasting blood glucose is higher than 15 mmol/L with ketones present, you should not exercise. It could cause you to develop worsening hyperglycemia and ketone production. Once your metabolic control is back in order, grab your running shoes and head for the door!

Consider these factors before you start exercising:

- ✔ **Whether or not you have heart disease.** Before you start exercising, your doctor may choose to send you for an exercise stress test (this is a test where your heart is monitored while you walk on a treadmill) to look for evidence of coronary artery disease (see Chapter 6) — even if you have no heart symptoms.

- ✔ **Whether or not you have high blood pressure.** Although exercise is good treatment for hypertension, it can be dangerous if you have severely elevated blood pressure.

✔ **The state of your blood glucose control.** Exercise is terrific therapy for elevated glucose levels, but it can be dangerous if you have severe hyperglycemia, in which case your blood glucose levels will have to be reduced to a safer level — generally under 15 or so — before you start an exercise program.

✔ **The state of your eyes.** Some forms of exercise can aggravate retinopathy (see Chapter 6). If you have not been to your eye doctor within the past year, you should have your eyes checked before you undertake any form of vigorous exercise or weightlifting.

✔ **Whether or not you have peripheral neuropathy.** You can still exercise if you have peripheral neuropathy, but it would be wise for you to read the section (in Chapter 6) on foot care and footwear first.

✔ **Physical limitations.** Things such as obesity, arthritis, peripheral vascular disease (see Chapter 6), and amputations may influence the nature of the exercise you undertake.

✔ **The medications you may be on.** Your doctor may need to adjust drugs such as oral hypoglycemic agents or insulin if you are going to be exercising.

How exercise works its magic

As you exercise and your muscles start to work, they require additional fuel. At first, glycogen, the storage form of glucose in the liver, begins to break down and release glucose which provides a source of energy to your muscles. With continued exercise, glycogen is used up, and the liver begins to make glucose from other substances in order to continue to provide energy.

With steady, moderate exercise, the body eventually turns to burning fat as the glucose production begins to diminish. This is a wonderful situation, especially because most people with type 2 diabetes have extra fat to offer.

If the exercise is very vigorous (or if you do not have sufficient insulin), the liver actually makes more glucose than the muscles can use immediately, and the blood glucose begins to rise. This explains some of the instances where the glucose is higher after exercise than it is before exercise. Vigorous exercise will not be continued for very long, and the extra glucose will be there to replenish the muscle tissue, once exercise ends.

The Hockey Heart Study

Where else but in Canada could a medical study come out by the name of the Hockey Heart Study? This study (published in 2002 in the *Canadian Medical Association Journal*; www.cmaj.ca/cgi/content/full/166/3/303) showed that a significant percentage of men playing recreational hockey had possible heart troubles develop while playing. The players wore portable electrocardiogram-type (EKG) devices that recorded their heartbeats during their games. When the recordings were analyzed afterward, there were quite a few abnormalities that showed up suggesting that the players may have been experiencing heart problems — such as impaired circulation to the heart — even though they had not had any symptoms. The full significance of these findings is not known, but it certainly suggests that the typical Canadian pastime of being sedentary for days, weeks (or months) on end and then going out for an hour of sprints up and down the ice may not be the best thing in the world to do.

Here are some other things to consider as you embark on your life-enhancing (and possibly life-saving) exercise program:

- Obtain (and wear!) a medical alert bracelet or necklace. This is important primarily if you are on medications that can cause hypoglycemia.
- Determine (with your educator) whether you will need to do more frequent blood glucose monitoring.
- Obtain (and wear) proper socks and shoes.
- Ensure that you consume sufficient water when you exercise.
- Bring treatment for low blood glucose if you are on medication that can bring this on.
- Arrange to have a companion join you when you exercise. It's not just the tango that is easier with two.

Finding the right type of exercise

People routinely ask us what "the best" exercise is. Whenever Ian is asked this, he recalls the time he asked the bicycle store owner what the best helmet was for his son. Her wise answer: "The one he will actually wear." So, too, with exercise. The type of exercise you do is far less important than simply finding one that you enjoy and will stick with.

We can classify exercise into two broad types: aerobic and resistance. During *aerobic* exercise your muscles use oxygen (such as when you walk). Your heart pumps faster to keep up with your muscles' demands. When we talk about cardiovascular conditioning we are referring to the benefits on the heart and circulation of aerobic exercise. *Resistance* exercise uses muscular strength to move a weight or to work against, well, a resistance. Examples of this would be weightlifting or exercising with weight machines. Resistance training will improve your muscular fitness and energy level and can also increase your metabolic rate.

Because the benefits of aerobic and resistance exercise are complementary, you should do both types.

Again, the most important thing in choosing an exercise is that you like it enough to carry on with it. Another factor that may influence your decision is the number of calories an exercise burns. Table 10-3 supplies this information.

Table 10-3	Exercise and the Amount of Calories You Burn in 20 Minutes at Different Body Weights	
Activity	*Calories Burned (57 kg/125 lb)*	*Calories Burned (80 kg/175 lb)*
Standing	24	32
Walking, 6.5 kph/4 mph	104	144
Running, 11 kph/7 mph	236	328
Gardening	60	84
Writing	30	42
Typing	38	54
Carpentry	64	88
House painting	58	80
Baseball	78	108
Dancing	70	96
Football	138	192
Golfing	66	96
Swimming	80	112
Skiing, downhill	160	224
Skiing, cross-country	196	276
Tennis	112	160

Everything you do burns calories. Even sleeping uses 20 calories in 20 minutes if you weigh 57 kilograms (125 lb).

When Rajeev, a 35-year-old dentist, found out that he had diabetes he decided to start exercising. Since his best friend golfed, he thought he would try that too. A couple of months later, despite playing golf several times per week, his glucose control and his weight had not shown much improvement. As it turned out, he had joined one of the few golf courses in Canada that require you to use a cart. He switched clubs (so to speak) and was soon walking up and down the fairways, burning calories with each and every step. Only 4 percent of golf courses in Canada have rules making cart use mandatory. That leaves you with 96 percent of courses in Canada to choose from. So the next time you are on the links, make sure the only driving you are doing is with your clubs. Fore!

You do *not* have to go out and spend a whole bunch of money on exercise machines, fitness clubs, and the like (though of course you are welcome to). We wish we had a dollar for every treadmill that now functions as a full-time clotheshorse or dust collector. Some comfortable clothes and shoes are all you need to begin your exercise program.

Virtually everyone can exercise. If you have a limitation that makes it difficult to do some types of exercise such as walking, try a different one such as swimming.

If we still haven't convinced you that you can start exercising regularly, we would suggest you consider joining a community centre or YMCA/YWCA where they have exercise programs. These are usually run by excellent fitness leaders who will be sensitive to your needs and can fit you into a class that is suitable for you. These facilities are often far less threatening (and far less expensive) than large, commercial fitness establishments.

The Diabetes Exercise & Sports Association (www.diabetes-exercise.org) is an organization dedicated to "enhancing the quality of life for people with diabetes through exercise and physical fitness." They have members who are exercise neophytes and they have world-class athletes within their ranks. Have a look at their site.

How to start exercising

Perhaps you have heard the famous Chinese proverb "A journey of a thousand miles begins with a single step." Proverbs are proverbs for a reason.

In our experience, there are two main obstacles to taking up exercise:

- ✔ Feeling overwhelmed by the task
- ✔ Inertia

Well, neither of these obstacles is insurmountable. We can assure you — in fact, we can guarantee you — it does not have to be too big a task. Set your sights low. Very low. Very, very, low. Get the point? If you never exercise, start your new program by simply walking to the end of your block and back. After a few days, circle the block. A few days later walk several blocks. Every week try to cover a slightly greater distance, and when you have succeeded with that, increase your pace. Once you have gotten into a routine, you will find that your inertia is a thing of the past.

A good rule of thumb is to increase your daily exercise by 5 minutes every week. Using this approach, you will be up to half an hour of daily exercise within a month and a half. Not too shabby.

If you think you may want to start getting out for a regular walk, but need something else to motivate you, consider buying a dog. Dogs love going for walks. And, just like you, they also need to exercise. Not sure you want the responsibility? Offer to take the neighbour's dog for a daily walk. Both your neighbour and their dog will be thrilled.

How much exercise is the right amount?

The Canadian Diabetes Association recommends that people with type 2 diabetes perform at least 150 minutes of moderate-intensity aerobic exercise each week, spread out over at least 3 non-consecutive days of the week. That is not to say that you have to rest on your well-deserved laurels if you have accomplished this. Indeed, the CDA encourages you to do at least 4 hours of weekly exercise. (In other words, about four times as much as your doctor is probably doing! Please don't tell your doctor we said that. We were just kidding; really.)

Examples of moderate exercise include the following:

- ✔ Brisk walking
- ✔ Biking
- ✔ Raking leaves
- ✔ Continuous swimming
- ✔ Dancing
- ✔ Water aerobics

Do you eat your entire week's calories in one meal? Do you do your entire week's breathing with one deep breath? No? Then remember, you should not try to do your entire week's exercise in one session either. It's simply not as effective if you do it that way.

There are several ways for you to determine if you are pushing yourself to the right extent:

- **The Talk Test:** You should be able to talk while exercising. (See the sidebar.)
- **The Breath Sound Check:** When you hear yourself breathing (not panting) you are going at the right pace. (Incidentally, this and the Talk Test were first developed by Dr. Robert Goode based upon pioneering research he did at the University of Toronto. See the sidebar for more information.)
- **Perceived Exertion:** Work at a level that feels moderate to somewhat hard, but not beyond that.

These three techniques are particularly helpful because they allow you to adjust your exercise according to your own needs.

Do not continue exercising if you have chest discomfort or severe shortness of breath. These can be symptoms of heart problems.

Resistance exercise

The Canadian Diabetes Association recommends the following for your resistance exercising:

1. Start with one set of 10–15 repetitions.
2. Progress to two sets of 10–15 repetitions.
3. Then progress to three sets of 8 repetitions three times per week.

If you choose to do resistance exercise, first meet with a qualified exercise specialist and then keep in touch with him or her periodically.

The Talk Test

The Talk Test has its origins in the mountain climbing community, where climbers would say to one another, "Climb no faster than you can talk." Dr. Goode took that phrase and applied it to exercise at sea level. He recognized that at sea level the limiting factor in allowing people to exercise is insufficient oxygen supply to the muscles. He and his team showed experimentally that if you have difficulty talking, you are close to or at your anaerobic threshold (that is, the point at which your muscles can no longer effectively extract oxygen from your bloodstream), which in turn makes your muscles fatigued. This observation allowed Dr. Goode and his team to set a "lid" on how much aerobic exercise you can comfortably do.

Exercise and oral hypoglycemic agent therapy

Taking oral hypoglycemic agent (OHA) therapy need not prevent you from exercising. In fact, your medicines will work much more effectively if you exercise regularly.

Both exercise and OHA medicines reduce blood glucose, so you could be at risk of developing hypoglycemia. In practice this seldom happens, but it is still important for you to carry appropriate treatment with you. (We discuss treatment for hypoglycemia in Chapter 5.) The OHAs that cause hypoglycemia are those (such as glyburide) that stimulate the pancreas to release insulin. (We discuss this in more detail in Chapter 11.) If you are on one of these agents and are running into problems with low blood glucose when you exercise, speak to your physician about either reducing your dose or switching to a different agent. We can't think of a greater disincentive to exercise than knowing it will bring on an episode of hypoglycemia!

Exercise and insulin therapy

Being on insulin should not stop you from exercising, but you will likely need to adjust your doses. If you do vigorous exercise but have insufficient insulin, your muscles will not be able to properly use the glucose in your blood and your glucose level will rise. Conversely, if you exercise and you have too much insulin in your system, you will develop hypoglycemia.

Your diabetes educator and your dietitian are the pros when it comes to helping you adjust your insulin doses and your nutrition plan to accommodate your exercise. Sometimes changing to a different type of insulin is required, in which case your diabetes specialist or family physician can assist you.

In almost all circumstances, you should have your insulin and diet adjusted to accommodate your exercise. You should rarely have to change your exercise to accommodate your treatment.

Chapter 11

Combating High Blood Glucose with Pills

In This Chapter

▶ Improving your glucose control with drugs taken by mouth ("oral hypoglycemic agents")
▶ Combining oral hypoglycemic agents

*I*n Chapter 6 we discuss bad things (like blindness, kidney failure and nerve damage) that you are doing your darndest to avoid (with our help) by keeping your glucose control in check. In Chapter 10 we look at the ways that you can improve your health in general (and your glucose control in particular) by making appropriate lifestyle changes. In this chapter we look at how, if you have type 2 diabetes, you can further benefit by taking pills to assist you in your battle against hyperglycemia.

The pills we use to combat high blood glucose are typically referred to as *oral hypoglycemic agents* or *OHAs,* although there is a trend toward calling them *oral antihyperglycemic agents.* This change in terminology actually makes good sense. After all, we are not trying to make you have low blood glucose (which is what hypoglycemic means); we are trying to prevent you from having high blood glucose (hence, anti-hyperglycemic). Nonetheless, since the majority of the time both physicians and patients still refer to them as oral hypoglycemic agents, that is the terminology we use in this book.

You may come across yet another term for oral hypoglycemic agents; *oral anti-diabetic agents (OAD's).* This is not our favourite term (in fact we don't like it at all) as it implies that diabetes is purely a problem with glucose - which is far from the case.

If you are like most people, you would rather not take pills, and who could blame you? Let's make a list of some of the possible reasons you may have for *not* wanting to take oral hypoglycemic agent therapy. We will take the liberty of quoting some things you might say (even though we probably haven't even met you. How presumptuous is that?) and we will even indicate if we agree with your concern or not.

Table 11-1   Reasons Not to Take OHA Medication

I don't want to take OHAs because:	*Our opinion:*
They are chemicals.	We agree.
They can have side effects.	We agree.
They are not as good a treatment as proper nutrition therapy and exercise.	We agree.
Some types can occasionally cause hypoglycemia.	We agree.
They can interact adversely with other medicines.	We agree.
They can be hard to remember to take.	We agree.
They are a sign that I am unable to control my blood glucose levels without them.	We agree.

Surprised that you are right (or at least that you are in agreement with us and so must be right!) on each point? But of course you are right. Who wants to take pills if you can avoid them? No one.

But now let's look at the other side of the coin. Let's make a list of some of the possible reasons you may have *for wanting* to take oral hypoglycemic agent therapy.

Table 11-2   Reasons to Take OHA Medication

I am willing to take OHAs because:	*Our opinion:*
They will help me reduce my blood glucose levels if nutrition therapy and exercise alone cannot do the trick.	We agree.
By improving my glucose control, they will help protect my eyes, nerves, and kidneys.	We agree.
They seldom have serious side effects.	We agree.
Minor side effects can usually be easily corrected by adjusting the dose or changing to a different OHA.	We agree.
With the appropriate drug and dose, I can usually avoid hypoglycemia.	We agree.
Serious drug interactions seldom occur.	We agree.
I know diabetes is a progressive disease and that is not my fault. Taking an OHA does not mean that *I* have failed, it simply means that *my pancreas* has.	We agree.

I am willing to take OHAs because:	*Our opinion:*
Remembering to take pills is a pain in the butt, but is a heck of a lot better than remembering to go for eye surgery and dialysis appointments.	We agree.
Dr. Blumer and Dr. Rubin are very persuasive.	We couldn't agree more.
Enough already. I give up!	'Nuff said.

For many years in Canada we had but two classes of oral hypoglycemic agent therapy from which to choose (could have been worse; in the U.S. they had only one). Thankfully, substantial strides have been made in recent years and we now have five different classes to choose from. (Well, to be perfectly accurate we have six, but more on that later in this chapter.)

In Chapter 4 we look at why people develop type 2 diabetes. We show that the underlying problem is twofold: insulin resistance (a condition where your tissues do not respond to insulin properly) and insulin deficiency (wherein your pancreas is unable to manufacture sufficient insulin to keep up with your body's needs). Knowing this, we can then understand how OHAs work to help you with your diabetes. Figure 11-1 illustrates how the different OHA's function.

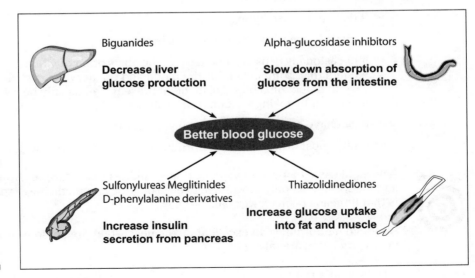

Figure 11-1:
How oral hypo-glycemic agents work.

Biguanides

Decrease liver glucose production

Alpha-glucosidase inhibitors

Slow down absorption of glucose from the intestine

Better blood glucose

Sulfonylureas Meglitinides
D-phenylalanine derivatives

Increase insulin secretion from pancreas

Thiazolidinediones

Increase glucose uptake into fat and muscle

The Oral Hypoglycemic Agents

All classes of OHAs have at least two things in common: they help to reduce blood glucose and they have unpronounceable names. In this section we take a look at the different types of oral agents that are available to assist you.

Biguanides

Metformin (Glucophage) is the only biguanide available in Canada. This drug has gained new popularity in recent years, ever since a large medical study (the UKPDS; www.dtu.ox.ac.uk/ukpds/index.html) showed it to be more protective of the cardiovascular system than sulfonylurea therapy, with, at the same time, equal ability to reduce blood glucose levels.

The Canadian Diabetes Association's new guidelines recommend that over-weight people with diabetes who require an oral hypoglycemic agent should use metformin (unless, of course, there is some reason it would be unsafe to use; see the warning below).

Metformin has the following characteristics:

- ✔ It lowers the blood glucose mainly by reducing the production of glucose from the liver.
- ✔ It does not cause hypoglycemia.
- ✔ It may reduce your risk of having a heart attack.
- ✔ It occasionally causes a decrease in the absorption of vitamin B12, a vitamin that is important for the blood and the nervous system. (This is easy to detect on a blood test and, if present, can usually be readily dealt with by taking a vitamin B12 supplement.)
- ✔ It can have a favourable effect on your lipids.
- ✔ Unlike most other OHAs, metformin does not cause weight gain.

 A new pill (Avandamet) is available that combines rosiglitazone (Avandia) and metformin. Its only advantage over taking the two medicines separately is that it means taking fewer pills per day.

Although metformin is an excellent medicine, certain precautions are necessary if you are taking it:

- ✔ It tends to cause nausea. This can be lessened if you take your metformin with food.
- ✔ It often causes diarrhea. One helpful way to avoid this (and nausea also) is to very slowly increase the dose. The dosing schedule Ian uses is available on his Web site (www.ianblumer.com/metformin%20handout.htm)

Metformin can cause — rarely — a serious adverse effect called lactic acidosis. For this reason, metformin should not be used if you have significant liver disease, heart failure, or kidney failure. *Mild* kidney malfunction does *not* prevent you from taking metformin. Your doctor should check your kidney function with a blood test that measures creatinine before prescribing this medication. Symptoms of lactic acidosis include nausea, vomiting, abdominal pain, poor appetite, and malaise.

If you are having certain types of X-rays where you will be given intravenous dye, your doctor will likely advise you to not take your metformin for a few days before and after the test. This precaution ensures that if the dye causes kidney problems, you will not have excess metformin accumulating in your body.

Thiazolidinediones

Thiazolidinediones (more easily referred to as TZDs and sometimes referred to as "glitazones") work by increasing glucose uptake from the blood into fat and muscle cells. They do this by reducing insulin resistance (see Chapter 4). The net result is lower blood glucose levels.

The Canadian Diabetes Association recommends that if you are overweight and on metformin but still have inadequate blood glucose control, that a TZD be added to your therapy. (If your control is particularly poor — as indicated by an A1C of 9 percent or higher — the CDA recommends that you be placed on both metformin and a TZD at the same time.)

There are two TZDs available in Canada, pioglitazone (Actos) and rosiglitazone (Avandia). These drugs share much in common and there is no proven superiority of one over the other. However, ongoing research *may* ultimately reveal one to have a better effect on lipids than its competitor. Stay tuned.

TZDs have the following characteristics:

- They can be taken once daily (though, for rosiglitazone, sometimes a better effect is seen if it is taken twice a day).
- It can take a few weeks of treatment before blood glucose levels start to improve. (Patience is a virtue with these drugs.)
- They do not cause hypoglycemia.

This class of drug is both effective and safe, but like any drug, there are some adverse effects that can occur:

- ✔ Fluid retention leading to swollen ankles

- ✔ Weight gain

- ✔ Anemia (This is usually mild and unimportant — except that if your doctor is not aware that TZDs can cause mild anemia, you could end up having unnecessary tests done.)

- ✔ Heart failure (This does not occur very often. It typically shows itself as shortness of breath.)

If you develop breathing difficulty while you are on a TZD you should seek immediate medical attention. It is also important that your doctor examine your heart *before* starting you on a TZD. If you have significant heart damage, you should not take a TZD.

There is virtually *no* evidence that either of the available TZDs causes liver problems; however, the original TZD (which is no longer available, having been removed from sale a few years ago) did cause severe liver injury in a few people. For that reason, current recommendations are that if you take a TZD, you should have your liver monitored (through a blood test) periodically. This precaution may well be removed in the not-too-distant future.

TZDs are excellent drugs and are being used with increasing frequency. In addition to their benefit of lowering blood glucose levels, there is rapidly accumulating evidence that they may help protect your pancreas's ability to produce insulin and possibly even reduce your risk of developing atherosclerosis (see Chapter 6 for a discussion of atherosclerosis). We do not yet have proof of these additional benefits, but we are heading in that direction. Like we said before, stay tuned.

Although TZDs are excellent drugs, they work best if used early on in your therapy. Unfortunately that is often not the way they are being prescribed. Most of the time, doctors are starting people on TZDs only *after* other OHAs have failed, which is, in fact, the least likely time for TZDs to meet with success. In our opinion, TZDs are grossly underused, and indeed, in Canada, less than 10 percent of OHAs prescribed are from this class. A significant reason for this may be their substantially greater cost compared to other, older oral agents.

TZDs can improve fertility in women who have a condition called polycystic ovarian syndrome. Accordingly, if you are a woman of child-bearing age, it is crucial that you take appropriate contraceptive precautions if you are prescribed a TZD.

Sulfonylureas

Scientists discovered sulfonylureas accidentally when they noticed that soldiers given certain sulfur-containing antibiotics developed symptoms of low blood glucose. Once scientists began to search for the most potent examples of this effect, they came up with several different versions of this drug. Sulfonylureas all have the following characteristics:

- ✔ They work by making the pancreas release more insulin.
- ✔ They are not effective in type 1 diabetes because in type 1 diabetes the pancreas is not capable of producing insulin.
- ✔ They can cause hypoglycemia.
- ✔ They can lead to weight gain.

As the name suggests, sulfonylureas are *sulfa* based, so if you are allergic to sulfa antibiotics, there is the (small) chance you could also have a reaction to this family of OHA. If you are prescribed a sulfonylurea, make sure you let your doctor know if you have a history of allergic reaction to other types of sulfa drugs.

Some sulfonylureas can interact with alcohol, causing unpleasant symptoms such as nausea and flushing (even if you are not inebriated).

Recent scientific evidence strongly suggests that if you are overweight and you need an oral agent, you should be placed on a biguanide and/or a thiazolidinedione (TZD) *rather than* a sulfonylurea unless there is some strong reason not to do so (see the discussion above on these other types of drugs). We agree and no longer use sulfonylureas as our "agent of choice," instead reserving their use as third-line OHA treatment.

Sulfonylureas available in Canada are gliclazide (Diamicron and Diamicron MR), glimepiride (Amaryl), and glyburide (Diabeta). Two other short-acting sulfonylureas (chlorpropamide and tolbutamide) are available in Canada but are rarely used.

Diamicron MR and Amaryl are long-acting agents and are taken once daily. Compared to the other sulfonylurea agents, these long-acting drugs are less likely to cause weight gain; however, a significant disadvantage is that government health plans are less likely to cover them.

Glyburide (Diabeta) is the most commonly used sulfonylurea in Canada, but it is also the OHA most likely to cause hypoglycemia. If you are having this problem, speak to your doctor about switching to a different drug.

Meglitinides

This new class of drug has but one member currently available in Canada, repaglinide (GlucoNorm). Like sulfonylureas, it stimulates the pancreas to secrete insulin.

These are the main reasons to choose a meglitinide over a sulfonylurea:

- ✔ They bring down glucose levels faster after meals.
- ✔ They are less likely (than short-acting sulfonylureas) to cause hypoglycemia.

These are the main reasons not to choose this over a sulfonylurea:

- ✔ It costs more.
- ✔ It has to be taken three times daily, while sulfonylureas are usually taken no more than twice daily.

D-phenylalanine derivatives

This is another new class of drug (almost always lumped together with the meglitinide family even though that is not technically accurate) with but a single, solitary member in Canada: nateglinide (Starlix). For all intents and purposes, it is almost identical in its method of action, potential side effects, and so on, as repaglinide, a meglitinide, with the significant exception that it is not as effective at lowering blood glucose levels.

At present, in our opinion, there is no compelling reason to use it.

Alpha-glucosidase inhibitors

Alpha-glucosidase inhibitors work by reducing the rate of glucose absorption from the small intestine into the bloodstream. The only agent in this family available in Canada is a drug called acarbose (Prandase). It works in the small intestine where it blocks the action of an enzyme that breaks down larger carbohydrates into smaller ones such as glucose. The result is that the rate of absorption of glucose into the blood is slowed.

There are two main advantages of this drug:

- ✔ There is virtually no risk of *serious* side effects.
- ✔ It does not cause hypoglycemia.

Does acarbose prevent heart disease?

Recent research (Canadian-led at that) may have uncovered a greater role for acarbose therapy. The STOP-NIDDM study (www.stop-niddm.com/home.htm) documented a 49-percent reduction in the risk of getting heart disease (or related problems) and a 34-percent lower risk of developing high blood pressure for people with impaired glucose tolerance (see Chapter 4) who took acarbose. We are keenly awaiting confirmation of these findings in subsequent medical studies.

There are also two main disadvantages of this drug:

- ✔ It is not particularly effective at reducing blood glucose readings.

- ✔ It tends to cause unpleasant gastrointestinal side effects (including gas, bloating, and flatulence). To avoid these it is often helpful to start with a very low dose and then slowly increase it. The dosing schedule that Ian uses is available on his Web site (www.ianblumer.com/acarbose%20handout.htm).

Given acarbose's side effect profile, you could say that the best candidates for this drug are those people who are "loud and proud."

If you develop hypoglycemia when you are on this medication, you must treat yourself with glucose or dextrose (such as Dextrosol), not sucrose. That is, you should not treat yourself with table sugar, fruit juice, or colas.

Because of the fairly small improvement in blood glucose control seen with this drug, and its unpleasant side effects, it is no surprise that there are not many people in Canada on this treatment. We do use it sometimes, but not very often.

Combining different oral hypoglycemic agents

The good news about glucose control is that shortly after your diabetes is diagnosed, there is a good chance you can achieve very good glucose control with intensive lifestyle therapy and often just one type of OHA. The bad news is that diabetes is a progressive disease, meaning that with time, your pancreas's ability to produce insulin peters out so that the therapy that worked so well initially works less well with time. That is *not* your fault! But it does mean you and your doctor should continually review your glucose control and reassess your treatment.

Mark on your calendar the day you found out you had diabetes. Consider that your starting point. Your goal is now to reach your target glucose control (see Chapter 9) within 6 to 12 months. Chart your progress by marking your A1C levels on your calendar. If they are not progressively improving, be sure to speak to your health care team to see what other strategies (lifestyle, medication, and so on) you can employ. As Eminem says, "Failure is not an option." (Well, he says it with, shall we say, more colourful language than we will use here.)

The great majority of people with diabetes end up requiring more than one oral hypoglycemic agent. In fact, as doctors have learned more and more over the past few years about the importance of excellent blood glucose control, we are introducing oral agents sooner in the management of diabetes and, equally importantly, we are increasingly often recommending *multiple* OHAs early on, sometimes from the day of diagnosis of diabetes (particularly if your blood glucose levels are especially high).

If you are treated with 2 or more oral hypoglycemic agents it is important that they work by different and complementary mechanisms. An excellent combination — our favourite, in fact — is metformin (which reduces glucose release from your liver as shown in figure 11-1) and a TZD (which helps move glucose into fat and muscle cells). If a third OHA is required we typically add a sulfonylurea or a meglitinide (which makes the pancreas release more insulin). There is no benefit in taking 2 different medicines that work the same way (for example, it is illogical to take the combination of a sulfonylurea and a meglitinide since they both have the same effect on the pancreas).

Though you may hate the idea of taking a whole bunch of pills, consider the alternative. Do you really want toxic levels of glucose poisoning your system day after day after day? (Now, we recognize that some people would say that they "don't want pills poisoning them either." True enough. All we can say to that is that the pills we use have proven themselves safe for the overwhelming majority of the millions of people that have used them, while high glucose levels are dangerous to everyone. And that includes you.)

It is always worth remembering that *no* oral hypoglycemic agent — or combination of agents — is likely to be particularly effective without appropriate lifestyle (nutrition, exercise, weight control) therapy also being used.

Our Preferred Way to Use OHAs

Wilson Chang, a 49-year-old small-business owner, had recently developed blurred vision and was drinking more water than usual. He saw his doctor and was found to have a fasting blood glucose of 11.2 mmol/L. Diabetes was diagnosed and he was sent to see Ian. Apart from being overweight (BMI 31; see Chapter 4 for a discussion of BMI), Wilson appeared healthy. This was how Ian and Wilson decided to proceed:

✔ **Day one:** On the day of Wilson's visit to Ian's office, he was referred to a diabetes education center, where he met with a registered dietitian and a diabetes educator (see Chapter 8). Lifestyle therapy (see Chapter 10) was started immediately. Because Wilson was having symptoms and because his glucose was quite high, he needed to be on OHA therapy right away. As Wilson was overweight, Ian prescribed metformin. Unlike glyburide, metformin would not cause Wilson to gain weight. And unlike a TZD, metformin would work right away. Wilson was instructed to gradually increase his metformin as per Ian's usual schedule (see above).

✔ **One month later:** Wilson was working with his diet and had lost a kilogram (2 lbs), but his glucose levels after showing some initial improvement had plateaued at about 9 to 10 mmol/L. Ian added a TZD to Wilson's OHA therapy.

✔ **Another month later:** Wilson was no longer having symptoms and had been doing some regular exercise, though not as diligently as he had hoped to. He had lost another kilogram (2 lbs) but was feeling a bit disappointed with his very modest success. His fasting blood glucose levels were now about 8 mmol/L. Ian reassured him that his weight loss, though not dramatic, was promising. As his blood glucose readings were still significantly higher than normal, Ian increased Wilson's TZD dose.

✔ **Another month later:** Wilson's weight had gone up half a kilogram (1 lb) and his running shoes were still whiter than Ian would have liked. Wilson's blood glucose readings were somewhat better, with fasting values averaging 7.0. Wilson promised to redouble his efforts at exercise and weight loss. No change was made to his OHA therapy.

✔ **Another month later:** Success! White running shoes no longer white. BMI 29. Blood glucose readings 4 to 7. Wilson happy. Ian happy. Dietitian happy. Educator happy. Local greasy spoon devastated.

The choice of OHA is important, but not nearly as important as getting the blood glucose levels down, regardless of the drug chosen to accomplish this. Indeed, one (possibly underutilized) option in the treatment of newly diagnosed type 2 diabetes is insulin; insulin is a particularly good choice if you are not overweight and your blood glucose levels are especially high.

We feel there is only one clear-cut mistake that doctors (and people with diabetes) make when selecting an oral hypoglycemic agent: not choosing treatment at all. All too often, doctor and patient delay necessary medication therapy far too long as all parties await lifestyle measures alone to bring glucose readings down to normal. Waiting a few weeks is almost always perfectly fine. Waiting more than two to three months is seldom a good idea. Waiting years is simply foolish.

The Canadian Diabetes Association recommends that target blood glucose readings be achieved by six to twelve months from the time of diagnosis of diabetes. Write a note with the date twelve months from when you found out you had diabetes. Stick the note on your fridge and look at it periodically; that's your due date (even if you're not pregnant!); the date by which you and your health care team are striving to deliver a healthy blood glucose level. And this is one delivery that is quite fine if it comes early.

The ADOPT study

The ADOPT study (*A Diabetes Outcome Progression Trial*), currently underway in a number of countries including Canada, should tell us which oral hypoglycemic agent class, if any, is superior to the others. In this investigation, people with recently diagnosed type 2 diabetes are being treated with either rosiglitazone, metformin, or glyburide. These patients will then be followed to see, in effect, whose glucose control will be better as time passes. We may even be able to determine if TZDs, as it is hoped, can help to preserve islet cell function (and hence, insulin secretion). If TZDs do "protect the pancreas," they will be the first drug proven to do so. And if that is the case, watch for use of TZDs to skyrocket in Canada — even though they cost more than other oral agents.

Chapter 12

Using Insulin Effectively

Dorothy Strait was 50 when she was diagnosed as having type 2 diabetes. Her initial treatment was lifestyle therapy and she was thrilled when a change in her diet, modest weight loss, and a daily walk brought her glucose levels down to normal. A couple of years later, however, despite being at a good weight and following a healthy lifestyle, her glucose levels started to climb and she began taking an oral hypoglycemic agent. That helped for a while, but her readings rose again and she started taking an additional oral agent. That also helped, but only temporarily, and her glucose readings had now risen to 11 and she was feeling fatigued. Her family doctor referred her to Ian to see if she should be on insulin. When Dorothy came to Ian's office, she was sad, angry, and frightened all at once. She felt "like a failure." She was "terrified of the needle" and told Ian, "I would hate jabbing myself. I simply couldn't do it. You can't convince me otherwise." As she spoke to Ian she was on the verge of tears.

"Dorothy," Ian said, "we will do whatever you want. I can't force you to do anything. And I wouldn't want to even if I could. *You* are the boss and *you* will decide what you want to do. But, I think you would be unfair to yourself if, whatever you decide, it wasn't an informed decision. So let's make sure you know the most important information to help you make your decision." Dorothy was certainly agreeable to that.

Ian said a few things to Dorothy that day. He remembers telling her, "It is crucial that you know that *you* are not a failure, your *pancreas* is, and that is not your fault. That happens to most people with diabetes. And as for 'hating jabbing yourself,' why would you like it? Who would? But you are *already* jabbing yourself each time you test your blood glucose. And doing a blood finger jab hurts a lot more than taking insulin. With the tiny needles we use nowadays, giving insulin is virtually pain-free. And as for not being able to do it, look at the other obstacles that you have overcome; you have changed your diet, you have lost some weight, you are exercising regularly, you are taking a whole bunch of pills that I'm sure you'd rather not have to, and you are testing your blood every day. You have managed all those things. And if you can handle all those things, I'm sure you could manage giving insulin also."

Dorothy became more at ease but was still apprehensive. "But, Doctor, when you start insulin, you are on it forever."

"That's usually true, Dorothy," Ian replied, "but not because insulin is addictive. It is because your pancreas is failing and it is not going to be rejuvenated. It can no longer make enough insulin, so we have to supplement it. We are simply giving your body back the hormone it is lacking. One other thing: medical science is always progressing. Other ways of giving insulin are being developed. Better pills are always coming along. I don't know if you will be on insulin injections 'forever.' Maybe in a few years you won't have to be."

Well, Dorothy still wasn't thrilled with the prospect of giving insulin. And of course there was no reason for her to be thrilled. But she met with the diabetes educator and was pleasantly surprised to find that giving insulin wasn't nearly as bad as she had thought. It wasn't fun by any means, but it wasn't horrible either. And as her glucose levels returned to normal and her energy improved she was very glad she had decided to take insulin after all.

What Is Insulin?

If you're a person with type 1 diabetes, insulin is your saviour. Simply put, without insulin you could not survive. And if you have type 2 diabetes, insulin may not very often be the difference between life and death (not in the short term, anyhow) but it often is the difference between good health and bad health. As we explain in Chapter 3, insulin is a hormone that is produced in the pancreas and released into the bloodstream, where it travels to different parts of your body. Insulin acts on certain cells (such as fat cells and muscle cells) to allow glucose to enter so that they can carry out their normal functions. (Ian vividly recalls one rather colourful speaker at a medical conference referring to insulin as the "Viagra of the cell.") If you do not have insulin in your body to allow glucose to enter into the tissues, the glucose hangs around in the blood and eventually starts to spill out into your urine.

We measure injected insulin in "units." Nowadays we have very scientific ways of determining the strength of insulin with laboratory machinery. We've come a long way from the time that a unit of insulin was based on how much insulin it took to cause a rabbit to have severe enough hypoglycemia that it would have a seizure.

Types of Insulin

Our pancreas normally functions on autopilot. When we eat, our blood glucose level goes up and our pancreas immediately responds by releasing insulin into the bloodstream, which promptly brings our glucose level back to normal. If your pancreas is malfunctioning and you require insulin injections, then our goal is to try to reproduce what your pancreas would normally do if it was healthy. We are aided by having a variety of different insulins to choose from, each with its own set of properties. When you are prescribed insulin, your doctor will try to match your body's needs with the most appropriate insulin. Since each person is different, it is possible that the type of insulin you are first started on will be changed to a different one depending on how your body responds.

The basic idea is to make sure you have the right amount of insulin in your body at all times. Therefore, we often use a quick acting insulin before meals to promptly bring down your post-meal glucose level. And, because our bodies *always* need some insulin, you will likely also be placed on an insulin that lasts longer to prevent your glucose level from going high inbetween meals.

Insulins (and their properties) available in Canada are listed in Table 12-1. Note that the times given are approximations and can vary significantly — even for the same person.

TIP

The terminology for insulins is very confusing. You may find *rapid-acting* and *fast-acting* used to mean one thing in one place and another thing in another place. You may also come across the term "short-acting" insulin with this term also being used in various (and inconsistent) ways. It's enough to drive one around the bend. To avoid becoming totally muddled, the best thing to do when reading about insulin is to look at the specific one being discussed and then refer back to Table 12-1 to see what properties that particular insulin has.

Another common misunderstanding is equating "Humulin" with "Humulin-N." Humulin is a trade name and refers to a *variety* of types of insulin marketed by one particular company (Eli Lilly in this case). Humulin-N refers to Eli Lilly's brand of NPH insulin. To say you are on "Humulin" conveys the same degree of information as saying you drive a Chevrolet — helpful, but only part of the story. More specific would be if you said you drove a Corvette or a Malibu or an Impala.

Table 12-1 Types of Insulin Available in Canada and Their Properties*

Classification	Generic Name	Trade Name(s)	Onset of Action	Peak Action	Duration of Action
Rapid-acting	aspart	Novorapid	5 to 15 minutes	60 to 90 minutes	4 to 5 hours
	lispro	Humalog			
Fast-acting	regular	Humulin-R Novolin ge Toronto	30 to 60 minutes	2 to 4 hours	5 to 8 hours
Intermediate-acting	NPH	Humulin-N Novolin ge NPH	1 to 3 hours	5 to 8 hours	14 to 18 hours
Long-acting	glargine	Lantus	90 minutes	None	18 to 24 hours
	detemir	Levemir	90 minutes	None	12 to 24 hours
Pre-mixed (the numbers after the names refer to the ratio of rapid- or fast-acting insulin to intermediate-acting insulin)		Humalog Mix25 Humulin (30/70) Novolin ge (10/90, 20/80, 30/70, 40/60, 50/50)	Depends on specific type	Depends on specific type	Depends on specific type

*This table is adapted from the CDA 2003 Clinical Practice Guidelines.

Rapid-acting insulin

There are two types of rapid-acting insulin available: aspart (NovoRapid) and lispro (Humalog). For all intents and purposes they are identical in their actions. Indeed, the only significant way in which they differ is that if you buy one type you help boost the share price of one company, and if you buy the other type you help the other company's valuation. These are the most important properties of rapid-acting insulin:

- ✔ You take it immediately before you eat.

- ✔ Its peak effect occurs at the same time as the glucose from your food is being absorbed from your small intestine, so the action of the insulin matches the rise in your blood glucose. That is what a healthy pancreas does too.

- ✔ It wears off within a short period of time (4 to 5 hours).

Compared with fast-acting ("regular") insulin, rapid-acting insulin is better at reducing post-meal blood glucose levels and is less likely to cause hypoglycemia. For these reasons, the new Canadian Diabetes Association Guidelines recommend the use of rapid-acting rather than fast-acting insulin.

If you have gastroparesis (a condition in which your stomach becomes less efficient at propelling food into your small intestine; see Chapter 6) and erratic blood glucose control, you may benefit from taking rapid-acting insulin an hour or so *after* your meal. Your diabetes specialist can help you determine if this would be a good option for you.

Fast-acting insulin

There is one type of fast-acting insulin. It's usually referred to as "regular" insulin. Perhaps of interest, it is called "Toronto" insulin everywhere in the world so long as your world is confined to Canada and, in particular, Toronto. (Ian can say that because he lives in Toronto.)

Here are the most important properties of fast-acting insulin:

- ✔ Because it does not have much action until 30 minutes after you inject it, regular insulin should be taken — you guessed it — 30 minutes before you eat. Because that can be such a hassle, most people end up taking it immediately before they eat anyhow. It will still work, but not as effectively.

- ✔ It has a longer duration of action than rapid-acting insulin.

- ✔ It is less expensive than rapid-acting insulin.

Intermediate-acting insulin

There is now only one type of intermediate-acting insulin being manufactured in Canada; that is, NPH (which is sometimes simply called "N"). Lente insulin, another intermediate-acting insulin, is no longer being manufactured in Canada and will be availabe in pharmacies only until existing supplies run out.

These are the most important properties of intermediate-acting insulin:

✔ Because it does not have much effect until a few hours after it is injected, intermediate-acting insulin does not help to reduce your blood glucose levels immediately after you eat.

✔ Because it has a fairly long duration of action, it is an excellent insulin to take at bedtime.

Long-acting insulin

Long-acting insulin works for, well, a long time. There are two types of long-acting insulin: detemir and glargine. Table 12-1 describes their properties.

These are the most important properties of long-acting insulins:

✔ They are "peakless" - meaning that they have the same effect on blood glucose levels 2 hours after the injection as they do 8 or more hours after the injection.

✔ Because they last up to 24 hours, they can often be taken just once per day.

✔ Because they do not have a peak or rapid effect, they do *not* effectively bring down glucose readings after meals. For this reason, long-acting insulins are usually supplemented with either a rapid- or fast-acting insulin given with meals (or, in the case of type 2 diabetes, sometimes with oral hypoglycemic agents).

✔ They are less likely to cause hypoglycemia than other types of insulin.

✔ They must not be mixed in the same syringe with any other insulin.

Detemir and glargine insulins are clear (hence, you can see through them). So are rapid- and fast-acting insulins. Because of this similarity in appearance, people have mistakenly given themselves one type of insulin when they had meant to give the other. It is crucial that you very carefully read the label before administering your insulin. (Since NPH insulin is cloudy it is not as likely to be confused with the other, clear types of insulin)

Intermediate (NPH, lente) and long-acting (ultralente, glargine) insulins are often referred to as "basal insulins" since they cover your baseline insulin requirements in between your injections of rapid- or fast-acting insulin.

Pre-mixed insulin

If you require insulin injections, you will almost certainly need to inject more than one type. Traditionally this was dealt with by mixing two types of insulin (fast-acting and intermediate acting) together in a syringe. That is a hassle, however, so manufacturers came up with pre-mixed insulins that combine rapid-acting or fast-acting insulin with intermediate-acting insulin. The most common type of pre-mixed insulin in use is called 30/70 and is a combination of 30 percent regular insulin and 70 percent NPH insulin. Pre-mixed insulin is often of value in treating type 2 diabetes, but because it does not allow the individual components to be adjusted, it is almost never the best treatment for type 1 diabetes.

Animal insulins

In very rare circumstances, people with diabetes are treated with animal insulins. The only ones still available in Canada are made by Eli Lilly and are Iletin II Regular Pork and Iletin II NPH Pork. At present only one-third of 1 percent of insulin used in Canada is pork insulin.

Insulin Treatment Strategies for Type 1 Diabetes

Our preferred insulin treatment strategies for our patients with type 1 diabetes are:

- ✔ Rapid-acting insulin with meals and intermediate-acting insulin at bedtime (and, often at breakfast time as well).
- ✔ Rapid-acting insulin with meals and detemir or glargine insulin at bedtime. (For those people taking NPH insulin who are experiencing hypoglycemia during the night, switching from NPH to detemir or glargine insulin is often highly effective at reducing — or sometimes completely eliminating — these insulin reactions.)
- ✔ Pump therapy (see below).

The reason why these strategies are so successful is that they closely mimic what a healthy pancreas does. In terms of the first two techniques, the intermediate-acting insulin (or glargine insulin) at bedtime prevents the blood glucose from rising overnight — by blocking glucose release from the liver — and the rapid-acting insulin taken with meals prevents glucose levels from rising too high as it gets absorbed into your blood after you eat.

We discuss insulin treatment strategies for people with type 2 diabetes later in this chapter.

How to Give Insulin

There is, in truth, only one way to learn how to give yourself insulin and that is by sitting down with a diabetes educator and having him or her teach you. You can no more learn how to give insulin by reading a package insert (or even this book, we are quite willing to admit) than you can learn how to drive a car without ever getting behind the wheel. This section will therefore address *general* principles of insulin administration.

Insulin delivery devices

Have you ever seen a movie where the actor says, "We can do this the easy way or we can do this the hard way. You decide." Well, the same applies to giving insulin.

Pens and syringes

For decades, the only way to give insulin was with a syringe and a bottle. Giving insulin this way is perfectly acceptable. But so is driving a 1982 Chevy. It may get you where you want to go, but it isn't quite the same as driving a 2004 Lexus. By far the easiest way to inject insulin (apart from using a pump, which we discuss later) is with an insulin pen device. And unlike a new Lexus, pen devices are free! Figure 12.1 shows a pen device. (There are other pen devices that look very different.) At present almost two-thirds of insulin used in Canada is given by pen injection. This number is rapidly growing and will likely be over 90 percent within a few years.

Figure 12-1:
The insulin
pen.

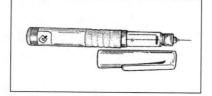

Insulin pen devices are supplied free of charge to diabetes education centres in Canada. All you need to do is ask for one. Most pharmacies will also give one to you free of charge. If a pharmacy advises you there is a charge, we would suggest you save your money and visit your diabetes education centre instead.

If you are on a dose of insulin that exceeds the amount that the pen can deliver with one injection, you do not need to remove the needle and inject yourself again. Instead, you can re-dial the pen while the needle is still inserted.

There are several different pen devices currently available, all of which are very good and very reliable. Your diabetes educator (or pharmacist) will give you the pen device that is designed for the insulin you have been prescribed.

Whether you have been taking insulin for 20 days or 20 years, there may well come a time when you accidentally give yourself either the wrong insulin or the wrong dose, or even forget to give a dose altogether. Fortunately, such a slip-up seldom leads to anything serious. Don't feel guilty or stupid if you make a mistake with your insulin; it happens to everyone. The way to deal with this type of oversight will depend on many factors, including the type of insulin you are taking (or, ahem, not taking), the dose, your blood glucose control, and the type of diabetes you have. Because there can be so many factors to take into account, it is best that you speak to your diabetes educator to formulate a plan of action in the event that you make an error with your insulin.

Jet injectors

If neither pen devices nor syringes suit your fancy, and if you don't mind spending a whole bunch of money (about $700), you can obtain a jet injection device (such as the AdvantaJet Injector — www.advantajet.com — distributed in Canada by Activa Brand Products; 800-991-4464). The idea behind these is that since they do not have needles, it will not hurt as much to give your insulin. Although that is true for some people, others find they experience just as much discomfort with a jet injector as they do from insulin given by needle. Jet injectors are not in common use in Canada.

Pumps

Not too long ago, insulin pumps were not much more than a novelty item. They were rarely used and were prone to malfunction. Nowadays, however, pumps are rapidly increasing in popularity, are much more reliable (though not always; see the Warning below), and for *some* people are an excellent treatment choice. Although people with type 2 diabetes can use pumps, it is usually people with type 1 diabetes who benefit the most from them.

Pumps have an insulin reservoir and are programmable so that a small amount of insulin is delivered from the pump through some tubing into a small plastic catheter inserted under the skin and kept in place for 2 to 3 days. (See Figure 12-2.) The insulin is administered 24 hours a day, and when you eat, you can instruct the pump to deliver an extra few units of insulin. Some pumps even have a remote control that you put on your key chain and when you need some extra insulin you just press a button (like opening your car trunk with a key-chain remote) and your pump delivers the additional amount. Pretty darn cool, if you ask us. There are currently about 4,000 pump users in Canada, but that figure is growing rapidly.

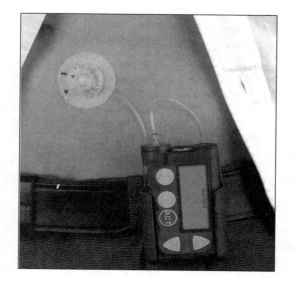

Figure 12-2: The insulin pump with its infusion set.

Pumps do not monitor your blood glucose levels. If you have a pump, you still have to do blood glucose testing. Also, a pump does not figure out how much insulin to give you; you have to tell it how much to give. (In the future this will change. See our discussion on bloodless meters in Chapter 9.) Pump therapy works best if you are carbohydrate counting (see later in this chapter).

Pumps are most suited to people with type 1 diabetes who are on four or more insulin injections per day. In virtually all cases, only rapid-acting insulin is used in pumps. Pump users do not use — or need — any intermediate or long-acting insulin.

If you have diabetes you already know that no aspect of treatment is perfect and that what is good for your next-door neighbour may not be good for you. This is true of pump therapy as well. There are good things about pump therapy:

- ✔ It is very convenient. You have less stuff (syringes, vials, pens, needles, and so on) to carry around with you and it is much easier to bolus (that is, give an extra quantity of insulin) with meals and snacks. It also allows for much greater flexibility regarding meal timing and exercise.

- ✔ It can help smooth out blood glucose levels, because problems with inconsistent and erratic insulin absorption of longer-acting insulins are no longer an issue. For some pump users, this results in improved A1C readings and fewer episodes of hypoglycemia.

And, of course, there are bad things about pump therapy:

- ✔ It is *very* expensive. A pump will cost you about $6,500 and supplies will run you $300 per month (and that does not even include the cost of insulin or blood glucose test strips).

- ✔ You and your pump are virtually inseparable. You can disconnect your pump for an hour or so such as when you shower or swim, but just like a teenager and a phone, separations must be kept to a minimum.

- ✔ It is lots of work. You must test your blood numerous times per day, the infusion rate has to be frequently reassessed, you have to spend many hours with your diabetes educator to learn how to use your pump, and so on.

When we first suggest pump therapy to our patients the usual response we hear is, "Doctor, I can't imagine having that thing attached to me all the time. It would make me feel like a prisoner." But we must say that these words are seldom, if ever, spoken by actual pump users; it's pretty well only people that haven't tried a pump who voice this concern. Indeed — and as surprising as this may seem — what we typically hear from our patients on insulin pumps is that they find pump therapy "liberating" and would "never" go back to conventional insulin pump injectors. Heck, we'd have to wrestle them to the ground to get them to give up their pumps. And as for the extra work involved with pump therapy, that is a trade-off that pump users are invariably happy to make.

Many private insurance companies will pay for most (or even all) of the cost of an insulin pump. Be sure to speak to them about this. They will likely require a supportive letter from your diabetes specialist. The pump companies themselves (see the contact information below) often offer financing as well as a several-month return policy so that if you decide you don't want to stay with a pump you can obtain a full refund. Be sure to find out all these details (in writing!) before you commit yourself to a pump purchase.

Tom, a 24-year-old accountant, was a very active man and was exceptionally attentive to his diabetes management. He would test his blood five, six, seven, or more times per day and was giving himself Humalog insulin with meals and NPH insulin at breakfast and at bedtime. In addition, when he would snack he would take a few extra units of Humalog. Some days he would take a total of seven injections of insulin. Tom's A1C was excellent at 6.8, but he was having frequent low readings overnight. "Tom," Ian said to him at the time of an appointment, "I think you should consider getting a pump." Tom was surprised and wondered why he should. "Because you are working very, very hard at managing your diabetes and I think you would find things are much easier for you on a pump," Ian replied. "We could also probably get rid of a lot of those overnight lows."

Tom tried the pump and within a week was back in the office. "How's it going?" Ian asked. "Well," Tom said, "I must admit I was a bit skeptical of your advice, but I decided to try the pump anyhow." Ian looked on expectantly. "And I have to tell you it was a *fantastic* decision. Oh, life isn't *easy*, but it is *easier*. When I need a bolus, presto, it's done. No one even notices when I give my insulin, not that that would bother me anyhow. And guess what; no more overnight lows." Ian asked Tom if he would ever go back to his insulin pen injections. "Not on your life. They'd have to shoot me to get this pump from me!"

Tom was an ideal candidate for an insulin pump. He was testing and injecting many times per day. He was motivated and interested in putting in the considerable time and energy necessary to learn how to use a pump. In the absence of this devotion, switching to a pump is no more likely to make your glucose control better than driving a Porsche rather than a Hyundai instantly makes you a better driver.

In our opinion, for those people who are appropriate candidates and have the financial resources, pump therapy is the way of the future until such time as a cure is found.

Following are the pumps available in Canada, along with their manufacturers, Web sites, and phone numbers:

Manufacturer	Pump Name	Contact Information
Animas Corporation	Animas IR 1000 Animas IR 1200 Animas IR 1250	www.animascorp.com 800-461-0991
Deltec Inc.	Deltec Cozmo	www.delteccozmo.com 866-662-6966
Disetronic Medical Systems Inc.	D-TRON plus H-TRON Plus	www.disetronic-usa.com 800-280-7801 ext. 5350
Medtronic MiniMed Inc.	MiniMedParadigm Paradigm 515 Paradigm 522 Paradigm 715 Paradigm 722	www.minimed.com 800-268-5346

Although some pumps are said to be waterproof, we feel that it is generally best to avoid taking the chance that water could get into your pump and interfere with its function. Briefly disconnecting your pump while you take a dip is usually a better option than swimming with it.

If you are trying to decide if a pump is for you — and, if it is, deciding which pump to choose — your diabetes educator is the best person for you to speak with. Not all educators have studied pumps, so your educator may refer you to an even more specialized teacher called a "pump trainer." It would also be a good idea for you to speak to a pump user to hear what they have to say. Your educator can likely provide you with the name of a "pumper" to contact (pump users are almost always more than happy to "spread the word").

How to Care for Your Insulin

Although insulin is not particularly difficult to look after, there are some "handling" issues that you should be aware of:

- ✔ Do not use insulin after the expiration date marked on the label.

- ✔ Before its first use, an *unopened* vial or cartridge of insulin should be stored in the refrigerator and may be used up to its expiration date. (Refrigeration helps to preserve the potency of the insulin.)

- ✔ After its first use, your vial or cartridge of insulin may be either refrigerated or kept at room temperature (see the tip below).

- ✔ After its first use, your vial or cartridge of insulin has a limited time (usually about 4 weeks) before it will need to be discarded. The package insert that came with your insulin will indicate the precise time recommended by the manufacturer of the particular insulin you are using.

- ✔ Insulin does not take well to excessive heat (such as being kept inside a car on a hot summer day) or, contrarily, to excessive cold (as Ian's patient found out when he returned to his car after his son's mid-winter hockey practice only to find his insulin bearing a surprising resemblance to a Popsicle). You should not use insulin that has been frozen or subjected to extreme heat.

- Many a person has successfully injected insulin through clothing, but we don't recommend you do it routinely.

- Most people reuse their needles, but because needles can get dull so quickly (which can both increase the discomfort of an injection and lead to skin damage including *lipohypertrophy* — which we discuss in Chapter 6) we don't recommend doing this routinely either.

- Dispose of used needles in a puncture-proof "sharps" container that is sealed shut before being discarded. Most pharmacies will accept these containers and will dispose of them for you.

- If you are using cloudy insulin (some insulins are clear and some are cloudy), roll the vial to mix the contents before you inject it. If there are clumps present, do not use the insulin.

You will find that injecting insulin that is at room temperature is more comfortable than injecting insulin you have just taken out of the refrigerator.

How to Adjust Your Insulin Dose

If you are taking insulin, you can pat yourself on the back; you have just been given the right to prescribe your own medicine. Well, not entirely, but to quite a significant extent. Insulin is unlike any other medicine your doctor will ever ask you to take. Unlike penicillin or heart medicines or, for that matter, oral hypoglycemic agents, insulin is, in general, *not* designed to be taken in a set dose day to day. If your pancreas was working properly it would constantly adjust how much insulin it was producing based on your body's requirements at any given moment. When you give yourself insulin, you are trying to mimic what your pancreas would normally do; so that means you, too, should be constantly adjusting your insulin dose. In fact when we ask a patient how much insulin they are taking, it is music to our ears when they reply; "oh, well that depends . . ." Precisely right. It depends. It depends on many things, including:

- What you are about to eat (If you have type 1 diabetes you may find carbohydrate counting — see the sidebar page 205 — very helpful.)

- Your current blood glucose level

- Your recent blood glucose levels

- Whether you will be exercising

- Which type of insulin you are using

The common denominator in this list is the need to make *pro-active* insulin adjustment. The single greatest reason for failing to achieve good glucose control is making *retroactive* insulin adjustment. To do this effectively, you should be like a soothsayer, trying to predict what your reading is likely to be in a few hours and taking the amount of insulin *now* that will anticipate your needs *later*. Far too often people simply say, "Oh, my reading is high, I need more insulin," or "My reading is low, I need less insulin." These statements are perfectly true, but they take into account far less information than is available and necessary.

Although insulin adjustment is essential for the great majority of people with diabetes, if you have type 2 diabetes and have excellent blood glucose control on the same daily dose of insulin, it would not be necessary for you to make routine changes.

Many, many people have the mistaken impression that their insulin dose correlates to the "severity" of their diabetes. In case you are one of these people, then, boy are we glad you are reading this paragraph. So there can be no chance of future misunderstanding let us make it perfectly clear: Your insulin dose tells you (and us) absolutely *nothing* about how "good" or "bad" your diabetes is. You can be on 10 units per day and have all sorts of complications and difficulties with your diabetes and you can be on 300 units per day and sail along very nicely, thank you very much. Just like you should wear the shoe size that your feet require, so should you take the dose of insulin your body requires. That's all there is to it.

Bill was a 65-year-old man with type 2 diabetes. He was taking 10 units of NPH insulin at bedtime. Although his readings were 5 to 7 mmol/L at bedtime, his fasting blood glucose readings were running 10 to 12 mmol/L. Bill blamed the high readings on eating too big a bedtime snack, but when he reduced his snack, it didn't help. Ian suggested to Bill that he increase his bedtime insulin dose by 2 units every 2 nights until his fasting readings came down to target. Within a few weeks, Bill was up to 22 units of insulin and his fasting readings were down to 5 mmol/L.

Bill's problem is a very common one. In the absence of sufficient quantities of insulin in your system, your blood glucose level will tend to rise overnight as your liver starts to release glucose into the blood (starting at about 3 a.m.) in response to increasing levels of other hormones (such as cortisol and growth hormone). This is called the *dawn phenomenon*. Intermediate-acting insulin (like NPH) taken at bedtime is the ideal way to combat this as it will be peaking just as your liver is about to start releasing glucose; however, the dose has to be adjusted to meet your body's demands, as Bill discovered.

If you have elevated fasting readings, but you are also having lows in the middle of the night, then you should *not* increase your bedtime insulin. Lows in the middle of the night indicate that you are taking too much insulin at bedtime. This is treated by *decreasing* your bedtime NPH (or lente) dose.

The *Somogyi phenomenon* (also referred to as a *Somogyi reaction*) refers to overnight lows followed by *rebounding* in which your liver pours out glucose but overshoots the mark and you end up having high fasting readings. The treatment for this is to reduce your bedtime insulin dose.

Mary was a 16-year-old girl with type 1 diabetes. She was taking NPH insulin at bedtime and was also taking Humalog insulin with each meal in order to prevent her blood glucose readings from climbing too high after she ate. Nonetheless, she found that sometimes her post-meal readings were excellent and other times they were poor, without any rhyme or reason. Mary met with the registered dietitian and discovered there was indeed a reason; her consumption of carbohydrate was varying quite a bit from meal to meal. Mary learned how to adjust her insulin based on how much carbohydrate she was eating (see the sidebar on carbohydrate counting) and soon there-after her readings were excellent.

If, like Mary, you are on multiple insulin injections per day, you are said to be on "intensive" or "intensified" therapy. Although we do use this term, we admit to not being overly fond of it, because *all* people with diabetes need to be treated intensively regardless of whether that means simply with diet and exercise, or oral hypoglycemic agents, or one, two, three, or more doses of insulin.

We have looked at a couple of ways in which insulin adjustment can help with blood glucose control, but there are, of course, many other situations that require different strategies. You can find more information on insulin adjustment by going to Ian's Web site and clicking the "insulin adjustment" link.

It is crucial that when you start insulin, you see it as just that, *a start*. You will need to stay in regular touch with your diabetes educator for ongoing dosage adjustment guidance. Without the educator's ongoing assistance, very few people ever master insulin adjustment and they typically end up feeling very frustrated. You may find it helpful to have a look at a handout Ian gives his patients who are about to start insulin (www.ianblumer.com/insulin%20initiation.htm).

Carbohydrate counting

Carbohydrates are *the* key nutrient in raising blood glucose readings after meals (see Chapter 10). You can take advantage of this by adjusting your insulin dose to fit with the likely effect on your blood glucose of the quantity of carbohydrates you are about to eat. This is called *carbohydrate counting* and it is a very effective strategy for many people with type 1 diabetes who are taking rapid-acting insulin (and, to a somewhat lesser extent, fast-acting insulin) with their meals.

The first step is to calculate how many grams of carbohydrate you are consuming and then to give a certain number of units of rapid-acting insulin based on that. It is somewhat a matter of trial and error. A common ratio is 1 unit of insulin for every 10 grams of carbohydrate, but it can range from 1 unit per 5 grams to 1 unit per 20 grams. And even that is not written in stone.

Bear in mind that not all carbohydrates will raise your blood glucose to the same degree (see our discussion on the "glycemic index" in Chapter 10). The fibre you eat should not be counted when totalling the number of "carbs" in your diet because, though it's a carbohydrate, it will not raise your blood glucose.

Carbohydrate counting may not be rocket science but it is not easy either and it is certainly not for everyone. If you are doing very well without carbohydrate counting, there is no reason you should feel you have to take on this additional task. If, however, things are not going all that well for you (and in particular if your glucose control is erratic and/or your A1C is not particularly good), you should contact your dietitian and diabetes educator to discuss whether carbohydrate counting may be the right thing for you.

Causes of Erratic Blood Glucose Control

There can be many reasons for glucose control to be erratic. One of these is called *brittle diabetes,* which is type 1 diabetes characterized by very frequent and unexplained hypo- and hyperglycemia, ketoacidosis, and repeated hospitalizations. Many people are labelled as having brittle diabetes, but in fact we usually find that the causes of wide swings in glucose levels and other difficulties are almost always correctable problems. Indeed, in our practices brittle diabetes is rarely seen. Here are some possible reasons for erratic blood glucose control:

- ✔ **Your nutrition plan:** Are you eating inconsistently? Do you eat almost nothing all day and then consume the bulk of your calories at suppertime? Do you "graze" from the time you get home in the evening until you go to bed? All these patterns can adversely affect glucose control.

- ✔ **Your exercise pattern:** Are you exercising for 10 minutes one morning and then 30 minutes the next evening and then 15 minutes the next afternoon? Consistent duration and timing of exercise is often helpful in maintaining consistent glucose control.

✔ **Your insulin regimen:** Are you on an insulin schedule that meets your needs? If, for example, you have type 1 diabetes but are only on twice-daily insulin, it is almost guaranteed that your blood glucose control will be erratic.

✔ **Insulin Absorption:** You may give yourself the same dose of insulin every day (something, by the way, that is seldom a good idea, as we discuss earlier in this chapter), but that does not mean that your bloodstream sees the same dose. Factors that can affect the rate of absorption of insulin from your injection sites include the following:

• Whether your injection sites have scar tissue

• Whether your injection sites have fat build-up (lipohypertrophy; see Chapter 6)

• Which part of your body you are injecting into (Fast-acting insulin will begin to work more quickly if injected into the abdomen than the arms or legs)

• Whether you exercise a certain part of your body after you inject there. (If you are about to go out for a run, you had best not use your leg as your injection site for your fast-acting insulin immediately beforehand.)

• Whether you are accidentally injecting into muscle. (This would cause the insulin to be absorbed faster.)

• Whether your insulin is beyond its expiry date (hint; it shouldn't be). (This isn't technically a problem with insulin absorption; rather it is that the potency of the insulin may not be the same once the expiry date has been reached.)

• Whether you have properly mixed the contents of your NPH, lente or ultralente insulin vial or cartridge.

Studies have shown the astounding fact that even if you inject the same amount of insulin into the same spot, the peak insulin level in your blood can vary by up to 40 percent! Which means that a 10-unit dose (for example) can have the effect of an 8-unit dose one time and a 12-unit dose another time. As we see it, the question isn't "Why are my blood sugars going up and down?" It should be "Why aren't my blood sugars going up and down even more?" Clearly, it would be a gross understatement to say that we are dealing with imperfect therapy. (Yet, even then, it still works remarkably well.)

✔ **Your stomach function:** Do you get full or bloated quickly? These symptoms can reflect poor stomach emptying called diabetic gastroparesis (see Chapter 6). With this condition, you may know how much carbohydrate you just ingested, but if your stomach isn't working properly, your blood glucose may not respond to your meal predictably.

✔ **Your small intestinal function:** People with type 1 diabetes are much more prone to a condition called *celiac disease*. If untreated, celiac disease leads to inadequate nutrient absorption from the small intestine.

✔ **Stress:** Stress does not cause diabetes, but it can certainly influence it. Stress causes the release of certain hormones in your body, including cortisol and adrenaline, both of which can make glucose levels rise. If you are on an emotional roller coaster, your glucose readings may be too.

✔ **Your menstrual cycle:** For some women with diabetes, where they are in their cycle can influence their glucose control. Some women find their glucose readings are higher around the time of their period and some find their readings are lower. Most women don't find much difference.

✔ **Work Schedule:** If you work a variable shift, you may find your readings are prone to fluctuating. As most people with diabetes quickly find out, diabetes loves consistency. Nonetheless, working variable shifts does not make excellent glucose control impossible, just more difficult.

If you are having wide and unpredictable swings in your glucose levels, it is essential that you get in touch with your diabetes educator and dietitian. They may be able to help sort out the reasons for the problem. If not, meeting with your family physician and diabetes specialist would be in order. It is rare indeed that erratic glucose control cannot be improved.

Having a honeymoon — whether or not you're married

The *honeymoon period* is a period of time after the onset of type 1 diabetes when the occasional individual has some recovery of their own pancreatic function and is able to stop giving themselves insulin injections. Typically this lasts for no more than a few weeks or months. All honeymoons are short, including — with rare exceptions — this one.

You're an award winner

Both companies that manufacture insulin in Canada give out awards to celebrate those individuals who have used insulin for 50 years. Eli Lilly (LillyforLife 50-Year Insulin Award) can be reached at 888-545-5972 and NovoNordisk (Novo Nordisk Half Century Award Program) can be reached at 800-465-4334.

Special Issues Regarding Type 2 Diabetes and Insulin Therapy

Unfortunately, insulin therapy for people with type 2 diabetes has typically been looked at as a sign of failure, a last resort greeted with equal parts doom and gloom. (See the anecdote that introduces this chapter.) What a shame! Insulin is simply one more treatment option and, indeed, one that is terribly underused. Goodness knows how many people might have been spared complications if only insulin had been used sooner in the course of their therapy.

The right time for you to start insulin if you have type 2 diabetes is when you cannot achieve appropriate blood glucose control without insulin. For some people that means starting insulin at the time of diagnosis; for others, after years of combined use of two or more oral hypoglycemic agents. The key point is that you and your health care team must always be looking at ways to improve your glucose control. If lifestyle change does the trick, great. If oral agents bring your readings into target, terrific. What we want to avoid is the all too common scenario where the person with diabetes and their physicians spend month after month, year after year, awaiting a magical improvement in glucose control that simply isn't going to happen without insulin administration.

There is no "best" insulin to be on if you have type 2 diabetes; however, most of the time twice-daily therapy with pre-mixed insulin (see Table 12-1) is a good choice. If you are very physically active then a better alternative may be rapid- or fast-acting insulin with your meals along with intermediate-acting insulin at bedtime. Your diabetes educator, family physician and diabetes specialist can help you decide which treatment program is best for you.

Sometimes, it is not an "all or none" strategy when it comes to insulin therapy for people with type 2 diabetes. If you are on oral hypoglycemic agents (see Chapter 11) and your glucose readings are good with the exception of your fasting value (which is likely up due to the dawn phenomenon, which we describe earlier in this chapter), the ideal solution is to continue your oral agents and to add a dose of intermediate-acting insulin (such as NPH) at bedtime. (One possible limitation with this solution is if you are using a TZD — see Chapter 11 — since in Canada it is not yet officially approved for use in combination with insulin.)

It is always worth remembering that for the great majority of people with type 2 diabetes, insulin resistance is a key underlying problem and the importance of adherence to a program of proper nutrition and exercise should never be minimized. It is astounding how often we see people who, despite being on huge doses of insulin and numerous oral hypoglycemic agent pills, are still having problems with glucose control — problems that improve virtually overnight once there has been appropriate dietary change and renewed efforts with exercise.

Donating blood

If you are on oral hypoglycemic agents you are still eligible to donate blood unless some other health problem precludes this. On the other hand, if you are on insulin therapy, the Canadian Blood Services' current policy is that you are not a candidate to give blood. The apparent rationale for this is concern that donating blood could make you feel unwell and in particular could lead to you having an episode of hypoglycemia. This policy is certainly well-intentioned, but we can't help but think it is perhaps unduly cautious.

Travelling with Your Insulin

We live in a mobile society, and if you use insulin, then where you go, your insulin goes too.

Airport security concerns

As you well know, airline security is now greater than ever. And this means you will need to take some additional measures when you are planning on travelling by plane.

Transport Canada has issued guidelines for when you are flying with diabetes supplies. The following information is from the Canadian Diabetes Association's reference to these guidelines:

- Advise the security personnel that you have diabetes and that you are carrying your supplies on board. Have available a letter from your physician indicating that you have diabetes and that you need to carry your diabetes medication and supplies.

- Organize your medication and supplies into one separate container and store it in your carry-on baggage.

- Your syringes must have the needle guards in place and must be accompanied by the insulin.

- Your insulin and any other medications must be in a container with a professionally printed pharmaceutical label identifying the medication. If the pharmaceutical label is on the outside of the box containing the insulin, the insulin must be carried in that original packaging.

- Your lancets must be capped and must be accompanied by a glucose meter imprinted with the manufacturer's name.

- ✔ If you have any difficulty throughout the screening process, you can request to speak to the screening supervisor.
- ✔ If you are travelling outside of Canada, consult with your airline for applicable international regulations.

There are at least three important reasons to take your insulin and supplies (injection devices, glucometer, hypoglycemia treatment, and so on) with you as part of your carry-on (not your checked) luggage:

- ✔ If you are going to London, England, for example, your carry-on luggage is not going to get mistakenly sent to London, Ontario.
- ✔ The baggage compartment temperatures may not be appropriate for your insulin.
- ✔ You will need it!

And although not technically an insulin "supply," make sure you take extra snacks with you on board in case your meals are delayed.

And on the subject of insulin supplies, if you will be travelling for any sort of extended period, make sure you have lots of extra insulin, blood glucose test strips, and so on. Better to have too much than to try finding a pharmacy at midnight in an unfamiliar city.

The Canadian Diabetes Association offers travel insurance to its members.

Adjusting your doses between time zones

Before you travel it would be wise for you to contact your diabetes educator to get advice specific to you, but in *general* terms:

- ✔ If you are heading east (meaning that you will be having a shorter day), you may need to take less insulin.
- ✔ If you are heading west (meaning that you will be having a longer day), you may need to take more insulin.

Travelling seldom causes big problems, especially if you are on a multi-dose treatment program with rapid- or fast-acting insulin taken with meals and intermediate- or long-acting insulin as your basal insulin. Often the best thing to do is to simply take your rapid- or fast-acting insulin at your new mealtimes, regardless of when they happen to be. If there is going to be a significant delay between meals take a snack and a small amount of your rapid- or fast-acting insulin halfway between those meals. Your educator can work out the specifics with you based on precisely how long your flights will be and how many time zones you will be crossing.

The insulin race is on

It may not be the Indy 500, but there is most certainly a race on to develop a way of giving insulin that does not require injections. Many companies are working to come up with a safe and effective product. A variety of techniques are being looked at, including insulin you administer by mouth (a pill, basically), insulin patches you wear, insulin you spray onto the inside of your cheek, insulin you spray into your nose, and, perhaps in the lead, insulin you take into your lungs by using a puffer (similar in concept to puffers used by people who have asthma).

Previous studies have tried (and failed) using insulin eye drops, rectal insulin, and even vaginal insulin. Suffice to say, if there is an orifice, researchers have tried giving insulin into it! Like most new medical products/devices/drugs, everything looks great at first (well, maybe not the rectal or vaginal insulin) and only with time do we find out the true benefits and the true risks.

Insulin injection therapy has been available for 80 or so years. We have a vast amount of knowledge about it. We know how it works. We know its risks and we know its benefits. To have a paradigm shift in the way in which we administer insulin will require doctors like us and persons with diabetes like you to be convinced that the "new and improved" treatment is truly both those things. We discuss new insulin delivery devices further in Chapter 22.

Chapter 13

Alternative and Complementary Therapies

*I*t is estimated that up to half of people with diabetes use some form of alternative or complementary therapy. Alternative and complementary therapy refers to non-traditional treatment, typically offered or recommended by people outside of the mainstream medical community. Suffice to say, a fair bit of controversy surrounds some (but not all) of these treatment options. Some alternative and complementary therapies have been around for many years, while others are fairly recent. In Chapter 10 we look at the role of vitamins and minerals as part of your nutrition plan. In this chapter we look at a variety of other treatments and see what role they may have in helping you with your diabetes.

We strongly recommend that you carefully evaluate non-traditional therapy in the same way that we hope you would consider prescription medication: know what it is supposed to do, what it is *not* supposed to do (that is, side effects), and, most important, whether there are certain health problems that would make it dangerous to take at all. In other words, you need to be an informed consumer. Never assume that because something is "natural" it must be safe. After all, arsenic is natural too.

Because some non-traditional therapies can interact with your prescription drugs, it is essential that you let your physician know if you are taking non-traditional therapies. Bring them (in their original bottles) to your doctors' appointments.

Determining the value of alternative and complementary therapies in managing diabetes is very difficult for several reasons:

- Very few scientific studies have investigated these treatments.

- Potential side effects have not been adequately assessed.

- The strength of non-traditional agents can vary enormously bottle to bottle, even if the label on the bottle says the same thing.

- The purity of non-traditional agents can also vary enormously. One survey of traditional Chinese medicines found potentially toxic substances or potent unlisted ingredients in up to 30 percent of bottles.

- Alternative and complementary therapies have not been required to pass much in the way of government scrutiny, so long as they are marketed as "foods," not drugs. (See the sidebar.) This is a surprise to most people, who think — quite understandably — that a company could not say their product performs in such and such a way without evidence to back their claim.

The new Natural Health Products Regulations

The Canadian government recognized the lack of oversight in alternative therapies and introduced new regulations (Natural Health Products Regulations) governing what are called "natural health products," effective January 1, 2004 (and to be phased in over the next 2 to 6 years). The new Regulations will require better labeling of herbs, vitamins, minerals and homeopathic treatments, and the company selling a product will have to be able to provide evidence that the product can perform as advertised. Companies will now require a product licence to sell "natural health products" in Canada. To get a licence, a company has to provide information regarding the products' medicinal ingredients, source, potency, non-medicinal ingredients, and recommended use. This is marvellous news as it means that patients, physicians, and alternative care practitioners alike will have more and better information available to assist us. (More information on the new Regulations is available at www.hc-sc.gc.ca/hpfb-dgpsa/ nhpddpsn/nhp_regs_e.html).

Aloe Vera

Many of us have applied aloe vera to treat sunburn and it is possible that in the future we will use it to treat diabetes as well. Indeed, in the Arabian Peninsula people ingest a form of aloe vera for this purpose. The inner portion of the aloe plant's leaves contains a type of fibre. If aloe vera reduces blood glucose levels, it could be because of this fibre. (We discuss the role of fibre in the treatment of diabetes in Chapter 10.) As with so many alternative and complementary therapies, we do not know if it is truly effective, but there is some evidence that it might be.

Coccinia Indica (Ivy Gourd)

Coccinia indica is a wild plant found in the India subcontinent. There are indications that it may be helpful in reducing blood glucose levels. So far, there have been no reports of adverse effects.

Fenugreek (Trigonella Foenum Graecum)

Fenugreek is a legume grown in India, the Mediterranean, and North Africa. Its use in treating diabetes goes back many centuries, and there is some evidence that it may be effective in reducing blood glucose levels. Once again, this is preliminary information.

Garlic

Garlic is used for many purposes. Sometimes, it is even used for cooking! There has been a suggestion that garlic could help lower glucose levels, though the evidence for this is contradictory. We can only hope that garlic does turn out to be helpful at lowering glucose levels; can you imagine the recipe possibilities? Garlic ice cream, garlic cheesecake . . . the list is endless. Anyone for a garlic brownie?

There is some evidence that garlic may increase your risk of bleeding during or after surgery. If you are going to be having surgery or if you are on blood thinners, be sure to speak to your doctor before you start taking garlic supplements.

Ginseng

Although we usually speak of ginseng as being one product, in fact there are several different plant species that share this name. There is Chinese or Korean ginseng as well as Siberian, American, and Japanese varieties. *American* ginseng has been found to improve glucose control to a small but significant degree; however, these observations must be considered preliminary (hopeful, but preliminary nonetheless).

Glucosamine

Glucosamine, a product derived from the outside skeleton of shellfish (such as crabs and shrimps) is commonly used to treat arthritis pain, not diabetes, but as it is used as an alternative therapy we thought it opportune to mention it here. There is some evidence that glucosamine can worsen insulin resistance and, as a result, could worsen your blood glucose control. Whether or not this happens to any significant degree remains to be proven. Because there are concerns that glucosamine could adversely affect your diabetes, the prudent thing would be to avoid it until we have more evidence about its safety.

Gymnema Sylvestre

Gymnema sylvestre is a tropical plant found in central and southern India. In Hindi, it goes by the name "destroyer of sugar," based on folklore that chewing the leaves results in the inability to taste sweet things. That, of course, would suggest that if it was effective in treating diabetes, it would be because it wrecks your appetite for dessert (maybe even for those garlic brownies we talked about earlier), but no, there is some *preliminary* evidence that, apart from suppressing appetite, it has the ability to reduce blood glucose levels; possibly by improving beta cell function.

"Pancreas Formula"

Pancreas formula is sold on the Internet as a mixture of herbs, vitamins, and minerals that help diabetes. No clinical or experimental evidence shows that pancreas formula does anything of value in the human body. Factual evidence does not support the claims that are made for this "treatment." The true *formula* here may simply be one that allows the sellers to get rich at others' expense.

Tea

There are three types of tea: green, oolong, and black. A recent study found that oolong tea consumption significantly reduced blood glucose levels. If you are going to try this, however, you had best *really* like oolong tea, because the test subjects drank 1.5 litres of it daily. Also, not all oolong tea is the same. In the study they used the variety found in China (because it is more strongly fermented). If further studies find oolong tea to be beneficial in controlling blood glucose levels, we may soon be recommending tea for two — 2 million Canadians with diabetes that is.

Vanadium

Vanadium is a mineral that is sometimes called a "non-essential nutrient." There is some hopeful data that it may assist with reducing glucose levels, but most people who have taken it during scientific studies ran into problems with nausea, flatulence, and diarrhea.

Laughter

You may have noticed that this chapter has been organized alphabetically. Except that is, for this little section on laughter. We thought we would save the best for last (you know what they say about the person who laughs last). A recent article in a major diabetes medical journal showed that doctors should perhaps be prescribing laughter — and we're not just talking Patch Adams here. Japanese researchers looked at a group of people with type 2 diabetes and assessed their blood glucose levels after the participants listened to a 40-minute lecture that was described by the researches as being "monotonous" and "without humorous intent." (Oh my, shades of medical school!) The next day these same subjects' blood glucose levels were measured after watching a comedy show. Well, you probably already figured out the punch line: the blood glucose levels were lower when the participants watched the comedy show than when they listened to the boring lecture. And that's no laughing matter. Then again, maybe that is exactly what it is.

The Bottom Line

Because of the limited scientific information available to guide our decision making, if you are considering taking an alternative or complementary therapy you will have to make your decision based as much on hope as on science. That is fine, of course, if we know the product has no potential for harm, but in the same way that we do not know about all the benefits that some remedies may hold, we do not know about all the potential downsides they may have. Thus, caution is required.

People with diabetes are not the only ones that need to consider both the good and the bad in complementary or alternative therapy. Their doctors too need to remain open-minded. Indeed, many drugs that doctors currently prescribe were discovered in nature, including antibiotics, potent anti-cancer drugs, and even aspirin — yes, that very aspirin that, interestingly, most doctors are now advising many people with diabetes to take. Ain't that something?

Miracle cures for diabetes

In your travels — especially of the cyber kind — you likely have come across promotions for products that are said to be a "miracle cure" for diabetes. We are all tempted by come-ons for products that seem to be the "magic bullet" for what ails us. But these magic bullets are more likely to be poison darts. The fraudulent nature of these false claims is clear if you watch for certain common themes to the promotions:

✔ A reliance on personal testimonials rather than hard science. Anecdotes are not proof of the value of a treatment or test. The favourable experiences of one or a few people are not a substitute for a scientific study. If they did seem to respond to the drug, it may be for entirely different reasons.

✔ References to scientific studies or journals that sound impressive and legitimate, but in fact are pseudo-scientific, obscure sources that cannot be readily reviewed to verify their accuracy.

✔ Lofty claims of benefit far surpassing any other available treatment.

✔ Allusions to conspiracies amongst the medical community in hiding something from the public.

One day there will be a cure for diabetes. And every person with diabetes will find out about it because every person in the diabetes health care field will be shouting with joy at the top of our lungs. You'll hear us. We guarantee it.

Part IV
Special Considerations for Living with Diabetes

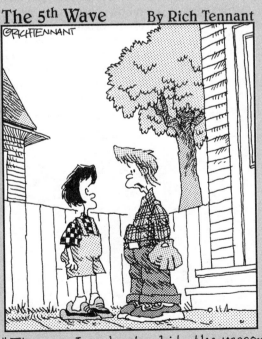

The 5th Wave   By Rich Tennant

"The way I understand it, the reason I was getting cold and tired was because my body wasn't making enough insulation."

In this part . . .

Diabetes in a child or an elderly individual poses special challenges and requires special management. In this part we look at the unique challenges that these groups have to contend with. Aboriginal communities have to tackle some special issues of their own, as you will discover. We also look at some very practical issues that confront people with diabetes, including employment, insurance, and driving. Those whose preferred means of locomotion is at the controls of an airborne vehicle will find answers to questions about piloting here.

Chapter 14

Your Child Has Diabetes

*W*hen a child has diabetes, it is a concern. When your child has diabetes, you may see it as a disaster. In this chapter we look at how you can keep your child healthy and prevent diabetes from ruling their life, and yours. You will find out how to manage diabetes in your child at each stage of growth and development from infancy up to and including early adulthood. And as we look at these issues, remember that you are not to blame for your child's diabetes. You did not cause it. And you should never have to feel guilty about it.

Your Baby or Preschooler Has Type 1 Diabetes

Although type 1 diabetes does not usually show up in babies, it can, and you should know what to expect when it does. Obviously, your baby is not verbal and cannot tell you what is bothering him or her. For this reason, you may miss the fact that your baby is constantly thirsty and urinating excessively in his or her diaper. The baby will lose weight and have vomiting and diarrhea, but this may understandably be attributed to a stomach disorder rather than diabetes. When the doctor finally makes the diagnosis, your baby may be very sick and require a stay in a pediatric intensive care unit. Do not blame yourself for not realizing that your baby was sick.

Once you have the diagnosis, the hard work begins. You must immediately learn to give insulin injections and to test the blood glucose in a child who will be reluctant to have either one done. You have to learn when and what to feed your baby to satisfy the child's appetite, to encourage growth and development, and to prevent low blood glucose.

At this stage, we are not aiming for tight blood glucose control. (Up to the age of 5, target pre-meal readings are 6.0 to 12.0 mmol/L; target A1C is as high as 9 percent.) Moreover, you must exercise extreme caution to avoid hypoglycemia. There are several reasons for this. First, the baby's neurological system is still developing. Frequent, severe low blood glucose will damage this development, so the glucose is permitted to be higher now than later on. Second, studies show that changes associated with high blood glucose leading to diabetic complications are not as critical until just before puberty, so you have a grace period during which you can allow your baby to have less tight control.

On the other hand, a small baby is fragile. Small losses of water, sodium, potassium, and other substances can rapidly lead to a very sick baby.

Here are some of the things you will need to know:

- ✔ How to identify the signs and symptoms of hyperglycemia, hypoglycemia, and diabetic ketoacidosis (see Chapters 4 and 5)

- ✔ How to administer insulin (see Chapter 12)

- ✔ How to measure the blood glucose and ketones (see Chapter 9)

- ✔ How to treat hypoglycemia, and how and when to use glucagon (see Chapter 5)

- ✔ How to properly nourish your child (Chapter 10 talks about general nutrition principles, but of course with a child this young you will need to get very detailed advice from a dietician.)

- ✔ What to do when your child is sick with another illness (see later in this chapter)

Your responsibilities as the parent of a baby or preschooler with diabetes are extensive and time-consuming, and the preceding list may seem rather daunting. But you can do it. Indeed, you must. But you should never feel you are in this alone. You should train family members and friends who can help out, even for a short time. Otherwise, you may end up feeling constantly emotionally and physically exhausted (as if being a parent isn't hard enough to begin with!).

Keeping in regular contact with a diabetes education centre is crucial if you have a child, especially an infant, with diabetes. A diabetes educator and dietitian can provide invaluable assistance. Also, these centres may allow you to access additional services such as that of a social worker, should it be necessary. Be aware that not all diabetes education centres specialize in children with type 1 diabetes, so ask them if this is their particular area of expertise; if it is not, they will gladly refer you to a centre that has this expertise. You should also have a pediatrician who has particular expertise in looking after young children with diabetes. Your family physician can refer you. If your family doctor is not familiar with one, your diabetes educator will certainly be able to recommend someone to you and your family doctor.

Your other children may resent the attention that you pay to this one child. If your other children start to misbehave, this may be the reason.

Diagnosing diabetes in your preschooler may be just as difficult as diagnosing it in the baby. The child is still running around in diapers, and may still be pre-verbal.

Preschoolers are beginning the process of separating from their parents and starting to learn to control the environment (by becoming toilet-trained, for example). This separation process makes it more difficult for you, the parent, to give the injections and test the glucose. You must be firm in insisting that these things be done. You'll need to do them yourself, of course, because a small child neither knows how to do them nor understands what to do with the information generated by the glucose meter.

Because a child's eating habits may not be very regular, the use of rapid-acting insulin (see Chapter 12) taken *after* meals is often helpful. You can first see how much of the meal your child ate and then give an amount of insulin based on that. Be sure to speak to your diabetes educator about this option.

Your Primary School Child Has Type 1 Diabetes

In some ways, managing diabetes gets a little easier with a primary school child, but in other ways, it gets more difficult. Your child can finally tell you when he or she has symptoms of hypoglycemia, so this is easier to recognize and treat. But you must begin to control the blood glucose more carefully because your child is reaching the stage where tighter control becomes necessary.

Your child is still growing and developing, so nutrition remains very important. You must provide enough of the right kinds of nutrients for this process.

When children go to school, they interact with other children and want to fit in. Children with diabetes may consider their condition a stigma. They may be very reluctant to share the fact of their diabetes with other children, or they may have told their friends and found that other children did not know how to handle the information. This is where your newfound expertise with diabetes can be invaluable as you can educate your child's friends about diabetes. You may need to speak to your child's friends' parents as well.

As time goes on, your child is going to separate from you further. He or she may insist on giving the insulin shots and doing the blood tests. Although you should encourage your child's involvement in these tasks, full duties for these should not be relegated to your child. Your ongoing supervision is important to ensure that things are being done properly. You should also be aware that because your child may feel uncomfortable letting peers know about the diabetes, he or she may avoid glucose testing and insulin administration when friends are around. In this circumstance, fast food may also tend to replace proper, healthy nutrition on a too frequent basis.

For children ages 5 to 12, target pre-meal blood glucose readings are 4.0 to 10.0 mmol/L and target A1C is 8 or less. The higher end of this target range is suitable for a 5-year-old, but you should aim for the lower end as your child advances through this age range. Because you are aiming for tighter control for children in this age range, hypoglycemia is more of a risk, especially at night. You can reduce the risk of hypoglycemia by taking any or all of the following steps:

- ✔ Give your child a bedtime snack. (A snack made with cornstarch is particularly helpful. Since cornstarch breaks down slowly, it provides glucose over a longer period of time.)

- ✔ Measure your child's blood glucose at bedtime and increase the amount of the bedtime snack if the glucose level is under target.

- ✔ Occasionally check your child's blood glucose at 3 a.m.

- ✔ Ask your child whether he or she has symptoms of nighttime low blood glucose, such as nightmares, headaches, and unexplained sweating.

- ✔ Be sure your child does not skip meals or scheduled snacks.

- ✔ Have your child check his or her blood glucose before exercising and, if below target, take extra carbohydrate according to the planned duration and intensity of exercise.

- ✔ If your child tends to not finish meals, speak to your diabetes educator about using rapid-acting insulin after meals, rather than taking it before meals. (We discuss insulin therapy in Chapter 12.)

Mature siblings and, of course, both parents should be aware of symptoms of hypoglycemia and know how to treat it (including knowing how and when to use glucagon). We discuss these issues in Chapter 5.

Seeing as your child spends so much time in school, it is essential that this environment be set up suitably. Schoolmates will likely not have much, if any, knowledge of diabetes and it is quite possible that your child's teacher may have only limited experience as well. As most any minority group member knows, overcoming ignorance is the surest way to prevent or undo stigmatization. For this reason as well as for reasons of safety and practicality we encourage you to meet with your child's teacher and the appropriate administrative people within the school to review issues such as these:

- ✔ When blood glucose monitoring will need to be done and whether your child will need assistance/supervision with this task. This discussion should also include where testing will take place and where lancets will be disposed of.

- ✔ When insulin is to be administered and whether your child will need assistance/supervision with this task.

- ✔ When your child is to eat meals (preferably with the rest of the class) and snacks. Younger children will require supervision (and no, not simply to make sure that food fights aren't about to break out! Rather, it is important to make sure they are actually ingesting the wonderful nutrients that are on their plate and in their glass).

- ✔ How to recognize and treat hypoglycemia, including, importantly, knowing how and when to use a glucagon kit.

- ✔ How to recognize hyperglycemia and what to do in the event that they suspect it. (Calling you — the parent — is an appropriate first step *if* your child is feeling perfectly well. But, if your child is *at all* unwell, the safest and best thing for the school to do is to immediately call an ambulance.)

- ✔ The need to allow your child to have a water bottle at his or her desk and to have permission to freely leave the classroom to go to the bathroom.

There is no reason that your child should not be able to participate in any and all school activities, including academics, sports, and field trips. This will require additional expertise, however, on the part of school officials and chaperones. Once again, you, the parent, can help out by teaching them what you yourself have already learned.

Your diabetes educator can serve as an invaluable resource in helping you familiarize your child's teacher and, most important, schoolmates about diabetes and how it affects your child. For example, Ian is blessed to work with wonderful diabetes educators (at the Charles H. Best Diabetes Centre for Children and Youth; www.charleshbest.com) who, in addition to their already myriad duties, have developed a school program where they will visit a child's school and give class presentations. This has been an overwhelming success. Ask your child's diabetes educator if they would consider doing the same. If they would like, have them call the Best Centre (905-666-7796) to learn more about the program.

Your Adolescent Has Type 1 Diabetes

Your adolescent with diabetes will provide some of your biggest challenges. (As if adolescence isn't tough enough even when you have perfect health.) The adolescent *can* achieve tight blood glucose control at this age, but it certainly is not easy. To have excellent control requires a high degree of adherence to proper lifestyle therapy (nutrition and exercise), and regular attention to glucose monitoring and insulin adjustment. As you can imagine, most adolescents, eagerly seeking independence and "freedom," would not be thrilled with this. (And who could blame them?) Yet, for all of that, adolescence and the teenage years do not have to mean that diabetes gets neglected.

Once your child reaches 13 years of age, target pre-meal blood glucose levels are 4.0 to 7.0 mmol/L, A1C 7 or less. When it can be safely achieved, we aim for even lower blood glucose (pre-meal target of 4.0 to 6.0) and A1C (6 or less) values. See Chapter 9 for a further discussion on this topic.

The hormonal changes that occur in puberty can result in worsening of glucose control; however, this can be compensated for by appropriate adjustment of insulin therapy. And speaking of hormonal changes, it is essential that adolescent girls be made aware of issues surrounding contraception and sexual health. Unintended pregnancy in an adolescent is always a problem; unintended pregnancy in an adolescent with diabetes is even more of a problem. Appropriate members of the health care team should address these concerns. We discuss diabetes and pregnancy in Chapter 7.

There are many ways you can help your adolescent child with his or her diabetes:

✔ Make sure that they know you have certain expectations — expectations born of love and concern — in terms of their management of the diabetes.

✔ Be supportive and understanding — even when they go through periods when they are less attentive to their diabetes than they should be. On the other hand, you want your child to know that you are far from indifferent to their inattention. Encouragement often works better than being authoritative or dictatorial (though, of course, these measures also have their occasional role, as any parent knows).

✔ Remind them that they need never be "ashamed" of diabetes. In its very essence, it is a simple shortage of a hormone. What shame is there in that?

✔ Keep an eye out for evidence of insulin omission. Teenage girls not infrequently skip insulin doses (with consequent hyperglycemia) because they have learned that it results in weight loss. (Also, see the tip below.)

✔ Review their blood glucose levels and assist them with insulin adjustment.

✔ As your child grows, gradually transfer responsibility for looking after the diabetes — based on your child's ability and interest — to your child. This may be the most important way in which you can help them in the long term. It is not an abdication of your responsibility, but the fulfillment of your ultimate responsibility: creating a responsible, mature individual who is able to look after him- or herself independently. (This is often the toughest task on this list to carry out.)

Up to ten percent of teenage girls (and some teenage boys) with diabetes have an eating disorder (such as anorexia nervosa or bulimia). This can result in malnutrition and, usually, poor blood glucose control. The child may deny that the problem exists. If your adolescent has erratic glucose control, the possibility of an eating disorder should be considered and discussed with the child and the child's doctor.

Sometimes, adolescents will share things with their diabetes educator that they may not so readily share with you, even though they know you love them dearly and care about their health. Indeed, diabetes educators often say that children of this age will spend the entirety of their first visit talking about everything in their lives *except* the specifics of their diabetes. But that is in no way a shortcoming. To help children with their diabetes it is essential to know them as people first, and people with diabetes second. Diabetes is, after all, but one component of their existence (and one they want to be far from front and centre). A diabetes educator who knows "how the adolescent ticks" will be in a far better position to know how best to help with the diabetes.

Your Young Adult Child Has Type 1 Diabetes

By the time your child reaches his or her late teens, he or she is a young adult and should be the one in charge of the diabetes. But even then, your son or daughter should not lack a support system.

Regrettably, what often happens is that teenagers "graduate" from a pediatric diabetes program (where they have started to feel very out of place as they sit amongst the younger — and smaller — children in the waiting room) and fail to hook up with an adult program or with an adult diabetes specialist. They "fall through the gaps" and it can take many years (all the while without proper supervision or guidance and without adequately controlled diabetes) before they end up seeking help. The single most important thing you can do to assist young adults is to find out if they have had their care transferred to an adult diabetes specialist and adult diabetes education centre *that has a special program for type 1 diabetes*, and to encourage them to establish these contacts if they have not done so.

Screening Tests for Organ Injury in Children and Adolescents with Type 1 Diabetes

The Canadian Diabetes Association recommends the following testing schedule for children with type 1 diabetes (see Chapter 6 for a detailed discussion on organ injury and how to test for it):

- ✔ **Kidney Testing:** At the onset of puberty (then annually), a first morning urine sample should be tested for albumin/creatinine ratio ("ACR") if your child has had diabetes for at least 5 years. Post-pubertal children should be tested yearly once they have had diabetes for 5 years.

- ✔ **Eye Testing:** At the age of 15 (then at least annually) your child should have an eye examination if he or she has had diabetes for at least 5 years.

- ✔ **Nerve Testing:** At the onset of puberty (then annually) your child should have his or her feet tested for the ability to feel a vibrating tuning fork or a thin nylon rod (a "10 gram monofilament") if he or she has had diabetes for at least 5 years. These painless tests can be done in the doctor's office and take but a moment to perform.

✔ **Lipids:** Testing of your child's lipids (including cholesterol and triglycerides) is required only if there is some additional risk factor present for cardiovascular disease.

✔ **Blood Pressure:** Your child's blood pressure should be checked routinely from the time diabetes is diagnosed.

Sick Day Solutions for Your Child with Type 1 Diabetes

Children with type 1 diabetes are susceptible to all the usual childhood illnesses, but diabetes complicates their care. An illness can affect glucose levels in opposite ways. An infection may increase the level of insulin resistance so that the usual dose of insulin is not adequate. Or it may cause nausea and vomiting so that no food or drink can stay down, and the insulin may cause hypoglycemia. For this reason, when your child is ill you will need to measure his or her blood glucose and ketone levels (see Chapter 9 for a discussion of meters that measure blood glucose and ketones) as often as every 2 to 4 hours. If the blood glucose levels are significantly elevated (above 12 mmol/L or so), the child may require additional rapid- or fast-acting insulin.

If your child's blood glucose levels are elevated — especially if ketones are present in the blood (0.6 mmol/L or higher) — the safest thing to do is to have your child promptly taken to the emergency department of the hospital. However, if you are fortunate enough to be working with a diabetes nurse educator that is both trained — *and* empowered — to deal with DKA *and* is immediately available, you can first contact him or her for detailed advice regarding the right type of fluids your child should take and how to properly adjust your child's insulin. Often times, with this type of intensive management, visits to hospital can be avoided. It is very important to be aware that there are *very few* educators that have this degree of expertise *and* authority. You should discuss these issues with both your educator and your diabetes specialist before your child gets sick so you will know what to do if and when your child becomes unwell.

The fact your child is not eating well does *not* necessarily mean that less insulin is required; Depending on blood glucose levels, he or she may need *more* insulin than usual.

Summer Camps for Children with Type 1 Diabetes

One resource that can be tremendously valuable for you and your child with type 1 diabetes is a diabetes summer camp. These Canadian Diabetes Association (CDA) camps are located in a variety of regions across Canada and provide a safe, well-managed place where your child can go and be in the majority. He or she can learn a great deal about diabetes while enjoying all the pleasures of a summer camp environment. (Certainly not a minor benefit is the opportunity for you to have time off for perhaps the first time in years.) A listing of diabetes summer camps is available on the Canadian Diabetes Association Web site (www.diabetes.ca) or by phoning the CDA (800-226-8464).

All CDA camps offer assistance with camp fees. The CDA advises that you contact the camp nearest you for more information.

Of course, you may be looking at sending your child to a regular day camp program. This is perfectly reasonable, but some advance planning is important. In particular, it would be wise to do the following:

- Speak to the camp director to make sure the camp can safely accommodate your child.

- Find out if the camp has a nurse on site.

- Arrange for your child to have a mature counsellor.

- Meet with the counsellor before the start of camp to make sure he or she has the necessary knowledge to look after your child. In particular, talk about how to deal with hypoglycemia and, especially, how and when to use a glucagon kit.

- Make sure that your child will receive the necessary snacks (and, of course, meals) at the appropriate times.

- Send a kit of important supplies with your child to camp. The kit should include glucose monitoring equipment, snacks, a glucagon kit, and, if your child will need to give insulin during the day, necessary insulin supplies.

- Make sure other staff — such as swim instructors and lifeguards — know that your child has diabetes.

- Find out if the camp has had other children in the past — or currently — who have had diabetes. If so, consider speaking to their parents to find out if things went well or, if not, why not.

- Ensure that your child wears a medical alert bracelet.

Your diabetes educator may have experience with regular day camps that have looked after children with diabetes. Give your educator a call and ask.

Your Child Has Type 2 Diabetes

The epidemic of obesity, which has spread to children in Canada (and elsewhere) in the past few decades, has led to a much higher prevalence of type 2 diabetes in children than has ever been seen before. Indeed, up to 25 percent (or, in some communities, considerably more) of children with diabetes have type 2 diabetes. This was virtually unheard of until recently.

The Canadian Diabetes Association recommends that obese children 10 years of age or older be considered for screening for type 2 diabetes every 2 years if they meet two or more of the following criteria:

- Are a member of a high-risk population group (Aboriginal, Hispanic, South Asian, Asian, or African descent)
- Have a family history of type 2 diabetes
- Have acanthosis nigricans (see Chapter 6)
- Have polycystic ovary syndrome (this is a condition associated with insulin resistance; see Chapter 4)
- Have high blood pressure
- Have abnormal lipids

Like children with type 1 diabetes, those with type 2 diabetes may be afraid of being stigmatized, and so may neglect the health issue so he or she can "be like everyone else" when it comes to eating, watching television, and so forth.

The key differences that suggest a child has type 2 rather than type 1 diabetes are as follows:

- Obesity
- Belonging to certain high-risk population groups (see above)
- A family history of type 2 diabetes
- No evidence of autoimmunity (see Chapter 4)
- Extremely rare ketoacidosis (see Chapter 5)
- Having acanthosis nigricans
- Evidence of ongoing insulin production in the body, as shown by a C-peptide level in the blood that is normal or elevated (C-peptide is made every time insulin is produced, so its presence indicates that the body is making insulin.)

The first therapy for a child with type 2 diabetes is intensive lifestyle measures (diet, weight control, exercise) however pills (in particular, metformin; see Chapter 11) and insulin may be necessary. The metformin can be withdrawn once the benefits of lifestyle measures have taken effect. Sometimes, even when insulin is used early in the course of diabetes, it can also subsequently be withdrawn.

You *must* help your obese child to lose weight, because most obese children will become obese adults. With the assistance of a dietitian, you can figure out the food that your child can eat to maintain growth and development without inappropriate weight gain. One of the most helpful techniques is to take the child into the supermarket and point out the difference between unhealthy foods (such as those rich in fat) and those that are nourishing. Another is never to use foods such as cake and candy as rewards. Finally, if you keep problem foods out of the house, there is much less likelihood that your child will eat them.

If your child with type 2 diabetes becomes unwell, you need to be sure that he or she is drinking enough liquids. Clear liquids (like tea and caffeine-free soft drinks) are usually best. As long as your child can hold down clear liquids, you can generally continue to take care of him or her — unless the blood glucose level is particularly high or your child is very unwell, in which case you will need to seek medical attention. If your child cannot keep down even clear fluids — in which case dehydration becomes a real concern — you will need to visit a hospital.

Your Child Has MODY

An unusual type of childhood diabetes goes by the name MODY, which stands for *m*aturity-*o*nset *d*iabetes of the *y*oung. This is a genetic condition leading to diabetes that has some features of type 1 diabetes and some features of type 2 diabetes. For example, affected children are not obese on the one hand, yet are not prone to ketoacidosis on the other. There are several forms of MODY and the treatment will depend on which of these types is present.

Although the term "MODY" remains in common use, it is being phased out in lieu of the names of the specific genetic defects present in the various types (for example, "Chromosome 20, HNF-4alpha" is the new name for "MODY1"). "MODY" may be not be as scientifically precise, but it sure is a heck of a lot easier to say (and remember)!

Chapter 15

Diabetes and the Elderly

*E*veryone wants to live a long time, but no one wants to get old. Nevertheless, as someone once said, getting old is better than the alternative! Woody Allen says the one advantage of dying is that you don't have to do jury duty. We think we would rather do jury duty.

Defining *elderly* is the first problem. Although some medical studies have defined elderly as being as young as 60 (egads!), and although we find that every year our definition seems to change, it's probably fair to say that about the age of 70 is the beginning of "elderly." By that definition, by the year 2020, more than 20 percent of the Canadian population will be elderly. And one-fifth or more of that group will have developed diabetes.

Elderly people with diabetes have special problems. They're hospitalized at a rate that is 70 percent higher than that of the general elderly population. Even without hospitalization, elderly people with diabetes have special problems. In this chapter, you find out about those problems and the best ways to handle them.

It is important to recognize that age by itself does not automatically create additional diabetes management difficulties. It is age *together with* failing physical or mental health that is responsible. An 80-year-old tennis-playing, bridge-tournament-winning, semi-retired engineer may be far better able to manage diabetes than a 60-year-old who has had two strokes and is confined to bed.

Diagnosing Diabetes in the Elderly

Like so much else in the world of medicine there is both debate and uncertainty (perhaps the one never exists without the other) about why diabetes becomes increasingly likely as we get older. It has been suggested that aging itself leads to diabetes, but it may well be that it is not so much the number of *years* we have under our belt that causes diabetes, but the number of *inches* under our belt. That, of course, is a very encouraging piece of news because it means that if we can keep our weight under control as we get older, we can help to protect ourselves from developing diabetes.

Depending on their mental functioning, elderly people who have developed hyperglycemia may or may not recognize the onset of typical symptoms such as increased urination and greater thirst. Instead, their main symptoms may be loss of appetite, weight loss, confusion, incontinence of urine, or weakness and lethargy. Because symptoms like weakness and lethargy are so non-specific, the cause can initially go unrecognized. And a doctor or patient may easily (and understandably) attribute urinary incontinence to prostate problems in elderly men or bladder problems in older women. (We have yet to see an elderly woman diagnosed as having an enlarged prostate!)

Evaluating Intellectual Functioning

Knowing the intellectual functioning of an elderly person with diabetes is extremely important because managing the disease requires a number of different skills. The patient has to follow a special diet, administer medications properly, and test the blood glucose. Studies have shown that elderly people with diabetes have a higher incidence of *dementia* (loss of mental functioning) than non-diabetics, making it much harder for them to perform those tasks.

If necessary, a physician can formally assess an elderly person's mental functioning by administering certain types of tests. If necessary, psychologists can conduct even more sophisticated testing. Testing makes it easier to tell whether the patient can be self-sufficient or will need help. Many older people now living alone with no assistance are a danger to themselves and would benefit from an assisted-living situation. Elderly people are often fiercely independent and — as millions of members of the "sandwich" generation know — changing their living situation can be very difficult.

Preparing a Proper Diet

In addition to the intellectual function required to understand and prepare a proper diabetic diet (see the preceding section), the elderly have other problems when it comes to proper nutrition:

- They may have poor vision and be unable to see to read or cook.
- They may have low income and be unable to purchase the foods that they require.
- Their ability to taste and smell may be decreased, so they lose interest in food.
- They often have a loss of appetite. This is especially likely if they live alone after the loss of a spouse or if they are depressed.
- They may have arthritis or a tremor that makes cooking more difficult.
- They may have poor teeth or a dry mouth, either of which make it more difficult to eat.

Any one of these problems may be enough to prevent proper eating, and as a result, their nutrition and, ultimately, their general health may suffer.

Dealing with Eye Problems

Elderly people with diabetes are more prone to eye problems that people without diabetes can also get, including cataracts, macular degeneration, and glaucoma. And they also are at risk of eye disease unique to diabetes: diabetic retinopathy. (See Chapter 6 for more information on these eye problems.)

Many elderly people do not receive the eye care they require. It is essential that everyone with diabetes — especially the elderly who can have a whole variety of different eye problems — see an eye specialist routinely. Removal of a cataract — a simple outpatient procedure nowadays — may make all the difference in the world.

Coping with Urinary and Sexual Problems

Urinary and sexual problems are very common in elderly people with diabetes and greatly affect quality of life. It is not uncommon for an older person with diabetes to have paralysis of the bladder muscle with retention of urine, followed by overflow incontinence when the bladder fills up. An older person may be unable to get to the bathroom fast enough. A chronically distended bladder can also lead to frequent urinary tract infections.

Almost 60 percent of men over the age of 70 have erectile dysfunction, and 50 percent have no *libido* (desire to have sex). The elderly take an average of seven medications daily, some of which may affect sexual function. Many elderly women with diabetes also experience sexual dysfunction. The causes for sexual dysfunction in both men and women are discussed in Chapter 7.

To have sex at any age, you need sexual desire and the physical ability to perform, you need a willing partner, and you need a safe, private place. For the elderly, any or all of these may be missing.

It is not always necessary to treat sexual dysfunction if you and your partner are okay with the situation as it is. If not, however, there are a number of effective therapies available (see Chapter 7).

There is a regrettable tendency for elderly people to be seen as asexual — even by members of the medical profession who should know better. For this reason you may have to take the initiative and bring up the issue of your sexual difficulties when you visit your physician.

Considering Treatment for High Blood Glucose

Goals for a very elderly, debilitated person with diabetes with a short life expectancy will be different from those of a person with diabetes who is elderly but physiologically young and could live for 15 or 20 more years. A person who has lived to age 65 has a life expectancy of at least 18 more years — plenty of time to develop complications of diabetes.

In a broad sense, blood glucose control in an elderly person has two main objectives. You can aim to maintain blood glucose levels in a range that will keep you free of symptoms of hyperglycemia (under 10 mmol/L or so) or you can aim for blood glucose levels that will minimize your risk of developing complications (under 8 mmol/L or so). The former is an appropriate target in an elderly person with a limited life expectancy and for whom any undue restrictions are inappropriate and, indeed, perhaps even cruel. The latter is appropriate if life expectancy and life quality are good.

Treatment always starts with proper nutrition and exercise, but an elderly person with diabetes may have limited ability to exercise. An elderly person who *can* exercise will derive many benefits from it, including improved blood glucose control, better blood pressure and lipids, and, importantly, a better sense of well-being. Because elderly patients have more coronary artery disease, arthritis, eye disease, neuropathy, and peripheral vascular disease, for some individuals exercise may not be possible. (See Chapter 10 for more on lifestyle therapy.)

Because nutrition is often not as robust or complete in elderly individuals, unless you are sure you are eating very well (see Chapter 10), it would be a good idea for you to take a daily multivitamin.

If lifestyle therapy with diet and exercise (see Chapter 10) have been found inadequate in controlling blood glucose levels, then oral hypoglycemic agents (see Chapter 11) or insulin (see Chapter 12) become necessary. This is complicated by a number of considerations special to the elderly:

- The patient may not be able to see the correct dosage.
- The patient may be mentally unable to take the medicine properly.
- Physical limitations may prevent the patient from taking medication, especially insulin.
- Patients often have decreased kidney function, making some drugs last longer.
- Poor nutrition may make the patient more prone to hypoglycemia.

For all these reasons, it is essential that you use the appropriate type and dose of therapy. Your physician will need to take into account these various factors in selecting a drug. Most important of all in an elderly person with compromised mental functioning (and therefore, less ability to detect and treat low blood glucose) is avoiding hypoglycemia.

Like younger people with diabetes, the elderly have several choices when it comes to selecting the best medicine to reduce blood glucose levels. There are also certain factors that may make one drug superior to another:

- ✔ If you are lean, a medicine that stimulates your pancreas to produce insulin would be a good choice. Because of their lesser likelihood of causing hypoglycemia, gliclazide (Diamicron) or glimepiride (Amaryl) are usually better choices than glyburide (Diabeta) for elderly individuals.

- ✔ If you are obese, a TZD (such as Actos or Avandia) is a suitable choice so long as your heart function is good and you keep a close eye out for evidence of fluid retention (such as the development of swollen ankles). Metformin therapy can be used, so long as you have good heart, liver, and kidney function and are not at significant risk of developing dehydration or other serious illness.

- ✔ If you have irregular eating habits, a good choice is an oral hypoglycemic agent that is taken only with meals and is short-acting (and so is not as likely as some longer-acting oral agents — like glyburide — to cause hypglycemia). Repaglinide (GlucoNorm) is one such drug.

- ✔ If you require insulin, the usual preferred approach — as it minimizes dosage errors — is to give a pre-mixed insulin with an insulin pen device.

As you can see, there are a number of factors to consider. It is important to note that despite some obstacles, *every* elderly person with diabetes can treat their blood glucose control successfully (even if not easily).

Remember too the importance of appropriate blood pressure and lipid control, which, among other helpful things, reduces the risk of heart attack.

Chapter 16

Diabetes in Aboriginal Peoples

● ●

In This Chapter

▶ Investigating the growing problem of diabetes in Aboriginal peoples

▶ Combatting diabetes in Aboriginal peoples

● ●

A boriginal peoples in Canada include First Nations, Inuit, and Métis populations. Although type 2 diabetes has become increasingly prevalent in all communities across Canada, the problem has reached truly epidemic proportions among Aboriginal peoples, with rates in some age groups as high as one out of every four people. Aboriginal leaders are tackling the challenge head-on, however, by rapidly developing and implementing strategies to deal with it. This chapter looks at the main elements of the problem and the solutions that Aboriginal leaders are pursuing.

Why Are Aboriginal Peoples More Prone to Diabetes?

No one knows definitively why certain groups of people are more prone to develop diabetes, but that they *are* more prone is not in question. Aboriginal communities throughout the world have been beset with rapidly rising rates of diabetes. Whether in Australia, South America, North America, or elsewhere, the trend has been the same. Given the widespread nature of the problem, clearly there must be a common thread. The leading proposal is what is termed the *thrifty gene hypothesis*.

As we discuss in Chapter 4, the thrifty gene hypothesis maintains that over the course of many generations, peoples that have lived without a consistent food supply may have genetically evolved a protective mechanism wherein they are able to use carbohydrates in a very efficient way metabolically. Thus, when food is scarce, they are protected. The unfortunate flip side to this is that when food is plentiful, their bodies end up readily storing the extra calories as fat, which, in turn, increases their risk of developing diabetes. Adding to the problem is that the Aboriginal diet has changed to one high in calories, saturated fat, and simple sugars, and that, like their fellow Canadians, Aboriginal peoples have become much more sedentary. Obesity rates have progressively risen and in some communities almost 50 percent of children are now obese.

The Extent of the Problem

An estimated 12 percent of First Nations peoples living on reserves have diabetes and 25 percent of those over the age of 45 are affected. These are rates far above those of the Canadian population as a whole (which has an average rate of 7.5 percent or so) and it is thought that the prevalence is going to increase further.

Inuit people actually have prevalence rates that are below average for the Canadian population, though even in this group, the number of people with diabetes is increasing.

Not only are diabetes prevalence rates high, but also there is evidence that the risk of the following complications is greater amongst Aboriginal peoples:

✔ Coronary artery disease

✔ High blood pressure

✔ Peripheral vascular disease

✔ Kidney disease

✔ Diabetic retinopathy

A number of factors compound the combined one-two punch of greater risk of having diabetes and greater risk of complications:

✔ Earlier age at onset

✔ Delay until a diagnosis is made

✔ Less access to diabetes education (Diabetes education is essential in helping you keep yourself healthy, yet less than 40 percent of First Nations with diabetes attend diabetes clinics.)

✔ Less access to other, important health care services such as dialysis (In some cases this necessitates travelling long distances to receive appropriate treatment and can require moving the entire family.)

How Aboriginal Peoples Are Combatting the Problem

Having recognized the extent and severity of the problem, Aboriginal communities are now tackling the problem on a number of fronts. Among initiatives in place in some regions are those that accomplish the following:

- Teach diabetes prevention programs in elementary schools

- Organize field trips to the local grocery store to teach about food selection

- Introduce programs to increase physical fitness (For example, the Sandy Lake community in northern Ontario has built a well-used and highly successful 6.5-kilometre (4.5-mile) walking trail. See the sidebar.)

- Establish health services programs geared specifically toward Aboriginal health issues and concerns

- Ban "junk food" from schools

- Get local stores to promote healthy foods over "snack foods"

Clearly, non-Aboriginal communities would be well served by following the lead set by these Aboriginal communities and adopting similar healthy-living strategies.

Aboriginal people living in larger urban areas can contact Native Friendship Centres (www.nafc-aboriginal.com), which can provide helpful advice regarding available treatment resources.

The Sandy Lake Health and Diabetes Project

Sandy Lake, Ontario, has one of the highest rates of diabetes in the country, but the community is in the forefront in the battle to fight the problem. Deputy Chief Harry Meekis said in an interview with the *Toronto Star* in April 2000, "We did it for the children. We want to be known, not just as the community with the third highest diabetes rate, but as the community that did something about it." They set up the Sandy Lake Health and Diabetes Project (www.sandylakediabetes.com), a multi-faceted program aimed at preventing diabetes. Components include classroom teaching on healthy eating and physical exercise, regular discussions on the radio, a cooking club and the promotion of healthy foods in local stores. As a result of this project, the community is stemming the rate of the rise of diabetes.

Chapter 17

Employment and Insurance Issues

. . . .

In This Chapter

▶ Dealing with workplace prejudice

▶ Knowing the law that's on your side

▶ Discovering recourse available to you

▶ Obtaining insurance

. . . .

After he found his very first job, one of Alan's young patients wrote to his mother, "Dear Mom, I'm working, even though my pancreas isn't." Most people need to work, and some people even want to work. People need to work for the same reason that a certain man did not turn in his brother-in-law who thought he was a chicken. We need the eggs (though not too many). Most of us, as adults, also require insurance, and this too can present obstacles. We look at these two subjects in this chapter.

Employing Both You and Your Rights

As a person with diabetes, you may run into various forms of discrimination when you try to get a job. As you can imagine, there are a number of reasons for this. Part of it is a seldom-justified concern on the part of prospective employers regarding the safety of having a person with diabetes working for them. Part of it has to do with their lack of understanding of the great strides that have been made in diabetes care, which mean that a person with diabetes often has a better record of coming to work than a non-diabetic. Like virtually all aspects of discrimination in society, discrimination against people with diabetes is based on ignorance.

Fighting for your rights

Canadians with diabetes have protections that citizens of other countries often do not. Section 15.1 of the Canadian Charter of Rights and Freedoms states: "Every individual is equal before and under the law and has the right to the equal protection and equal benefit of the law without discrimination and, in particular, without discrimination based on race, national or ethnic origin, colour, religion, sex, age or mental or physical disability." Although it is not particularly appealing to consider diabetes as being a "disability," this designation does give you certain legal protections under the Charter.

Other groups and organizations actively campaign for your rights, including the Canadian Medical Association, which has an official policy position that "previous blanket discrimination in the workplace . . . should now be replaced with a case-by-case review."

The Canadian Diabetes Association's position statement states that:

- ✔ A person with diabetes should be eligible for employment in any occupation for which he or she is individually qualified.

- ✔ A person with diabetes has the right to be assessed for specific job duties on his or her own merits based on reasonable standards applied consistently.

- ✔ Employers have the duty to accommodate employees with diabetes unless the employer can show it to cause undue hardship to the organization.

Employers cannot say that *any* cost they incur is an "undue hardship." This provision is *not* meant to be used as an excuse to avoid hiring people with diabetes. As you know, most people with diabetes — including yourself — require minimal accommodation on the part of their employer. Usually all that is necessary is the allowance of a few extra minutes per day for blood glucose testing and the taking of medicines, as well as appropriate breaks for snacks and meals.

When you are going for a job interview, you do not have to inform your prospective employer that you have diabetes, or, for that matter, tell him or her anything else about your health unless the health issues are directly related to a specific job requirement or you are applying for a "safety-sensitive" position such as working as a police officer or firefighter (see the very next section). As well, after you are hired, you do not need to provide medical information unless your employer needs to know certain things in order to make appropriate accommodation to your specific needs.

The Canadian Human Rights Commission (www.chrc-ccdp.ca) document, "A Place for All: A Guide to Creating an Inclusive Workplace," is designed to assist both employers and employees in understanding their legal rights and responsibilities in setting up an accommodating workplace.

Will they hire you?

In part because of the now established rights that people with diabetes have achieved, there are virtually no organizations that will issue an outright "ban" on hiring you just because you have diabetes. There are people with diabetes who work just about anywhere and everywhere. And they function as effectively and efficiently as anybody else. Of course!

As we mention in the previous section, however, there are *some* (not many, mind you, but some) exceptions to your usual employment rights. If you are applying for a safety-sensitive position (such as firefighting or police work), the inherent unpredictability of these jobs (are fires or robberies ever predictable?) may work against your being hired. Nonetheless, there is no blanket or uniform policy across Canada, and each fire department and police force determines its own hiring practices.

There are many police officers, firefighters, and paramedics among our patients; however, most of these individuals were diagnosed after they had been hired. Would they have been hired anyway? Impossible to know. Will diabetes potentially jeopardize their jobs? That too is impossible to answer, although our personal observation is that a shift in job description is not unusual (for example, a firefighter being moved to a supervisory role).

In the end, the following factors, among others, may influence your ability to obtain and retain a safety-sensitive job:

- ✔ The policies of a given force
- ✔ Whether a force has set earlier precedents
- ✔ How knowledgeable and comfortable the health staff and administrators are about diabetes
- ✔ How well controlled your blood glucose levels are and, in particular, how often you have hypoglycemia (especially, severe hypoglycemia) and what your general state of health is
- ✔ How able you are to perform the required tasks

The last two items on this list seem far and away the most important to us. Each person is different. And that includes each person with diabetes.

The Canadian Forces have the wise policy of making decisions on a "case-by-case basis," which of course is as it should be. Their *general* policy, however, is that:

✔ If you already have diabetes when you apply for a position with the Canadian Forces, they will be unlikely to hire you.

✔ If you develop type 2 diabetes *after* you are already enrolled, you will likely be "retained without career restrictions."

✔ If you develop type 1 diabetes after you are already enrolled, you will "normally be released" or you "may be accommodated for a 3 year period, then released." The rationale for this is that Canadian Forces members must be not only "employable" but "*deployable*." (The Canadian Forces points out that the "type of care required might not always be offered in a theatre of operation — such as in Kabul.")

The most important point is that, with a few exceptions such as those described above, there is almost nothing you cannot do if you have diabetes. You can climb mountains — in both the literal and the figurative sense. And when it comes to employment, there are almost no jobs in Canada that you cannot both obtain *and* perform.

What recourse do you have?

If you feel you have been discriminated against because of your diabetes regarding employment or prospective employment, you have several avenues of recourse:

✔ If discrimination occurs in federal jurisdiction, you can file a human rights complaint with the Canadian Human Rights Commission. Information on this is available on their Web site (www.chrc-ccdp.ca).

✔ If discrimination occurs outside of federal jurisdiction, you can file a complaint with the human rights commission in the appropriate province or territory.

✔ The Canadian Diabetes Association (CDA) has created a National Advocacy Council, composed of both volunteers and staff, mandated primarily to "act on broad policy matters which can have a positive impact for many people affected by diabetes." The Council "offers advice and guidance," but in general is looking at the "big picture," and unless your concern has national implications, given their limited resources, they may not be able to take on your particular case. If you have a concern you want addressed it is best to start by contacting your local CDA branch and go from there.

Sometimes you can rectify a situation resulting from discrimination by lifting the veil of ignorance from your employer's eyes. You may find the quickest remedy to your concerns is to educate your employer. If you do not have success with your own efforts at teaching them about diabetes, you may wish to refer them to the CDA document "Diabetes in the Workplace: A Guide for Employers and Employees." (This document is available at the CDA Web site: www.diabetes.ca.)

Insuring Your Health

Most of this book is about doing our best to insure your good health. As hard as *that* can seem at times, obtaining the other type of insurance you may want is often the harder of the two.

Thankfully, Canadians have a publicly funded, universal health care program, so fundamental health care will be available to you regardless of your income. When it comes to life, disability, and travel insurance, things get more difficult. The protections offered to you by human rights laws that we talked about earlier in this chapter do not apply in the same way when it comes to insurance policies. Indeed, when you are applying for insurance you can expect to be asked if you have diabetes, and you must tell the truth; otherwise, any policy you are granted may be subject to revocation or non-payment of benefits.

Life insurance

Having diabetes does not automatically exclude you from obtaining life insurance, though it does make it more difficult. Of course, if you develop diabetes while you are already covered, you will have an easier time than if you are applying for insurance (or an increase in your coverage) *after* you have been diagnosed (what insurance companies refer to as having a "pre-existing condition").

Insurance companies make their determination about your insurability on a "case-by-case" basis, meaning that they will look at you as an individual and make their decision on more than the simple fact of your having diabetes. They will look at what kind of therapy you are receiving, what kind of glucose control you have, whether you have complications from your diabetes, and so forth.

If you are approved for a policy, you will likely find that your premiums are higher, for the same level of benefits, than those of a person without diabetes.

If you look after your health well, there is a good chance you will live longer (and healthier) than non-diabetics who don't look after themselves well. Hopefully, insurance companies will take into account all the rapidly accumulating data about how healthy people with diabetes can be. Can you imagine the surprise if insurance companies were ever to charge people with diabetes less than others because of their good habits?

It is worth bearing in mind that different insurance companies have different policies (so to speak), so if one place turns you down, try somewhere else. Another thing you can do is to go through a licensed insurance broker who can act on your behalf, deal with multiple insurers, and try to help you obtain an appropriate policy.

Disability insurance

Unless you had disability insurance before you were diagnosed as having diabetes, it's unlikely that you will find an insurance company that will offer you a policy.

Travel insurance

Travel insurance is much easier to obtain than disability insurance; however, you will need to carefully scrutinize any policy you are offered to see what is excluded from coverage. You may find that if you become ill with a diabetes-related condition, you will not be covered. The Canadian Diabetes Association offers travel insurance (see the next section).

Where you can find help getting insurance

To assist people with diabetes in fulfilling their insurance needs, the Canadian Diabetes Association offers its members travel insurance and "credit life" insurance that covers your credit or loan obligations so that, in the event of your death, a monthly benefit will be paid out until the end of the coverage term. Unlike certain types of insurance offered by banks, for example, the CDA policy is not tied directly to an individual. You can find out more information from the CDA (800-226-8464) or from their partner in this venture, AIG Life Insurance Company of Canada (www.centreunion.ca).

Chapter 18

Driving and Piloting When You Have Diabetes

Few adults in Canada get by without ever having to drive somewhere. (And of course if you are a teenager you have to drive everywhere!) We are so dependent on our cars to get us to work or the movies, grocery shopping or the hardware store, doctors' appointments or dentists' appointments, that for most people, losing your licence is not just inconvenient, it can be downright devastating. In this chapter we take a look at the measures you can take to help preserve your licence, and, if you have lost it, what steps you can take to regain it. We also look at the issues surrounding piloting a plane if you have diabetes.

Are You Medically Fit to Drive?

To most people it would seem self-evident that if you have diabetes you would be at much higher risk of having a car accident. Of course, at one time it was self-evident to most people that the world was flat, too. The truth of the matter is that medical studies do *not* show convincing evidence that having diabetes increases your risk; in fact, one study even showed that people with type 1 diabetes had a lower risk than non-diabetic drivers under the age of 30. How about that! Nonetheless, provincial and territorial bodies have the important and appropriate task of ensuring that drivers are safe to operate motor vehicles, so there are a number of hurdles you are going to have to overcome.

Your ability to obtain and retain a licence will depend on a number of factors, including the means by which your diabetes is being treated. This section looks at those issues specific to your diabetes (of course, non-diabetes factors may also impact on your fitness to drive). The recommendations in this section are based on those established by the Canadian Diabetes Association (CDA). Note that these are *recommendations*, not legally binding rules or regulations. Also be aware that these recommendations have been newly revised in 2003 and as such not all licensing bodies may have reviewed them and incorporated them into their practices.

Steps for all drivers with diabetes

The CDA recommendations include that all drivers with diabetes should do the following:

- Have your fitness to drive assessed based on your personal situation (that is, the decision about your suitability to drive should be made on a case by case basis).

- Have a periodic medical examination with special attention being paid to determine if you have any serious complications from your diabetes.

- Test your blood glucose level routinely and keep a log of your results.

- Ensure that you are up-to-date on how to avoid hypoglycemia and how to treat it if it occurs.

- Measure your blood glucose level immediately before and at least every 4 hours during long drives. If you have hypoglycemia unawareness (see Chapter 5) you should test more often.

- (We would recommend testing hourly, even though that may seem like quite a hassle; trust us, it would be much more of a hassle if you got into an accident because of hypoglycemia.)

- Always have your hypoglycemia treatment nearby. (The trunk of your car isn't nearby!)

- Don't drive if your blood glucose level is less than 4 mmol/L. If your level is between 4.0 and 5.0, ingest some carbohydrate before you resume driving. (If you are a commercial driver, you should never drive if your blood glucose level is less than 6.0 mmol/L.)

- Don't resume driving until at least 45 minutes have passed since you treated an episode of hypoglycemia.

Pull off the road and stop at a safe area if you think you may be hypoglycemic. Don't keep driving!

Applying for a commercial licence

As you might imagine, it is much trickier to obtain and maintain a professional driver's licence if you have diabetes, especially if you are taking insulin therapy. Nonetheless, your suitability to drive should be judged on a case-by-case basis, and indeed, licensing bodies increasingly recognize this, we are pleased to say.

When you first apply for a commercial licence, the appropriate government body will review your request and base their decisions on many different factors, including, importantly, your blood glucose control (especially whether or not you are having problems with hypoglycemia) and whether you have complications from your diabetes.

To assist both governments and individuals with diabetes, the CDA has developed *recommendations*. Like the CDA recommendations in the preceding section, these are not legally binding rules or regulations. If you want to apply for a commercial licence you should contact the appropriate licensing body to see what their specific requirements are, but it is a safe bet that they will want — as a minimum — the following things as suggested by the CDA:

- ✔ Complete a questionnaire that pays particular attention to both your risk of having hypoglycemia and how often you may have been experiencing hypoglycemia. (You can get a sample questionnaire from the CDA.)
- ✔ Have your diabetes specialist perform a full assessment of your health status.
- ✔ Have a full eye exam performed by your eye specialist.
- ✔ Obtain documentation from your diabetes education centre proving that you have attended their program.
- ✔ A recent A1C result.
- ✔ Have a record of your blood glucose measurements (taken at least twice daily) dating back 6 months (or less, of course, if you were diagnosed less than 6 months ago).

The licensing body will likely be more impressed with a downloaded log from your glucose meter than a handwritten record.

Exclusion criteria for maintenance of a commercial licence

The Canadian Diabetes Association's exclusion criteria (that is, those things that, if present, would prevent you from holding a commercial licence) include your having:

- An episode of severe hypoglycemia within the past 6 months (see Chapter 5)

- Ongoing, hypoglycemia unawareness (see Chapter 5)

- Poorly controlled glucose levels (hyperglycemia *or* hypoglycemia)

- The recent introduction of insulin or, if you are already on insulin, a change in your type of insulin or the frequency that you give it

- Significant visual impairment

- Peripheral neuropathy or cardiovascular disease (see Chapter 6) that is severe enough that it could affect your ability to drive

- Inadequate frequency of blood glucose monitoring

- Inadequate knowledge of the causes, symptoms and treatment of hypoglycemia (Don't worry, we have yet to see this determined by a quiz or essay! It is an *impression* that your health care providers would make based on your discussions. It is essential that you — and anyone with diabetes — know all about hypoglycemia anyway. If you don't, read Chapter 5 and, in addition, be sure to ask your health care team to review this crucial subject with you.)

Keeping Your Driver's Licence

If you have diabetes and lose your licence, the most likely reason would be that you had an episode of hypoglycemia while you were driving that led either to a collision or to your being pulled over by police because of erratic driving. (This, of course, is one of the most important reasons for you to wear a medical alert, so that those who come to your aid would quickly recognize that you had diabetes and were not intoxicated.) Hypoglycemia bad enough to lead to this situation is almost only seen if you are treated with insulin (rather than oral hypoglycemic agents) and is much more likely to occur if you have type 1 diabetes.

There are many unfair things about having diabetes, but perhaps least fair of all is that the better your glucose control is, the more prone to hypoglycemia you will be. Nonetheless, that is a fact of diabetes life and you have to work around that to protect you and your licence. Fortunately, most of the time you can avoid episodes of severe hypoglycemia while driving by taking a few relatively simple steps. The measures recommended by the CDA are listed earlier in this chapter. In our experience these are the two most important measures you can undertake to avoid losing your licence:

- ✔ *Never* drive your vehicle unless you have checked your blood glucose level immediately before you are about to drive, to ensure that it is not low.

- ✔ Check your blood glucose levels very frequently. It may be a hassle to keep interrupting your driving, but if you test *every hour* you substantially reduce your likelihood of running into problems. You would readily determine if your levels were dropping and could equally readily deal with it before it got out of hand. Of course there are exceptions, and your level could drop quickly even if you checked half an hour before, but for the majority of people hourly testing is a good protective manoeuvre.

When you are driving, *never* assume your blood glucose levels are normal just because you "do not feel low." You must test to be sure. And *never* say to yourself, "Oh, I think I might be getting low; if I start to feel worse I'll pull off the road." If you think you are low, get off the road immediately! Your licence may depend on it. More importantly, your life (and the lives of others) may depend on it.

Regaining Your Driver's Licence

Though each area of the country has its own policies, if you lose your licence because of an incident that occurred when you were hypoglycemic, *in our experience* the following are the two most important things the licensing body will look for in considering your request for reinstatement of your licence:

- ✔ Evidence of satisfactory blood glucose control as reflected by a carefully kept and accurate log of your readings for the preceding few months, with this record revealing an absence of frequent or severe hypoglycemia. (*Note:* Hyperglycemia is not as dangerous when it comes to the safety of your driving.)

- ✔ A letter from your diabetes specialist or a copy of your diabetes specialist's records with this documentation reflecting your ongoing co-involvement in your management (remember, you are a part of your health care team; see Chapter 8) and your adherence to therapy.

Your physician's duty to report

Physicians are trained always to look out for the best interests of their patients. And that is as it should be. Physicians are also bound — quite rightly — by rules of confidentiality. There are, however, exceptions to the way that physicians normally practise. Indeed, in most areas of Canada it is *the law* that doctors have to report (to the appropriate licensing body) a patient that the physician feels is unsafe to operate a motor vehicle. This is a terribly difficult position for physicians to be in, as the person being reported is invariably and understandably very upset. Even worse, it is often emergency room physicians who have to make this report and they do not have the benefit of a previous relationship with the patient. Reporting patients is one of the most difficult and unpleasant tasks that doctors face.

Flying High with Diabetes

Certainly one of the most remarkable examples of how prejudices are diminishing when it comes to diabetes is the recent change in the rules governing the suitability of pilots to maintain a licence after they develop diabetes. These changes, however, have not come easily or quickly.

Stephen Steele vividly remembers the day back in May 1986 when his life turned upside down. At the time he was a successful pilot with a major Canadian airline with over 14 years of safe flying under his belt. Then, in the spring of 1986, he recognized worrisome symptoms and was soon diagnosed as having type 1 diabetes. His career instantly evaporated as he was immediately and permanently grounded from flying. No country in the world would permit a person with insulin-treated diabetes to pilot an aircraft. Stephen's career was over.

Or was it?

In 1992, Transport Canada's Civil Aviation Medicine Branch initiated a review of the implications of diabetes on piloting in the context of modern diabetes therapy. The Branch created new guidelines wherein people with insulin-treated diabetes could be considered for medical certification based on their individual situation. This gave new hope to Stephen and he set his sights on regaining the pilot's seat he had been forced to relinquish. Driven by passion and conviction, he poured his energies into upgrading his skills to meet the needs of contemporary aircraft, all the while paying meticulous attention to his health. This was no flight of fancy; this was a mission.

Stephen did everything within his power to rule his diabetes. He monitored his blood glucose readings numerous times per day, he exercised regularly, he avoided those things in his diet that could unfavourably affect his blood glucose control, and he made it a practice to adjust his insulin to suit his needs.

After 15 long years, in November 2001, Stephen Steele regained his Airline Transport pilot's certification. His unfailing efforts had finally paid off in what was both a personal victory and a victory for all people with diabetes.

Your success in being allowed to pilot an aircraft will depend on a number of factors including your blood glucose control and the nature of your diabetes therapy. We discuss these issues in the next 2 sections.

Piloting with non-insulin treated diabetes

Although the Aviation Medicine Review Board now decides each individual's case on its own merits, Transport Canada Civil Aviation guidelines (www.tc.gc.ca/CivilAviation/Cam/TP13312-2/diabetes/menu.htm) include statements to the effect that:

✔ If you are able to control your blood glucose levels with diet alone, you may be considered fit to have a licence so long as you do not have other, serious health problems that could interfere with your ability to perform your duties.

✔ If you require oral hypoglycemic agents to control your blood glucose levels you may be considered for medical certification so long as.

  • You have not experienced any recent severe hypoglycemia.

  • Your oral agent has not recently changed in type or dose.

  • You have stable blood glucose control.

  • You do not have any serious complications from diabetes.

Piloting with insulin-treated diabetes

Once again, each individual's case will be treated on its own merits; however, the most important element that is considered in determining your suitability to be able to pilot an aircraft is whether you meet Transport Canada's definition of "low risk" for hypoglycemia. Low risk criteria include:

- ✔ No history of severe hypoglycemia
- ✔ Stable blood glucose control
- ✔ No problems with hypoglycemia unawareness

Because hypoglycemia is the single greatest concern for pilots with diabetes, it is mandatory for pilots to maintain blood glucose levels at a level higher than is generally considered best in terms of preventing long-term damage to the body. As such, it obliges the pilot with insulin-treated diabetes to make the uncomfortable trade-off between optimal blood glucose control and job preservation.

Part V
The Part of Tens

The 5th Wave   By Rich Tennant

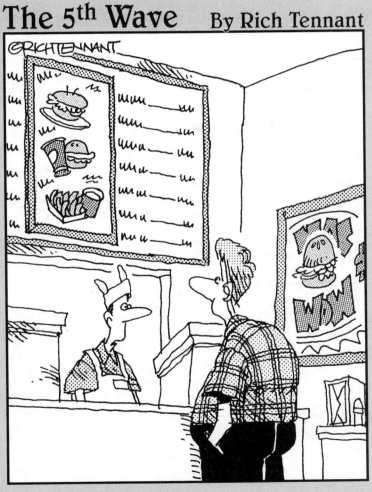

"Sorry sir—we don't currently offer a 'Happy Hemoglobin Meal'."

In this part . . .

Just ahead, a potpourri of tips that will help you achieve good health and steer your way through the health care system. We also look at frequently asked questions posed by people with diabetes. Rounding off our discussion is a look into a crystal ball, as we peer into what future directions diabetes care might take. Could there be a cure on the horizon? In this part we look at possible candidates.

Chapter 19

Top Ten Ways to Prevent Complications (The Seventy-Percent Solution)

Although we may not yet have the means to cure diabetes (though we do have a number of ways to help prevent or delay type 2 diabetes, as you can find out in Chapter 4), we do have the means to reduce the likelihood of complications from it. In fact, with currently available therapy we can lessen your risk of organ damage by a whopping 70 percent (or more). Unfortunately, most people with diabetes do not know this (hey, what a good reason for reading this chapter!) and many physicians do not know this either (hence the need for people with diabetes to be well-educated about their condition and actively involved in their health care). This chapter looks at the top ten ways you can prevent complications from developing.

Eat Earnestly

If you are what you eat, then it is plain to see how you can have a hand in shaping your destiny. If you gain excess weight, you gain insulin resistance too, but it does not take a lot of weight loss to reverse the situation. Even losing small amounts of weight can favourably influence your glucose control and your health in general. The most important point about following a diabetes meal plan is that a "diabetic diet" is a healthy diet for anyone, whether they have diabetes or not. You should not feel like a social outcast because you're eating the right foods. And you should not feel guilty if occasionally you eat the "wrong" foods either, for that matter. Remember; there is no such thing as "cheating." A healthy diabetes meal plan is not a crash diet, a high-protein diet, a grapefruit diet, or any other recent fad diet. A diabetes meal plan is a lifelong program of healthy, well-balanced eating.

You can follow a diabetic diet wherever you are, not just at home. Every menu has something on it that's appropriate for you. If you're invited to someone's home, let them know you have diabetes and that you are limited in terms of the amount of carbohydrate and fat you can eat. If that fails, then limit the amount that you eat. And if that is somehow not possible, then accept the fact that your diet will not always be perfect (and whose is?) and go on from there.

Follow a healthy diet designed by *both* you *and* your dietitian and you will have an excellent foundation in your plan for good health. Ignore proper nutrition and you will be destined to have poor glucose control; indeed, both the pills and the insulins we use to control blood glucose are much less effective in the absence of proper dietary therapy. Your destiny is in your hands — and in your mouth.

See Chapter 10 for more on your diet.

Exercise Enthusiastically

If we were to tell you that we had a treatment for you to take that would cost you nothing, that would only have to be taken once per day, that could help keep your glucose levels under control, reduce your blood pressure, improve your lipids, reduce your stress level, help prevent heart attacks, and could lower your risk of dying over the next ten years by one-half, you would not only be wanting it, you would be demanding it! Okay then, it is yours. *Exercise.*

Preferably daily (or at least most days of the week). Preferably for at least 25 minutes at a time. Make exercise as much a part of your life as breathing. The key to success with exercise? Finding the type you like and sticking with it. There is no need to run the Boston Marathon or swim across Lake Ontario (though you are welcome to if you want); something as simple (and inexpensive) as a daily walk is highly therapeutic.

See Chapter 10 for more on exercise.

Learn for Life

Every day, the two of us read professional journals or attend lectures or go to conferences, all with the express purpose of educating ourselves about how best to look after people with diabetes. And the diabetes educators we work with do the same. As do the dietitians. As do the podiatrists and the pharmacists and all the other professionals whose mission it is to help you stay healthy. Your whole diabetes team is always learning. You, too, are a part of your diabetes team. So that means *you* have to do your share of leaning.

The more you know, the better are your odds of being healthy. In Ian's waiting room hangs a large banner that reads: "Rule your diabetes; don't let it rule you!" Your continued education is the single most important factor in allowing you to do this. Don't be in the dark. Know what you should eat. Know how you should exercise. Know what your blood pressure is and what it should be, what your lipids are and what you are aiming for. The ancient precept "Know thyself" remains as true today as when it was written 2,500 years ago.

Don't be a passive partner in your diabetes care; be actively involved. You can learn from the other members of your health care team (especially from your diabetes educator and dietitian). You can learn by reading this book, reviewing (reputable) Web sites such as that of the Canadian Diabetes Association (www.diabetes.ca), and attending meetings of your local CDA branch. Your learning should only stop when you no longer have diabetes.

Remember that there is a lot of misinformation on the Web, so you must be careful to check out a recommendation before you start to follow it. Even information on reliable sites may not be right for your particular problem.

See Chapter 8 for more on education and the health care team.

Give the Heave-ho to Harmful Habits

You win a lottery . . . but lose your ticket. You buy a brand-new car . . . and minutes later, lock your keys inside. You have a breakaway . . . and mishandle the puck. We all have our missteps — golden opportunities that we manage to make a mess of. But most of these are small miscues or, at worst, temporary setbacks. Having diabetes may be no piece of cake (well, actually, you can have a piece of cake, but that is another story), but with careful management you can lead a full, active, and long life. What a shame that smoking can wreck all that. Smoking is bad enough in a non-diabetic, but if you have diabetes, smoking makes almost every complication more likely to occur. You place yourself at enormous risk of a heart attack or a stroke, blindness or amputations; the list goes on and on. But you can change the odds. Quit smoking now and you can markedly improve your odds of avoiding these complications. Some things in life are beyond our control. Smoking isn't one of them. Millions of Canadians have quit smoking. So can you.

Does it seem unfair that once you were diagnosed as having diabetes, all those good-meaning people (family, friends, doctors, nurses, dietitians . . .) asked you to change your diet, your exercise, your weight, and, if you smoke, your tobacco use too? Well, if you think so, then you may also think it unfair that we will now ask you to moderate your drinking. No more than one (for women) or two (for men) a day. Tops. Your health is our *raison d'être*. No apologies for that.

See Chapter 6 for tips on quitting smoking. See Chapter 10 for more on alcohol and diabetes.

Go for Great Glucose

It is a proven fact that high blood glucose levels are toxic to your body. They can lead to blindness, kidney failure, and nerve damage. But you are clearly not just waiting around for bad things to happen; if you were, you wouldn't be reading this book right now. To prevent high blood glucose from damaging your body, be sure to test your blood regularly. Compare your readings with your targets (see Chapter 9 and the Cheat Sheet at the front of this book). If your values are too high, speak to your health care team about what changes can be made to your treatment plan to help get your blood glucose control where it should be. Excellent control is within your grasp, but don't feel that you have to do it on your own.

Contain Cholesterol and Tame Triglycerides

Elevated LDL cholesterol, low HDL cholesterol, elevated triglycerides, and high total cholesterol/HDL ratio are bad things. Low LDL, high HDL, low triglycerides, and a low total cholesterol/HDL ratio are good things. Now which package do you want for your birthday? Got the wrong gift? So trade it in. There is no reason to accept poor lipids. Optimal lipids will reduce your risk of cardiovascular disease. So optimal lipids are what we are after. Your physician should check your lipids routinely (refer to the Cheat Sheet and Chapter 6 to find out how often and to see what your targets are). Make sure you and your doctor review your lipid test results (they're yours, after all), and, if they are not where they should be, establish a plan of action to *get them* where they should be. Remember, it is nice, but not enough, to find out that your lipids are "good" or "okay" or "all right." Find out the exact numbers. And write them down. (The Cheat Sheet at the front of this book has a space to do just that). One other thing — recent research suggests that you may be able to reduce the risk of damage to your body by taking cholesterol-lowering medicine *even if your lipids are already within target*. Speak to your doctor about the Heart Protection Study (which we discuss in Chapter 6) to see if you should be on therapy even if your lipids are perfect.

Beat Back Blood Pressure

Among the nasty things that high blood pressure causes are strokes, eye damage, heart attacks, and kidney failure. Quick: What was your blood pressure the last time your doctor checked it? And was that considered perfect for you? If you knew these two answers, congratulations. If you did not, then reread this chapter after your next visit to the doctor and congratulate yourself next time around. Your doctor should routinely check your blood pressure, and, just as with your lipids, you should make sure you find out the specific measurement. If your value is higher than it should be (see Chapter 6 for a discussion on high blood pressure), speak to your doctor about a plan of action to achieve your target blood pressure.

Eye Your Eye Doctor

You may have 20/20 vision; heck, you may be able to see a speck of dust on the back of a gnat on the tail of a bird on the top of a tree on the peak of a mountain — but what you *can't* see is the back of your eyes. Only a skilled eye professional can determine the true health of your eyes. Don't be misled into thinking that your visual acuity (that is, what kind — if any — of prescription lenses you wear) has anything to do with the health of your eyes. It doesn't. See your eye doctor regularly so you can, well, continue to *see* your eye doctor.

See Chapter 6 for more on eye care.

Fuss Over Your Feet

We walk, on average, about 184,000 kilometres in our lifetime. That's over four trips around the equator (well, okay, we realize that those darn oceans would keep getting in the way, but you know what we mean). So if we want to keep those lovely lower appendages of yours up to this task, you gotta look after 'em. Having diabetes means that your feet are at risk of damage including ulcerations, infections and even frank gangrene and, potentially, amputation. But these devastating complications are largely avoidable. Show your feet you care by looking after them with all the helpful measures we discuss in Chapter 6. Go ahead, love your feet. It's okay; *really*. In fact, it's essential.

Master Medicines

You may have noticed that your success with diabetes is based on a combination of things, including knowledge, lifestyle treatment, and medicine use. Although no one wants to take medicines, you cannot underestimate their importance. Indeed, with each passing year physicians are asking people with diabetes to take more and more pills. The reason is simple: the medicines we use can keep you healthy and even save your life. Most people with diabetes both need to take and should take medicines to accomplish the following:

- ✔ Optimize blood glucose (this usually requires two, and often three different types of medicine)
- ✔ Optimize blood pressure (this usually requires two or three, and sometimes four different types of medicine)
- ✔ Optimize lipids (this usually requires one and sometimes two different types of medicine)

✔ Prevent blood clots (Aspirin — also known as ASA — is typically used to reduce your risk of having a heart attack. Unless there is some reason you cannot take ASA — such as being under 21 years of age — it should be a part of your daily routine.)

✔ Prevent heart attacks and strokes (If you are at high risk of cardiovascular disease, *angiotensin-converting enzyme inhibitors* — thankfully abbreviated as "ACE inhibitors" — are often a good thing to take to reduce this risk. Most people with diabetes who are 55 years of age or older should be on an ACE inhibitor. Many people with diabetes who are younger than 55 years of age should also take them.)

✔ Prevent kidney failure (If you have *any* evidence of diabetes-related kidney malfunction, taking ACE inhibitors or angiotensin receptor blockers — "ARBs" — can help keep those wonderful filters of yours performing wonderfully.)

✔ Prevent pneumonia (Ah, at least this isn't a pill you have to remember to take.) Many people with diabetes fall ill each year from pneumonia. But you can markedly reduce your risk for developing influenza pneumonia by the simplest of measures: have an annual flu shot. You should also have another type of vaccination to protect you against a different form of pneumonia called pneumococcal pneumonia (revaccination is sometimes given 5 years after the initial vaccination).

See Chapter 6 for the inside scoop on these measures and more.

"My goodness!" you might *(and should)* say. "That could be seven or more different types of medicine to take every day." No one should tell you that is not a big deal. It *is* a big deal. But lying in a hospital bed with a stroke or an amputation or a dialysis machine at your side is, by far, a bigger deal. We have the means to keep you healthy and to help you live a long, full life. And those means include medicines. Don't think of the pills you need to swallow each day as a weight upon your shoulders. Think of them as a life preserver!

And there you have it — the ten most important ways that you can reduce your risk of developing complications from diabetes. These measures are readily available to each and every person with diabetes, and if they were followed, thousands upon thousands upon thousands of people with diabetes could lead healthier and longer lives. Most importantly, *you* can! And remember one other crucial point. If you do not meet all your targets, that does not mean you have failed and it does not mean it was all for naught. *Any* improvement in your weight or exercise or blood pressure or glucose levels or any of the other items listed above will help you reduce your likelihood of developing complications. This is not an "all or none" issue.

The Cheat Sheet at the front of this book summarizes this top ten list.

Chapter 20

Top Ten FAQs (Frequently Asked Questions)

- -

- -

Though every person with diabetes is unique — and needs to be treated as such — there are some questions that do come up remarkably often. Sometimes it's because the answer is not obvious (for instance, why in the world would blood glucose levels go up overnight even if you have not been eating?), and sometimes it's because the answer is not easy to find (for example, how to get your doctor to be a more effective communicator). This chapter looks at the ten most commonly asked questions that we hear in our offices. (And we even supply the answers!)

Why are my sugars higher when I get up in the morning than when I go to bed?

This can seem like quite a conundrum. Did you take an unremembered stroll to the fridge at 3 a.m.? Not likely, unless you are one very hungry sleepwalker. Was it an overly big snack at bedtime that made your readings go up? Improbable, unless your snack was so huge that it would make Dagwood Bumstead proud. No, the answer lies within your body, not within your fridge or pantry.

Beginning about 3 a.m. your body starts to increase production of hormones such as cortisol and growth hormone, which are important for normal metabolism, but which can, in a person with diabetes, lead to the release of glucose from the liver. This is called the *dawn phenomenon*.

Although this is a common problem, it is not one we, ahem, take lying down. The most successful strategy to fight this problem is to take a dose of intermediate-acting insulin (like NPH) at bedtime. Evening doses of metformin can also help but are often less effective.

Another, less common, but very important cause is a "rebound" after an episode of overnight hypoglycemia. This is called the *Somogyi phenomenon*.

If you are already on bedtime, intermediate-acting insulin, then it could simply be that your insulin has worn off and you need to increase your dose.

We discuss insulin issues in detail in Chapter 12.

Why are my blood sugars yo-yoing?

If you are like most people with diabetes, you will have experienced times when, despite your best efforts, your glucose control seemed a mess. High one minute, low the next. High for a couple of days, low for the next two. Up and down, down and up, for no apparent rhyme or reason.

But of course there is a reason; it's just a matter of detective work to figure out what that reason is.

Sometimes doctors and patients naively think that all we have to worry about in terms of glucose control is what you eat, how you exercise, and what medicines you take. Although these are the most important factors, there are, in fact, *many* other things that can influence blood glucose control, including your stress level, your stomach and bowel function, your menstrual cycle, and more.

We discuss these issues in detail in Chapter 12.

Why are my sugars getting worse, even though I'm following my diet and taking my pills?

Few things are as frustrating to the person with type 2 diabetes as finding that despite following a proper diet (with occasional indiscretion — which is perfectly fine, by the way), taking more and more pills, and exercising regularly (okay, maybe *irregularly*, but doing *some* anyhow), his or her blood glucose levels are progressively worsening. If you have been in this situation, you probably asked yourself, "What am I doing wrong?"

The answer is, you are probably doing *nothing* wrong.

The problem is, diabetes is a progressive disease. We wish it wasn't, but it is. Which means that despite your (and our) best efforts, your pancreas is going to have a hard time keeping up. In fact, the day you were diagnosed as having type 2 diabetes your pancreas was already running at only one-half normal function. The net result is that, with all likelihood, you are going to require more and more medicines to control your glucose levels as time goes by. Worsening pancreas function is also the reason that the majority of people with type 2 diabetes will eventually require insulin therapy. That is not a sign that *you* have failed; it is a sign that *your pancreas* has. And that, of course, is not your fault.

It is *theoretically* possible that certain types of oral hypoglycemic agents may have the ability to preserve the pancreas's ability to produce insulin. The ADOPT study is looking this issue. (See Chapter 11 for details.) We should have the results in a few years.

What's the difference between an A1C level and a blood glucose level?

One of the most important tests in assessing overall glucose control is also one of the least understood. Your A1C (or "hemoglobin A1C") helps us know what your average blood glucose level has been over the preceding 2 to 3 months. It is measured in different units than blood glucose (percentage, not mmol/L) and represents the proportion of your hemoglobin (the substance in your red blood cells that carries oxygen) that is permanently attached to glucose. The higher your average glucose readings over the preceding few months, the more glucose your hemoglobin is exposed to and the higher your A1C will be. Because it is an entirely different test than the one for blood glucose level, an A1C of 7 percent, for example, does not mean that your average blood glucose level is 7 mmol/L.

We discuss this in detail — and provide a graph comparing average blood glucose to A1C — in Chapter 9.

Since I used to be on pills, but now I'm on insulin, does that mean I've developed type 1 diabetes?

No, you still have type 2 diabetes. We can say that you have "insulin-treated" diabetes, but that is *not* the same as having type 1 diabetes where you would be absolutely dependent on insulin to stay alive, not just to maintain good blood glucose control.

(The one exception to this is if you have a relatively uncommon condition called LADA, which is a slowly developing form of type 1 diabetes that can often be treated in its early stages with pills.)

We discuss these issues in detail in Chapter 4.

Do I really need to be on insulin — once you're on insulin you're on it forever, right?

If you have type 1 diabetes, then yes, you need to be on insulin and for all intents and purposes it will be forever (or until we have a cure).

If you have type 2 diabetes and despite appropriate lifestyle and oral hypo-glycemic agent therapy your blood glucose control is still not what it should be, then yes, you *really need* to be on insulin, and yes, it will likely be forever. But if you are starting out with much to improve in your lifestyle, then there is a significant chance that with diet, exercise, and weight loss, oral hypo-glycemic agent therapy will start to work better and, sometimes, effectively enough that you may end up being able to come off insulin.

The other thing to consider is that there may soon be ways to give insulin without your having to inject yourself. See Chapter 22 for the inside scoop.

Probably the single greatest management failure that people with type 2 diabetes and their physicians make is inappropriately delaying insulin therapy. The person with diabetes may say to his or her doctor, "Let's give it more time. I'll work on my diet, lose some weight and take pills." The doctor in turn may say, "Okay, we'll wait and see." That would be perfectly fine if the period of waiting was brief, but regrettably, it often stretches into many months or even years — and all the while, high blood glucose levels are progressively damaging your organs.

I'm watching my diet and avoiding fatty foods, so why is my cholesterol level still high?

Some people can eat a bacon double cheeseburger and have normal cholesterol levels. And other people could order a veggie burger and have abnormal cholesterol levels. The difference? Genetics. Some people are simply genetically programmed to have livers that manufacture excess cholesterol. Indeed, *all* of us produce the bulk of our cholesterol within our bodies. If you have a body that tends to over-produce cholesterol, you can combat this by following a proper diet, exercising, and getting your blood glucose control in order — but often this is not sufficient. Our genes are very strong. Often that helps us. Sometimes it does not.

We discuss cholesterol levels in detail in Chapter 6.

Why do I need blood pressure pills if my blood pressure is good to start with?

Because "good" is seldom good enough. If you have diabetes, then your risk of cardiovascular, kidney, and eye disease is high enough that your blood pressure can't just be "good" or "okay." It has to be perfect. Great. Excellent. Spectacular. Marvellous. Stupendous . . . Optimal blood pressure will go a lot farther at keeping you healthy than will "good" blood pressure. And to achieve optimal blood pressure (usually this is less than or equal to "130 over 80"), high blood pressure medicines are often required.

We talk more about high blood pressure in Chapter 6.

How can I get my doctor to start telling me what's going on?

Congratulations. That you have asked this question tells us that you want to be an active participant in your health care. You are not content to assume that "everything must be okay" since your doctor hasn't told you otherwise. You want to know your blood pressure and your cholesterol. You want to know your last A1C and whether your eye doctor observed any retinopathy.

Even if he or she does not necessarily always show it, you can be quite confident that your doctor is absolutely *thrilled* that you are interested enough in your health that you want to be actively involved in your diabetes management. Nonetheless, there are some doctors that, at times, are not particularly good communicators.

If you are feeling in the dark, there are several steps that you can follow to obtain more information. We would suggest trying these in the order they are listed, proceeding to the next step if the earlier one did not meet with success:

1. **Let your doctor know you are interested:** Perhaps your doctor simply doesn't realize that you want to know the specifics of your results. Your first step should always be to simply let your physician know that you are keenly interested in your health and would like to know as much as possible about how you are doing. He or she will likely be overjoyed.

2. **Ask *specific* questions:** "Doctor, what is my blood pressure?" is more likely to get you a specific number than is asking "Doctor, how's my pressure?" which would likely be met with an "It's fine."

3. **Ask for copies of your lab results:** When you ask for these, make sure you word your request in a non-threatening way; otherwise, your doctor may feel that you are second guessing his or her judgment (which you *may* be, but there is no benefit to you if your doctor is made to feel defensive). Try something like "Doctor, I like to keep tabs on my lab results. Would it be a problem for me to have a photocopy for my records?"

4. **Ask other members of your health care team:** If none of the previous steps has succeeded, try asking other members of your health care team. It may well be that if one of your physicians (say, for example, your diabetes specialist) is not readily forthcoming, another one may be (for example, your family physician). Your diabetes educator is another person to try, since he or she may have received copies of lab results or consultation letters from your physician(s).

Will I always have diabetes?

We're sure you can tell why we saved this question for last; it is far and away the most difficult question we ever have to answer.

The quick answer is a simple "we don't know" — and, of course, we don't. The more complicated answer is (and this is our personal and highly subjective guess) the following:

- ✔ If you have type 1 diabetes you are *unlikely* to have it forever. It is only a matter of time before a cure is found (perhaps islet cell transplants, perhaps gene therapy or some other innovative treatment; see Chapter 22). Sure, you may have heard this prophecy year after year and may be frustrated by the eternal wait (and who could blame you?). Nonetheless, we can tell you that we would never have used the word *cure* 10 years ago, but in the new millennium we dare to mention it. When will a cure be found? That we cannot say. But that there will be one, we have no doubt.

- ✔ If you have type 2 diabetes, the situation is much trickier, and we suspect that there will not be a cure in the foreseeable future. The factors leading to type 2 diabetes are complex and far from completely understood. It is highly unlikely that we are dealing with a single cause for which there will be a single cure. On the other hand, more and better treatment options are rapidly emerging. Even if we cannot undo your diabetes, it is likely that we will be able to offer such effective therapy that your diabetes will become less and less of a hassle for you to deal with.

As diabetes specialists we are always full of hope. Every day, research comes out revealing new insights into the condition. And the pace with which new and better therapies are emerging is simply astounding. The single greatest advantage to you in having a disease that is rapidly becoming more common is that this stimulates research scientists and drug companies to put tremendous resources into finding ways to help you. When we look back at our careers and see what medical science knows now that it did not when we first began our practices, we can only marvel at the progress we have made in our quest to keep people with diabetes healthy. Our 70-percent solution (see Chapter 19) will, no doubt, soon be an 80-percent solution, then a 90-percent solution, then . . .

Chapter 21

Top Ten Tips for Getting the Best Possible Health Care

*I*n medical school you learn lots about anatomy and physiology. You learn lots about pathology and statistics. And you learn lots about diseases and how to treat them. But one thing that you don't learn is how to help your patients get the most out of their visits to their health care providers and from the health care system in general. In this chapter we share with you some key tips that we have learned over the years — tips that will help you when you see your health care team, save you time and aggravation, and help you stay healthy.

Prepare for Your Visit

If you were going to be travelling to the Caribbean for a holiday, you would make sure you packed the right things and dressed appropriately for your destination. Well, when you are going to be seeing a member of your health care team it is a good idea to be similarly prepared. The evening before your appointment is a good time to make sure everything is ready. Let's say, for example, you were going to see your diabetes specialist. Here's what you'd be wise to do:

> ✔ **Make sure your glucose logbook is ready** (and don't leave it behind on the kitchen counter!). If you don't usually write down your readings — and, by the way, we think you should — transcribe them from your meter's memory into your book. If your doctor has readings to review it will be a lot easier for him or her to give you advice regarding your glucose control.

✔ **Take your medicines with you.** Put all your medicines in a bag and take them with you to your appointment. Your doctor will likely want to review them with you. If you prefer to carry a list, it is essential that it be up-to-date and include, for each drug, the name, the dose, and how often you take it. If you are taking alternative or complementary therapies (see Chapter 13) take those with you too.

✔ **Check to see if you will be needing any prescription renewals.** Some doctors will renew prescriptions only while the patient is with them in their office. If that is true of your doctor, save yourself the hassle of a return visit just to get a prescription: ask your doctor for one while you are there.

✔ **Dress for the occasion.** It is much easier to be a diabetes specialist in Canada in mid-July than in mid-January. In summer, shirts having replaced sweaters and sandals having replaced boots, it is a piece of cake to check a blood pressure or examine a foot or assess some other part of anatomy. But alas, in Canada summer lasts about 2 weeks (okay, maybe longer in Victoria and, perhaps, even Vancouver). Still, there is no reason for you to not get the physical examination you require just because it is −30°C outside. When you are getting dressed, make sure that you wear clothes that will allow:

  • Your neck to be readily exposed so that your thyroid can be examined.

  • Your arm to be easily accessed to allow for a blood pressure measurement. Avoid wearing sleeves that cannot be rolled up easily.

  • Your feet to be exposed readily so that they will get checked. Pantyhose, for example, may help keep you warm, but also they may prevent your feet from being examined. (A simple yet highly effective way to make sure that your feet get examined is to remove your shoes and socks while you are waiting for your doctor to come in the examining room.)

✔ **Think ahead about what questions you want to ask.** If there are certain things that you have been waiting to ask your doctor, write them down and bring the paper with you. Otherwise, you may forget your questions, only to remember them after you have left the office. And that can be very frustrating!

✔ **Plan to bring two sets of ears.** If you feel that you want the support of a friend or family member, or, equally important, the benefit of two memories, then plan on bringing someone with you to your doctor's appointment.

If you are going to bring someone with you to your appointment, make sure you ask your doctor if it is okay to have them join you *before* your companion walks, unannounced, into the examining room. Otherwise, you may severely regret bringing your teenage daughter with you when your doctor asks you whether you are experiencing erectile dysfunction. (Reversing generations — and perhaps more disconcerting to you — your teenage daughter with diabetes may be far less likely to talk to her doctor about her need for birth control if you are sitting there.)

If you will be seeing your dietitian and if you are not the person in charge of food preparation in your house, it is essential that you *and* your partner both go. Oh, by the way, do *not* announce to the dietitian that you do not have to know the information because you do not do the cooking. It is unlikely that you will be eating 100 percent of your meals at home, and besides, the food will be going in *your* mouth — don't you want to know why?

Plan for Your Next Visit

Your diabetes specialist and ophthalmologist likely have their appointment schedule drawn up many months in advance. Indeed, some specialists are fully booked for well over 6 months. So if you realize on April 1st that, say, you haven't seen your eye doctor for a year and you want an appointment for the next day, the receptionist will likely tell you that you sure are in the spirit of April Fool's Day and wasn't that a good joke you just made.

A much better idea is to book your *next* appointment *before* you leave the *present* one, even if the next appointment won't be for another year. If you are told that you should call to book an appointment because they do not know what the doctor's office hours will be that far in advance, ask *when* you should call and then mark the date in your calendar so that you don't forget.

Tired of waiting an hour or more in your doctor's waiting room? Try booking your next visit for the first appointment of the day.

A Requisition for Success

If you have diabetes, you and your forearm are no stranger to the local laboratory. Typically, your doctor will give you a requisition as you leave his or her office, ask you to go to the lab, and tell you that you will be contacted if there is a problem. Well, we can tell you we immediately see a problem! The problem is that you will have missed out on a golden opportunity to review your test results face-to-face with your doctor. And if you won't be seeing your doctor again for 6 months, that's a long time to be in the dark.

A much better system is to get a requisition as you are leaving your doctor's office not for tests that you need *then*, but for the tests you will need *later* (that is, at the time of your next appointment). Go for the tests 2 weeks or so before your next visit and that way, when you arrive for your appointment, your doctor will already have the results and you can review them together.

Healthy Numbers

You will get a lot more out of your visit to your doctor — and work more effectively with him or her — if you are familiar with what your "numbers" are. The Cheat Sheet at the front of this book summarizes these for you. Here are the key numbers to know:

- Blood pressure
- A1C
- Blood glucose levels
- Lipids (total cholesterol [TC], LDL cholesterol, HDL cholesterol, TC/HDL ratio, and triglycerides)
- Urine albumin/creatinine ratio ("ACR")

Remember that knowing what your numbers are is of little value unless you know what your *targets* are supposed to be. Additionally, it is crucial that if your numbers are not within target, you and your health care team undertake measures to achieve your goals.

Has It Really Been That Long?

Okay, quick — we're going to have a little quiz. Tell us the following:

- When is the last time you saw your family physician and when did he or she want to see you next?
- When is the last time you saw your diabetes specialist and when did he or she want to see you next?
- When is the last time you saw your diabetes educator and when did he or she want to see you next?
- When is the last time you saw your dietitian and when did he or she want to see you next?
- When is the last time you saw your eye doctor, podiatrist, and the rest of your health care team and when did they want to see you next?

We're easy markers so we'll consider a pass to be 40 percent. So, did you get the necessary two questions right? If you did, congratulations! If you did not, try this test again in a few weeks. Since the average member of your health care team looks after several thousand people whereas you look after just you, no one is in a better position than you to keep track of when you are supposed to see a health care team member. If your health care provider hasn't told you when you are to return, ask.

Not every member of your health care team is necessarily involved in your ongoing health care. Your diabetes specialist, for example, may have seen you a few times, given you and your family physician a suggested treatment program, and then handed your care back to your family doctor. Nonetheless, if you feel you would like to see your specialist again, you can ask your family physician if he or she feels it necessary. This becomes especially important if, despite your and your family physician's best efforts, you are not reaching your targets (Canadian Diabetes Association recommended targets are listed on the Cheat Sheet at the front of this book).

Know Who Does What

Having read the previous tip, you have now arranged all the necessary follow-up appointments you need with the various members of your health care team. As we discuss in Chapter 8, each of them has a special role to play; however, sometimes it can be confusing for the person with diabetes to know who is going to be doing what and when. Indeed, sometimes (thankfully, not often) the various members of the team mistakenly assume that another member of the team is going to be doing something, and as a result no one does it. You can avoid this by having a look at the Cheat Sheet at the front of this book, where we note how often different parts of you (such as your eyes and your feet) need to be examined and how often certain laboratory tests should be performed. If you are due for one of these procedures but you are unclear who will be arranging things, ask your health team members. They may well appreciate the reminder.

No News Is Good News. Not!

If your doctor tells you that you will be called if your test results come back abnormal, you can rest assured that he or she will. Unless, of course, the lab report gets sent to the wrong doctor, or gets lost in the filing, or gets accidentally discarded, or the lab did the wrong test, or the lab didn't do the test at all, or the lab did the right test on the wrong patient, or . . .

If you are sent for a test, make sure that if you do not hear back from your physician's office with the result, you contact the office to double-check that everything was all right. You do not need to speak directly to the doctor; simply ask the receptionist to check for you. The receptionist may well tell you "We would have called you if there was a problem." In which case you can tell them that you read this book by Drs. Blumer and Rubin called *Diabetes For Canadians For Dummies* and they said to call. Blame us; we can handle it.

Here's a far better way to avoid the uncertainty of waiting for a call about your results. Have your tests done — when feasible — in advance of your appointment. That way, the results are available for review at the time of your doctor's appointment (see "A Requisition for Success" earlier in this chapter).

Oil and Water Sometimes Mix Better than Hospitals and Diabetes

We can assure you that if you have severe ketoacidosis or hyperosmolar hyperglycemic state (both of which we discuss in Chapter 5), there is no better place for you to be than in the hospital. Indeed, your life could depend on it.

On the other hand, if you are hospitalized with a problem *not* directly related to your diabetes, your diabetes may not get the same degree of attention as the condition that landed you in hospital. Although this is understandable, it remains important that your diabetes get the attention it requires.

The following tips will help when you are hospitalized:

- ✔ If you are in hospital with a major illness (such as a heart attack), make sure your glucose readings are tested regularly and that your control is maintained at a good level; as we discuss in Chapter 6, this can directly influence your prognosis.

- ✔ If you are well enough to use them, bring your diabetes supplies (including your glucose meter, insulin administration devices, and even your insulin) with you to hospital. Nurses in hospitals are terribly overworked and may find it a huge relief to know that you are able to assist with looking after your own basic diabetes needs. (You will likely need to get permission from your attending doctor in hospital to be allowed to do this.)

- ✔ Most of the people looking after you will be very knowledgeable and helpful when it comes to your diabetes. Recognize, however, that you may encounter certain health care providers that are not quite so familiar with diabetes issues, and you may have to spend some time explaining your diabetes management to them.

The following tips will help you if you are having *outpatient* surgery:

- ✔ Ask for your case to be scheduled for "first case of the day," as this will make it easier for you to get promptly back on your usual insulin or oral hypoglycemic agent schedule.

- ✔ Ask your doctor what to do with your insulin (or oral hypoglycemic agents) the night before your surgery, the morning of your surgery, as well as later on that day. If it is anticipated that you may not be eating properly for a few days (such as after dental surgery), check with your physician (or your diabetes educator) and your dietitian about how to adjust your diet and your insulin (or oral agents) for that few days.

Often, what works well in preparation for outpatient surgery is to take one half of your usual bedtime intermediate-acting insulin the night before your surgery. When you arrive at the hospital in the morning, check your blood glucose and, depending on the result, give yourself anywhere from no insulin to a full dose of your rapid- or fast-acting insulin. It is essential that you do not do any of this without first checking with your physician.

Know Your Drugs

Anytime you are handed a prescription, you are being given a medicine that is supposed to enhance your health. But as you likely know (perhaps all too well) medicines can have their downsides too. Sulfonylureas (such as glyburide), for example, can help bring down high blood glucose but can also lead to low glucose. ACE inhibitors are great at protecting the kidneys, but can also lead to bothersome coughing. Statins can prevent heart attacks, but can cause muscle damage. We could go on and on. Fortunately, the numbers of people that benefit from these and other drugs are vastly greater than the numbers of people that have serious adverse effects.

Here are some important things you should know about any medicine you are prescribed:

- ✔ How often you are to take it
- ✔ Whether it needs to be taken with food or on an empty stomach
- ✔ Whether you can consume alcohol if you are taking it
- ✔ What you should do if you forget a dose
- ✔ What the most *common* side effects are
- ✔ What the most *serious* side effects are
- ✔ What the likelihood of you experiencing a side effect is
- ✔ What you should do if you believe you are experiencing a side effect

> ✔ What laboratory tests (if any) are to be done to monitor for toxicity. (Some drugs require periodic testing of, for example, your liver.)
>
> ✔ Whether one of your other drugs can interact adversely with another of your drugs
>
> ✔ Whether you are to repeat your prescription after the initial supply has run out

A commonly made — and potentially dangerous — error is to assume a drug was "finished" after the pill bottle is finished. You will need to take most medicines used to treat diabetes (including those for glucose control, high blood pressure, and high cholesterol) on an ongoing basis.

It is not only unhelpful, it is downright counter-productive for you to simply be given a long list of all the possible side effects that a particular drug can cause. Such lists do little more than frighten or intimidate people — or else they are simply ignored. What you want to know are the *key* things to look for. One particularly good Web site in this regard is MEDLINEplus Drug Information (www.nlm.nih.gov/medlineplus/druginformation.html). This is an American site, but it lists Canadian-brand drugs as well.

Remember that your alternative or complementary therapies may have their own set of risks, including the way they interact with your prescription drugs. Be as informed about your alternative and complementary therapies as you are about your prescription drugs.

Know How to Stay "In the Know"

As we mention earlier in this book, you will no longer have to stay current about diabetes treatment when you no longer have diabetes. Until that day comes, it will be crucial for you to stay abreast of new developments and, in particular, new therapies that will help you stay healthy.

The simplest and often most effective way for you to stay "in the know" is to be in regular contact with your health care team. In addition, reading the publications (such as Diabetes Dialogue) of the Canadian Diabetes Association is very helpful, as is having a look from time to time at high-quality, well-maintained Web sites (see Appendix C).

Even if you do not need *routine* contact with a diabetes specialist, it is often a good idea to see one from time to time. This is particularly helpful if you have heard about (or if your diabetes educator has told you about) some new therapy that has come out and you are wondering if it may be appropriate for you. Your family physician may be knowledgeable about it and be able to guide you, but if not, he or she would likely be happy to send you back to see your specialist.

Chapter 22

Top Ten Future Directions in Diabetes Care

*W*hat an exciting time to be diabetes specialists! It seems that not a day goes by that we do not read or hear about some new advance that will help us help people with diabetes. With recent innovations, our patients are living longer and, equally importantly, living healthier. Not only that, but with each successive generation of new technology, glucose monitoring and insulin administration becomes easier (not easy, mind you, but easier). And things are going to keep getting better. There are many terrific developments on the horizon. In this chapter we look at what we can expect over the next few years.

More Power to You

It may not seem as glamorous as some other innovations, but not to be overlooked (and indeed, worthy of being first on this top ten list) are the huge strides being made in recognizing the key role that you, the person with diabetes, has to play — in particular regarding dietary therapy and exercise.

Over the next few years, look for further research to help sort out the existing controversies. Will Dr. Atkins's diet be found to have a role in diabetes management, or will it turn out, as presently thought, to possibly help glucose control, but at the expense of potentially hurting organ function? Will the glycemic index turn out to be a useful tool or simply a hassle? Are we over-emphasizing fats and cholesterol in the diet or under-emphasizing them? Look for trans fatty acids to become more and more of a hot topic; the same goes for omega-3 fatty acids.

Look for more sophisticated and more accurate food labelling to assist you in making appropriate food selections. We look forward to a change in the often misleading way that foods are promoted as being "low fat" or "low cholesterol" or "lite" with scarce mention that they may be rich in calories. Similarly, we look forward to greater awareness that just because a product is said to be "natural" does not necessarily mean that it is safe, beneficial, or healthy (poison mushrooms are natural, are they not?).

Look for further changes in exercise recommendations. We anticipate ongoing efforts to determine the respective roles of aerobic versus resistance exercise. As well, the recommended frequency and amount of exercise will, no doubt, be a source of ongoing discussion.

Blood Test, What Blood Test? New Ways to Test Glucose Levels

One of the few good things about the diabetes epidemic is that corporations see a multi-billion dollar market open to them if they can perfect a non-invasive means of reliably checking glucose levels. In the United States the Glucowatch is available (see Chapter 9), but it has its shortcomings (including causing skin irritation, not giving real-time glucose results, and being very expensive). Here are some other technologies under development:

- **Near-infrared spectroscopy:** Using this technique, a beam of light is shone on an earlobe, a lip, or certain other readily accessible parts of your body, revealing the glucose content of the tissues. An implantable version of this has been tried — with some success — in dogs.

- **Far-infrared spectroscopy:** Particularly appealing with this method is that no external energy source is required; instead, it harnesses your body's own heat production. Similar technology is used in the devices you may have seen that measure body temperature using the eardrum.

- **Photo-acoustic spectroscopy:** This technique uses a beam of light to heat (gently, we hope) tissues and produce a pressure wave that is measured by use of a special microphone. Instrumentation then converts this into a glucose measurement.

- **Laser skin punctures:** A company is working on a device that uses a laser to painlessly produce microscopic punctures in the skin. Small amounts of fluid can be extracted and deposited onto a patch, where the glucose level would be measured.

- **Ultrasound:** A research team has found that low-dose ultrasound applied to the skin can make it easier to obtain fluid (not blood) through the skin. They envision an ultrasound device used together with a sensor worn on the wrist that would display your glucose level.

- **Continuous Glucose Monitoring System:** We talk about this device in Chapter 9. It is still not suitable for long-term use, and, at present, it does not give real-time readings, but if these issues are sorted out, this system or some version thereof may have a big role to play.

- **A tear-able idea:** The proportion of glucose in your tears is roughly the same as that in your blood. Researchers are working on ways to take advantage of this, including placing chemical sensors around the edges of contact lenses that would change colour depending on your glucose level.

This list is but a partial sampling of technologies and devices under development and, in some cases, already at the prototype stage.

Preventing Diabetes

A slew of recent studies have shown that preventing (or at the very least, delaying) type 2 diabetes appears possible. As we discuss in Chapter 4, a number of drugs have shown promise in this regard. Additionally, there is an exciting ongoing study called DREAM (*Diabetes Reduction Assessment with ramipril and rosiglitazone Medication*; www.diabetes.ca/Section_About/dreamstudy.asp) which is looking at whether people with a high risk of developing type 2 diabetes can reduce that risk by using ramipril (Altace) or rosiglitazone (Avandia).

But who wants to take drugs if they don't have to, eh? Regardless of which drugs we have available to try to prevent diabetes, we know they are all inferior to what *you* can do for *you* (or what you can recommend to a loved one). Following a healthy lifestyle with good nutrition, achieving and maintaining a proper weight, and exercising regularly — now, that's where it's at. The future is here.

For type 1 diabetes, we look forward to the results of the TRIGR study (we discuss this in Chapter 4), which is seeking to determine if early exposure to cow's milk may be a factor leading to this form of diabetes. As well, the recently formed TrialNet organization (which we also discuss in Chapter 4), composed of researchers who will be working on collaborative research projects on type 1 diabetes, offers hope of future success.

Stem Cell Research

Stem cells are at the top of the pyramid when it comes to all the different cells we have in our bodies. Stem cells transform into (or lead to the creation of) a variety of other cell types and eventually become our blood cells or our liver cells or our muscle cells or a whole host of others, including — and this is where it is so key in terms of potential diabetes therapy — our islet cells. Research pioneered by Dr. Lawrence Rosenberg of McGill University in Montreal has determined that a naturally occurring human protein called *islet neogenesis associated protein* causes stem (or stem-like) cells in the pancreas to transform into new insulin-producing islet cells. There is currently a preliminary study underway in which people with diabetes are receiving this therapy. The idea that we can regenerate islet cells is truly revolutionary, and if the current research is successful it could lead to similarly revolutionary treatment for diabetes. You can read more about Dr. Rosenberg's research online at ww2.mcgill.ca/uro/Rep/r3116/rosenberg.html.

Moving southward, at the University of Florida, researchers have taken stem cells from the livers of adult rats, exposed the cells to high levels of sugar and, lo and behold, the stem cells began functioning like islet cells and started to make insulin. The cells were then inserted back into the pancreases of diabetic rats and the rats no longer had elevated glucose levels!

If stem cell research does meet with success, it will most likely be of benefit in those situations where the main problem is insulin deficiency (such as is seen with type 1 diabetes) rather than insulin resistance (such as is commonly seen with type 2 diabetes). Nonetheless, since many people with type 2 diabetes do, in fact, have a substantial reduction in their ability to produce insulin, it could be that this therapy would have a role there too.

Gene Therapy

Our genes are those parts of our DNA that are responsible for giving us brown eyes or blue, tall stature or short, red hair or blond (or, if your hair is blue, maybe your genes influenced your choice of hair colouring!). As we discuss in Chapter 4, some genes can put us at risk of acquiring certain health problems, such as diabetes. So it follows that if our genes can make us susceptible to diabetes, maybe we can manipulate genes to protect ourselves from getting diabetes or to even reverse diabetes.

✔ Recent research at the University of Calgary under the guidance of Dr. Ji-Won Yoon (www.ucalgary.ca/UofC/faculties/med/webs/microinfect/Yoon.html) has involved inserting insulin DNA into laboratory animals' liver cells, "tricking" these cells into acting like islet cells of the pancreas and starting to produce insulin. This research may ultimately lead to an abundant supply of insulin-producing human liver cells to overcome the shortage of donor pancreases available for islet cell transplants (see later in this chapter).

✔ Also at the University of Calgary, a team of scientists led by Dr. Norman Wong has discovered that by injecting certain growth factors into rat intestinal cells, these cells started to produce insulin.

✔ Dr. Timothy Kieffer (of the University of British Columbia) and Dr. Anthony Cheung (of the University of Alberta in Edmonton) have led research efforts wherein certain cells ("K-cells") in the gut were genetically altered so that they could produce insulin. Early success has been achieved in laboratory animals whereby diabetes was prevented despite loss of the insulin-producing pancreatic beta cells. You can read more about Dr. Kieffer's work at www.ahfmr.ab.ca/publications/newsletter/Spring01/spring01/inside/insulin.feat.htm.

✔ Dr. Gerald Prud'homme at the University of Toronto has been experimenting with the injection of a certain gene into muscle tissue in mice. The muscle cells absorb the gene and start to manufacture insulin.

Thank goodness for Canadian researchers! (And we have yet to speak about the Edmonton Protocol; see later in this chapter.)

Gene therapy and stem cell research are amazing, exciting fields of research that may one day lead to a cure for some people with diabetes. Bear in mind, however, that the encouraging results obtained so far are primarily in laboratory animals and many issues remain to be sorted out. Nonetheless, there has never been a time deserving of greater optimism.

PKC Inhibitors

That high blood glucose damages the body is not new information, nor is it news. What *is* news is the fact that we now have strong evidence that the *way* in which this occurs is by high glucose leading to activation of a protein called PKC (*Protein Kinase C*) and that preventing this activation may prevent this damage.

Although ideally we would keep blood glucose levels in a perfect range and prevent complications *that* way, the truth is that avoiding any and all hyperglycemia (even with the best of therapy) is as difficult as avoiding any and all mosquitoes during a Winnipeg summer (even with the best of therapy!). And that is where a medicine that could block stimulation of PKC would prove so useful. Whereas PKC inhibitors do not prevent high blood glucose, they may prevent its consequences.

Scientists are actively researching PKC inhibitors, and we should have a clearer idea of their place in therapy, if any, in the not too distant future.

Amylin (and Pramlintide)

Amylin is a recently discovered hormone produced by the same (beta) cells in the pancreas as secrete insulin. It has been found that people with type 1 diabetes are markedly deficient in amylin (which makes sense if you consider that their manufacturing plant — the beta cells — are severely damaged) whereas people with type 2 diabetes can still produce amylin, but not in sufficient quantities. This situation mirrors that of insulin production in type 1 and type 2 diabetes.

Amylin does the following:

- Slows down the rate at which the stomach propels food into the small intestine (which, in turn, reduces the rate at which glucose gets absorbed into the blood)
- Reduces glucagon levels after meals. Glucagon is a hormone made in the pancreas that causes the liver to release glucose into the blood stream. (We talk more about glucagon in Chapter 5.)

These two actions are complementary in that glucose from both the gut *and* from the liver are kept in check.

It sounds like amylin therapy would be ideal to help control glucose levels in people on insulin therapy, and there are many millions of pharmaceutical company dollars riding on this hope. One downside to amylin therapy is that it cannot be taken orally. Researchers have developed an injectable form (pramlintide) that is taken with meals and is the subject of very active investigation.

Get a GLP on Yourself

GLP-1 is the easier-to-say handle for a substance called *glucagon-like peptide-1*. As we explain in the previous section (and more in Chapter 5), glucagon is a pancreatic hormone that causes glucose to be released from the liver. GLP-1 is a hormone that, though related to glucagon, has very different properties. GLP-1 is produced in the small intestine in response to eating. After being secreted, GLP-1 travels to the pancreas where it stimulates the beta cells to release insulin.

Now you might think, "So what; we've already got a whole bunch of other medicines that do the same thing." And of course, you would be right; drugs such as glyburide also stimulate the pancreas to release insulin. The difference, however, between GLP-1 and these other drugs is that GLP-1 turns on the pancreas only when blood glucose levels are elevated, which makes GLP-1 a lot smarter than agents such as glyburide that don't have the sense to know to turn off their action if you are hypoglycemic.

 Other properties of GLP-1 include its ability to reduce glucagon levels, to slow down the rate at which food is expelled from the stomach into the small intestine, and to suppress appetite. It could turn out that these properties are as important as its ability to stimulate insulin secretion.

One significant downside to GLP-1 therapy is that it must be given by injection. Another is that its action is very brief, so it has to be given several times per day. Needless to say, researchers are hard at work trying to develop longer-acting, oral forms of GLP-1. More (*much* more!) information on GLP can be found at www.glucagon.com (a site maintained by Dr. Daniel Drucker of the University of Toronto).

New Ways to Give Insulin

Wouldn't it be nice if insulin could be given as conveniently as taking a pill or using a nose spray? Well, if you answered yes — and we bet you did — you aren't the only one that feels this way. Indeed, pretty well everyone feels this way. And that's where the old expression "necessity is the mother of invention" comes into play. (As does the equally old expression: "You can never be too rich . . ."). We can assure you that people who adhere to both expressions are working diligently at finding a solution. We aren't there yet, but progress is being made on a number of fronts:

✔ **Oral insulin:** The difficulty with taking insulin by mouth is that it is a large protein and proteins of this size are broken down by digestive enzymes in the gut. If you simply took a gulp of insulin, it would be destroyed before it even had a chance to get into your bloodstream. To take insulin by mouth, you need a way to protect insulin from those digestive enzymes. One method would be to package the insulin in *biologically erodable microspheres*. These are tiny round packages that can carry insulin through the intestinal lining, where the insulin is released in an active form into the circulation. The packages then break up and leave the body.

✔ **Inhaled insulin:** Inhaled insulin has held out great promise, but has had false starts and isn't likely to be on your neighbourhood pharmacy shelf for a while yet. There are a variety of inhaled insulin products under development, including the following (manufacturers' names are in brackets):

  • Aerodose® (Aerogen, Inc.)

  • AERx® (Aradigm Corporation)

  • AIR® (Alkermes, Inc.)

  • Exubera® (Nektar Therapeutics)

  • Spiros® (Elan Pharmaceuticals, Inc.)

  • Technosphere™/insulin (Pharmaceutical Discovery Corporation)

Most studies to date have been very encouraging, though they have encountered some problems with coughing. See the sidebar for more information.

- ✔ **Intranasal insulin:** This technique holds promise and some early studies have shown similar glucose control to that achieved with insulin injections; however, we will need proof of its long-term safety and effectiveness before it will be ready for prime time.

- ✔ **Buccal insulin (insulin applied to the inside of the cheek):** Researchers have developed a variety of systems for buccal administration of insulin, including a Canadian one (Oralin). As with most all of the potential therapies we discuss in this section, preliminary data look promising, but we will need more knowledge before we can say whether buccal insulin will ultimately have a place in diabetes therapy.

- ✔ **Topical insulin (insulin applied to the skin):** Some people already use this method of delivering medicine into the body in the form of nicotine patches (used to help people quit smoking) and nitroglycerin patches (used to treat angina). At present, insulin absorption is not yet consistent enough or predictable enough for this form of insulin administration to be put into practice.

- ✔ **An implantable insulin pump:** This device is implanted under the skin and delivers insulin either into the abdominal cavity or into a vein. The major problem has been obstruction of the tube carrying the insulin, but this has been managed without surgery in most cases. More work needs to be done before this device is ready for general use.

Why choose the lungs for insulin delivery?

"Why the lungs for insulin delivery?" you might ask. The answer lies in the lungs' anatomy. Our lungs have hundreds of millions of little sacs ("alveoli") that function to extract oxygen from the air and to rid our bodies of carbon dioxide. These sacs are rich in blood flow and have a very extensive surface area over which inhaled substances can be absorbed. How extensive? The size of a tennis court! Now, even if the closest you've ever come to a racquet is when your neighbours have an overly loud party, you would still have to admit that's pretty impressive. But unlike Mount Everest, "because it's there" does not necessarily mean that we should tackle it. After all, if insulin was meant to be in the lungs, that's where our islet cells would be located. (Then again, our pancreases aren't located under our skin, yet we've been giving insulin there for 80-odd years.) The bottom line is that inhaled insulin holds much promise, but before it becomes part of our therapy we need to be certain that it is not just effective, but safe as well.

The ultimate goal (next to having a cure, of course) is to connect a reliable insulin sensor by a feedback mechanism to an insulin pump. That way your blood glucose readings could be monitored routinely and insulin administered when needed, without your even having to be aware of the process. This would be a true artificial pancreas. This is not all just a pipe dream. In fact, researchers in Australia have studied a prototype of such a device. We look keenly forward to seeing published studies emerge on this type of treatment option.

(We discuss existing insulin administration methods in Chapter 12.)

Islet Cell Transplants

Dr. James Shapiro and his colleagues at the University of Alberta in Edmonton have gained worldwide attention through their pioneering work on a new form of diabetes therapy. Using the "Edmonton Protocol," they have removed islet cells (which, you may recall, are the insulin-producing cells of the pancreas) from cadavers and injected them into the livers of people with type 1 diabetes, and, in many cases, rendered these participants free of the need to inject insulin. (About 85 percent of patients treated in Edmonton are free of insulin injections 1 year after islet cell transplantation and about 70 percent after 2 years; however, significantly lower success rates have been achieved at other research centers.) Islet cell transplants have been tried for a number of years, but never with this kind of success. Exciting news, indeed.

This technique has many advantages over transplanting an entire pancreas, including, importantly, avoiding major surgery (and its potential for complications). The islet cells are given by a needle inserted into the liver; it does not require an incision or general anesthetic.

One major problem with organ transplants (including islet cell transplants) is that the recipient needs to take anti-rejection drugs. Without these, your immune system would see the new organ as being a foreign invader and try to destroy it. Unfortunately, anti-rejection drugs can cause their own problems, including making you more prone to infections, causing kidney damage, and, importantly, making glucose control worse. Having said all this, the Edmonton Protocol uses a new combination of anti-rejection drugs, a combination that does *not* have the same likelihood of serious adverse effects.

As with all new treatments (and old ones too for that matter) it is essential to look at both the pluses and the minuses. (Whatever you do, don't stop reading this section before you have read *both* — doctors' orders!)

Why might islet cell transplants *be a good treatment* for you?

✔ There is a good likelihood you will no longer need to give yourself insulin injections.

✔ The procedure is quite safe.

Why might islet cell transplants **not** *be a good treatment* for you?

✔ Significant numbers of recipients have needed to go back on insulin injections.

✔ You would need to take anti-rejection drugs. (Thus, in our opinion it is inappropriate to consider islet cell transplants a "cure.")

✔ *Quite* safe is not necessarily safe enough. Complications have occurred due to both the islet cell administration procedure itself as well as from the anti-rejection drugs that are used. These include:

- Bleeding
- Blood clots in a vein in the liver
- Injury to the gallbladder
- Mouth ulcers
- Acne
- Worsening of lipids
- Elevation of blood pressure
- Deterioration in kidney function

✔ There is the *theoretical* risk that your immune system, once activated by having received the foreign islet cells, will attack any future islet cell or pancreas transplant you might receive.

✔ Very few people have undergone the procedure and the Edmonton Protocol began just a few short years ago. As such, we do not know what its long-term safety or effectiveness will turn out to be.

Another important consideration is that there is a tremendous shortage of donor islet cells, so wanting an islet cell transplant and being able to receive one are not necessarily the same thing.

Dr. Shapiro himself — for good reason — has said (in *The Lancet* medical journal), "The procedure can . . . only be justified in patients at great risk from their diabetes; ie, those at risk of severe recurrent hypoglycemic coma or metabolic instability despite compliance with an optimum insulin regimen."

The question we ask ourselves whenever we consider islet cell transplantation as a possible option for one of our patients is this: "Would we simply be trading one set of problems for another?" So far, our answer is a qualified "yes," perhaps we would be.

You should consider this form of therapy to be experimental at this stage in the game.

If you would like to find out more about your possible suitability for an islet cell transplant, have a look at the Edmonton Protocol Web site (www.med.ualberta.ca/islet/).

Another approach to islet cell transplantation is the use of *microencapsulated pancreatic islets,* which are injected into the person requiring insulin. The idea is to surround the insulin-producing cells with a protective capsule so that the cells in the body that want to destroy these injected foreign cells cannot get to them. So far, this approach has not been very successful. Although the cells continue to work and make insulin, they become covered with a layer of other cells. The process is called *fibrosis.* The result is that the blood glucose cannot get in to trigger insulin production and release, and the insulin cannot get out.

As anybody who has ever drawn up a top ten list knows all too well, such a list is inherently subjective and usually controversial. So if you have an item you feel *should have* been included on this or the previous chapters' lists, or if you disagree with one that we *have* included, we won't take it personally. In fact, we invite you to e-mail Ian (he's willing to take the fall for both of us) with your suggestions. Ian can be reached at diabetes@ianblumer.com.

Part VI
Appendices

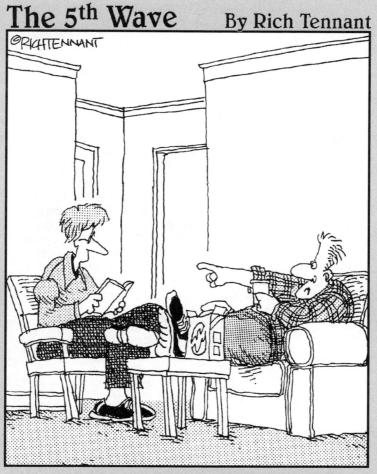

The 5th Wave   By Rich Tennant

"C'mon, Darrel! Someone with diabetes shouldn't be lying around all day. Whereas someone with no life, like myself, has a very good reason."

In this part . . .

Although your body may have but one appendix, *Diabetes For Canadians For Dummies* has four! In the first appendix we look at the food group system. After you have digested that (or before, if you prefer), you can pull out the pots and pans, fire up the stove, and cook up one of the delectable recipes in Appendix B that have been submitted by dieticians from coast to coast. To quench your appetite for even more information, Appendix C lists some particularly satisfying Web sites. Lastly, Appendix D provides a quick glossary reference so you can look up the meaning of those words — both obscure and not so obscure — that you may be uncertain about.

Appendix A

The Food Group System

In This Appendix

▶ Looking at the Canadian Diabetes Association Food Group System

▶ Using food choices to create your diet

*I*n this appendix, you discover the method that dietitians in Canada are using to help their clients to eat the right number of calories from the correct energy sources while permitting them to vary their foods. Although many thousands of different foods are available, each one can be broken down on the basis of the energy source (carbohydrate, protein, or fat) that is most prevalent. This basic feature underlies nutrition planning, as you will see.

Here we look at the *general* principles of meal planning (and snacks, too!); you will need to see a registered dietitian to create a nutrition program that fits with your *specific* needs. We discuss the role of registered dietitians as part of your health care team in Chapter 8.

The Food Group System

To assist people with diabetes to choose healthy foods for their meals and snacks, the Canadian Diabetes Association has developed "The Good Health Eating Guide." In this system, foods are divided into seven groups according to the amount of carbohydrate, protein, and fat they contain. Here are the groups:

 ✔ Starch foods

 ✔ Fruits and Vegetables

 ✔ Milk

 ✔ Sugars

 ✔ Protein foods

 ✔ Fats and Oils

 ✔ Extras (This refers to things such as low-sugar vegetables — examples being asparagus or broccoli — and small portions of Canadian delicacies such as ketchup and relish.)

You may have noticed certain symbols on the packaging of many products you purchase at the grocery store. These symbols, designed to assist with recognizing the different food groups, are being phased out and replaced with more detailed, more consistent, easier-to-understand product labelling. These labels will include information on 13 nutrients (fat, saturated and *trans* fats, cholesterol, sodium, carbohydrate, fibre, sugars, protein, vitamins A and C, calcium, and iron) as well as the number of calories for a specified amount of food. You can find a wealth of information on the new labeling system on the Web at "Healthy Eating is in Store for You" (www.healthyeatingisinstore.ca).

Within each group there are many different *food choices*. The amount specified beside each food in the tables that follow represents one choice from that group and can be interchanged with any other choice in the same group. This system is highly effective, so long as you are keeping track of the amounts you are eating from the different groups.

Listing all food sources in this space isn't possible, but you can obtain a list of just about all the foods you might eat by ordering "The Good Health Eating Guide Resource" from the Canadian Diabetes Association (800-226-8464).

In the United States they use a similar concept, but they use the word *exchanges* rather than *choices*.

Starch Foods

The Starch food choices are listed in Tables A-1 and A-2. Each choice contains about 15 grams of carbohydrate, 2 grams of protein, and 68 calories. The Guide recommends high-fibre starch choices. On food labels, look for 4 grams or more of fibre per serving.

Table A-1	Starch Food Choices	
Cereals, Grains, Pasta	*Bread*	*Dried Beans, Peas, Lentils (higher in fibre and protein)*
Bran cereals, 125 mL (½ cup)	Bagel, small, ½	Beans and peas (cooked), 125 mL (½ cup)
Cooked cereals, 125 mL (½ cup)	Breadsticks, 2	Lentils (cooked), 125 mL (½ cup)

Cereals, Grains, Pasta	Bread	Dried Beans, Peas, Lentils (higher in fibre and protein)
Shredded wheat biscuit, 1	English muffin, ½	Baked beans, 125 mL (½ cup)
Wild rice (cooked), 75 mL (⅓ cup)	Wiener, ½ bun	Falafel, 2
Pasta (cooked), 125 mL (½ cup)	Hamburger bun, ½	Lima beans, 125 mL (½ cup)
Puffed wheat, 375 mL (1½ cup)	Pita, 15cm (6"), ½	Hummus, 125 mL (½ cup)
Rice (cooked), 75 mL (⅓ cup)	Raisin bread, 1 slice	
Shredded wheat, bite size, 125 mL (½ cup)	Tortilla, 20cm (9"), 1 round	
	White bread, 1 slice	
	Whole wheat bread, 1 slice	

Table A-2	More Starch Food Choices	
Crackers/Snacks	**Starchy Vegetables**	**Starchy Foods with Fats**
Soda crackers, 6	Corn, kernel, 125 mL (½ cup)	Waffle, 1
Graham crackers, 3	Corn on the cob, ½ medium	Tea biscuit, 1
Matzoh, 15cm (6"), 1	Potato, baked, ½ medium	French fries, 10
Melba toast, 4 slices	Plantain, ⅓ small	Muffin, 1 small
Popcorn (no fat added), 750 mL (3 cups)	Yam, sweet potato, 125 mL (½ cup)	Pancake, 15cm (6"), 1
Pretzels, 7		Croissant, 1 small
Rice cakes, 2		Potato chips, 15
Rusks, 2		Mashed potatoes, 125 mL (½ cup)

Fruits and Vegetables

All fresh, frozen, and canned fruits as well as unsweetened juices are in this group. However, not all vegetables are listed here. Those with a higher carbohydrate content such as corn and potatoes are found in the Starch Foods list. Very low-carbohydrate vegetables such as spinach and cabbage are in the Extras group. Each Fruit and Vegetable choice (see Table A-3) contains about 10 grams of carbohydrate, 1 gram of protein, and 44 calories of energy.

Table A-3	Fruit and Vegetable Choices		
Fruit	*Dried Fruit*	*Fruit Juice*	*Vegetables (fresh, frozen or canned)*
Apple, ½ medium	Apple, 5 pieces	Apple, 75 mL (⅓ cup)	Beets, 125 mL (½ cup)
Applesauce, 125 mL (½ cup)	Apricots, 4 halves	Carrot, 75 mL (⅓ cup)	Carrots, 125 mL (½ cup)
Apricots, 2	Dates, 2	Grapefruit, 125 mL (½ cup)	Parsnips, 125 mL (½ cup)
Watermelon, 250 mL (1 cup)	Pear, ½	Grape, 50 mL (¼ cup)	Peas, 125 mL (½ cup)
Banana, ½ small	Prunes, 2	Orange, 125 mL (½ cup)	Rutabaga, 125 mL (½ cup)
Blackberries, 250 mL (1 cup)	Raisins, 25 mL (2 tbsp)	Pineapple, 75 mL (⅓ cup)	Squash, 125 mL (½ cup)
Blueberries, 125 mL (½ cup)	Banana flakes, 25 mL (2 tbsp)	Prune, 50 mL (¼ cup)	Turnip, 125 mL (½ cup)
Cantaloupe, 175 mL (⅔ cup)		Pineapple, 75 mL (⅓ cup)	Mixed vegetable, 125 mL (½ cup)
Cherries, 10		Tomato, 250 mL (1 cup)	Tomatoes, (canned), 250 mL (1 cup)
Cherries (canned), 75 mL (⅓ cup)			
Figs, 1 medium			
Fruit cocktail, 125 mL (½ cup)			

Fruit	Dried Fruit	Fruit Juice	Vegetables (fresh, frozen or canned)
Grapefruit, ½			
Grapes, 125 mL (½ cup)			
Honeydew, 175 mL (⅔ cup)			
Kiwi, 1			
Mango, 75 mL (⅓ cup)			
Nectarine, ½ medium			
Orange, 1 small			
Papaya, 125 mL (½ cup)			
Peach, 1 large			
Peaches (canned), 125 mL (½ cup)			
Pear, ½			
Pears Halves (canned), 1 half			
Persimmon, 1			
Pineapple, 125 mL (½ cup)			
Pineapple (canned), 125 mL (½ cup)			
Plum, 2 small			
Raspberries, 250 mL (1 cup)			
Strawberries, 250 mL (1 cup)			
Tangerine, 1 medium			

Milk

The different kinds of milk available nowadays vary only in their fat content. The carbohydrate and protein content remain the same. One Milk choice contains about 6 grams of carbohydrate, 4 grams of protein, and from 0 to 4 grams of fat (skim milk, 0 grams fat and 40 calories; 1% milk, 1 gram fat and 49 calories; 2% milk, 2 grams fat and 58 calories; homogenized milk, 4 grams fat and 76 calories).

One Milk choice equals:

✔ Milk (skim, 1%, 2%, or homo): 125 mL (½ cup)

✔ Buttermilk: 125 mL (½ cup)

✔ Evaporated milk: 50 mL (¼ cup)

✔ Powdered milk: 25 mL (2 tbsp)

✔ Plain yogurt: 125 mL (½ cup)

Sugars

Sugar and food with added sugar such as candy, Popsicles, and regular jam can be part of a healthy meal plan. Current recommendations suggest no more than 10 percent of the total calories you consume be supplied by these foods. For example, if you are on a 1,500-calorie meal plan, your Sugars allowance would be about four choices because each Sugars choice contains about 10 grams of carbohydrate and 40 calories.

One Sugars choice equals:

✔ Cranberry sauce: 25 mL (2 tbsp)

✔ Honey/molasses/corn/maple syrup: 10 mL (2 tsp)

✔ White or brown sugar: 10 mL (2 tsp)

✔ Regular jam, jelly or marmalade: 15 mL (1 tbsp)

✔ Hard candy: 2

✔ Popsicles: 1 stick (½ Popsicle)

✔ Marshmallows: 2 large

✔ Cranberry cocktail: 75 mL (⅓ cup)

Likely in 2005, the Good Health Eating Guide is going to be adopting a 15 gram carbohydrate value for each choice within the fruits and vegetables, milk and sugars groups.

Protein Foods

One choice contains no carbohydrate, about 7 grams of protein, 3 grams of fat, and 55 calories of energy. Only lean Protein choices are listed here. All foods listed are cooked.

Meat and poultry:

- Beef: round, sirloin, flank, tenderloin, ground: 30 grams (1 oz)
- Pork: fresh, canned, cured, or boiled ham, ground: 30 grams (1 oz)
- Veal: All cuts except for cutlets: 30 grams (1 oz)
- Poultry; chicken, turkey: 30 grams (1 oz)

Fish and shellfish:

- All fish, fresh and frozen: 30 grams (1 oz)
- Crab, lobster: 50 mL (¼ cup)
- Oysters: 3 medium
- Canned in water (tuna or salmon): 50 mL (¼ cup)
- Canned sardines: 3 small
- Fresh shrimp: 5 large

Cheese:

- Low fat (about 7% milk fat): 1 slice, 30 grams (1 oz)
- Cottage cheese: 50 mL (¼ cup)
- Ricotta cheese: 50 mL (¼ cup)

Egg:

- Medium egg: 1

The following Protein choices are high in fat. Choose them less often.

- Bologna: 1 slice
- Canned luncheon meat: 1 slice
- Sausage: 1 link
- Weiner, hot dog: 1
- Salami: 1 slice
- Peanut butter: 15 mL (1 tbsp)
- Regular cheese: 1 slice, 30 grams (1 oz)

Fats and Oils

These foods (see Table A-4) have 5 grams of fat and little or no protein or carbohydrate per portion. The calorie count is, therefore, 45 calories. The important thing in this category is to notice the foods that are high in cholesterol and saturated fats — and avoid them.

Table A-4	Fat Choices
Unsaturated Fats	**Saturated Fats**
Avocado, ⅛ medium	Butter, 5 mL (1 tsp)
Salad dressing, regular, 10 mL (2 tsp)	Bacon, 1 slice
Margarine, 5 mL (1 tsp)	Coconut, dried, 15 mL (1tbsp)
Salad dressing, low fat, 25 mL (2 tbsp)	Cream, 25 mL (2 tbsp)
Margarine, diet, 15 mL (1 tbsp)	Cream, sour, 25 mL (2 tbsp)
Mayonnaise, 5 mL (1 tsp)	Cream, heavy, 15 mL (1 tbsp)
Almonds, 8	Cream cheese, 15 mL (1 tbsp)
Cashews, 5	Gravy, 25 mL (2 tbsp)
Pecans, 5 halves	Lard, 15 mL (1 tbsp)
Peanuts, 10	Pâté, liverwurst, 15 mL (1 tbsp)
Walnuts, 2 whole	Shortening, 5 mL (1 tsp)

Unsaturated Fats	*Saturated Fats*
Sunflower seeds, 15 mL (1 tbsp)	
Pumpkin seeds, 20 mL (4 tsp)	
Oil (corn, olive, soybean, sunflower, peanut), 5 mL (1 tsp)	
Olives, small, 10	

Extras

The foods listed in this group contain very small amounts of carbohydrate or none at all, with no fat or protein.

Extra vegetables

Extra vegetables contain some carbohydrate; however, unless you eat them in large amounts, they do not need to be counted as part of your meal plan. They include the following:

Asparagus

Beans, string, green, or yellow

Bok choy

Broccoli

Brussels sprouts

Cabbage

Cauliflower

Celery

Lettuce

Mushrooms

Okra

Onions

Peppers, green, red, and yellow

Spinach

Tomato wedges

Zucchini

Free foods

These foods do not contain significant amount of calories, so you can eat as much of them as you want without worrying about serving size (though, of course, if you eat a pound of chili powder you may regret it for other reasons!).

- ✔ **Drinks:** Bouillon, sugar-free drinks, club soda, coffee, and tea (but remember that excess consumption of caffeinated products can raise blood pressure)
- ✔ **Condiments:** Horseradish, mustard, pickles (unsweetened), and vinegar
- ✔ **Seasonings:** Basil, lemon juice, celery seeds, lime, cinnamon, mint, chili powder, onion powder, chives, oregano, curry, paprika, dill, pepper, salt, flavouring extracts (vanilla, for example), pimiento, garlic, spices, garlic powder, ginger, soy sauce, herbs, wine (used in cooking), lemon, and Worcestershire sauce

As we discuss in Chapter 10, sugar-free candy, sugar-free gum, sugar-free jam or jelly and sugar substitutes can be consumed fairly liberally, however bear in mind that sugar alcohols vary in the degree to which they are absorbed into the body and, also, in high doses they can cause unpleasant gastro-intestinal symptoms such as abdominal cramping and diarrhea.

Using "The Good Health Eating Guide" to Create a Nutrition Plan

Having different foods in each group that can be interchanged makes it easy to create a nutrition plan with great variation. The following menus show the amounts for diets of 1,500 (Table A-5) and 1,800 (Table A-7) calories.

Table A-5	1,500 calories
Breakfast	*Lunch*
2 Starch choices	2 Starch choices
2 Fruits & Vegetables choices	2 Fruits & Vegetables choices
2 Milk (1%) choices	2 Protein choices
1 Protein choice	1 Fats & Oils choice
2 Fats & Oils choices	Extras as desired

Dinner	Snack
2 Starch choices	1 Starch choice
2 Fruits & Vegetables choices	2 Milk (1%) choices
3 Protein choices	
2 Fats & Oils choices	
Extras as desired	

This menu provides 190 grams of carbohydrate, 78 grams of protein and 47 grams of fat, keeping it in line with 50 percent of energy from carbohydrate, 20 percent of energy from protein, and 30 percent of energy from fat.

Translating this into food, you can have the menu in Table A-6 on one day:

Table A-6	A Sample Menu
Breakfast	**Lunch**
2 slices toast	2 slices bread
1 pear	125 mL (½ cup) carrots & 1 peach
250 mL (1 cup) 1% milk	1 slice cheese (low-fat) & 1 slice ham
1 egg	5 mL (1 tsp) margarine
2 tsp margarine	Extra vegetables (such as lettuce, cucumber for sandwich)
Dinner	**Bedtime Snack**
1 medium potato	1 shredded wheat biscuit
125 mL (½ cup) peas	250 mL (1 cup) 1% milk
125 mL (½ cup) grapes	
90g (3 oz) lean beef	
20 mL (4 tsp) regular salad dressing	
Salad or Extra vegetables	

For an 1,800-calorie diet, you could have the menu in Table A-7:

Table A-7	1,800 Calories Sample Menu
Breakfast	**Lunch**
2 Starch choices	3 Starch choices
2 Fruit & Vegetable choices	2 Fruit & Vegetable choices
2 Milk (2%) choices	2 Protein choices
2 Protein choices	2 Fats & Oils choices
2 Fats & Oils choices	Extras as desired
Extras as desired	
Dinner	**Snack**
3 Starch choices	1 Starch choice
2 Fruits & Vegetable choices	2 Milk (2%) choices
3 Protein choices	
2 Fats & Oils choices	
Extras as desired	

This diet provides 219 grams of carbohydrate, 89 grams of protein, and 59 grams of fat, again maintaining the 50:20:30 division of calories. Using the example of the 1,500-calorie diet, go ahead and try to make up an 1,800-calorie diet at this point.

Appendix B

Recipes: A Tasty Trek from Coast to Coast to Coast

. . . .

In This Chapter

▶ Caribou Stew from the Yukon

▶ Caribou and Lentil Spaghetti Sauce from N.W.T.

▶ Arctic Char Chowder from Nunavut

▶ Oatmeal Bannock from B.C.

▶ Corn Chowder and Potato Soup from Alberta

▶ Chuckwagon Chili and Berry Breakfast Drink from Saskatchewan

▶ Beef Kabobs and Turkey Rolls from Manitoba

▶ One-Pot Easy Chicken Rice from Ontario

▶ Lentil Rice Casserole from Quebec

▶ Madawaska Ploye from New Brunswick

▶ Heart-Smart Biscuits from Nova Scotia

▶ P.E.I. Potato Chili from — you guessed it — P.E.I.

▶ Steamed Partridgeberry Pudding and Fish Cakes from Newfoundland and Labrador

. . . .

As a lifelong Canadian, Ian finds that every time he travels across Canada he finds more reasons to love this country. And as a lifelong eater, Ian finds that when he thinks back on places he has visited, often the first thing that comes to mind is the food he has eaten. Whether it was fish 'n' chips in Twillingate, a crepe in old Quebec City, a steak in Calgary, Arctic char at the Wildcat Café, or a salad at Roundhouse Lodge, memories of the place and the food are often inextricably linked. (These are, of course, Ian's fond memories. He has opted not to share the details of his crummy burger from an anonymous province, his stale chocolate cake from another unnamed province . . .!)

This appendix takes you on a tastebud-tantalizing journey across Canada as we look at recipes that have been submitted by some of the country's dietitians.

Yukon Territories

Caribou Stew

¾ kg (1½ lb) diced caribou meat*

1½ L (6 cups) water

15 mL (1 tbsp) vegetable oil

175 mL (¾ cup) diced celery

375 mL (1½ cup) diced carrots

250 mL (1 cup) diced potatoes

250 mL (1 cup) diced onions

5 mL (1 tsp) garlic powder

10 mL (2 tsp) Worcestershire sauce

420 mL (14 oz) canned tomatoes

* Lean ground beef can be substituted for caribou meat.

1 In stewing pot, heat oil.

2 Place diced caribou meat, water, salt, and pepper into the pot.

3 Brown the meat.

4 Add diced vegetables and continue to cook until tender.

5 Add tomatoes, garlic, and Worcestershire sauce.

6 Mix 15 mL of flour in 250 mL of ice-cold water to make a paste.

7 Add paste gradually to the stew.

8 Cook slowly until stew reaches desired thickness.

Yield: *6 servings*

Each serving *contains 152 calories, 12 grams carbohydrate, 19 grams protein, and 3 grams fat. It constitutes 3 Protein choices and 1 Fruit and Vegetable choice.*

Contributed by: Sharlene Clarke, R.D.N., Elisa Levi, R.D., First Nations Health Program, Whitehorse, Yukon Territories

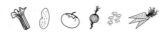

Northwest Territories

Caribou and Lentil Spaghetti Sauce

15 mL (1 tbsp) vegetable oil

¼ kg (½ lb) ground caribou meat*

½ medium onion

2 medium carrots

125 mL (½ cup) dried, red lentils

798 mL (28 oz) spaghetti sauce (jar or can)

5 mL (1 tsp) dried oregano (optional)

2 mL (½ tsp) garlic powder (optional)

125 mL (½ cup) cold water

¼ of a small box frozen, chopped spinach (thawed)

* Lean ground beef can be substituted for caribou meat.

1 Get all your ingredients together. Chop the onions. Grate the carrots.

2 Heat oil in large pot over medium-high heat. Add ground caribou meat and cook well.

3 Add onion, carrots, and cook 10 minutes until soft.

4 Add lentils, spaghetti sauce, dried oregano and garlic powder, and 125 mL cold water.

5 Bring mixture to a boil, stirring well, Reduce heat, cover pot, and simmer 20 to 30 minutes. Add a little water if mixture is too thick.

6 Add frozen spinach. Cook 10 minutes longer.

Yield: 6 servings

Each serving *contains 280 calories, 36 grams carbohydrate, 16 grams protein, and 8 grams fat. It constitutes 2 Starch choices, 1½ Protein choices, ½ a Fruit and Vegetable choice, and 1½ Fat and Oil choices.*

Contributed by: Mabel Wong, R.D., Healthy Choices Cooking Club, Yellowknife, Northwest Territories

(Mabel notes that "We first used this recipe in Taloyoak with muskox!")

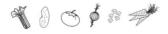

Nunavut

Arctic Char Chowder

1 kg (2 lbs) Arctic char

50 mL (¼ cup) finely diced salt pork or bacon

125 mL ½ cup) chopped onion

250 mL (1 cup) diced potatoes

500 mL (2 cups) water

250 mL (1 cup) skim milk powder

2 385-mL cans evaporated milk

2 mL (½ tsp) salt or salt to taste

0.5 mL (⅛ tsp) pepper or to taste

5 mL (1 tsp) garlic powder

15 mL (1 tbsp) parsley (optional)

1 Fry the salt pork or bacon in a heavy pot until crisp.

2 Sauté the onions until tender in the bacon fat, then add the potatoes.

3 Mix together water and skim milk power, and add to pot.

4 Cover and simmer for 30 minutes or until potatoes are tender.

5 Add the raw Arctic char, cubed, evaporated milk, salt, pepper and garlic powder. Bring to a simmer but do not boil. Simmer for half an hour to cook the char. (The flavour of the chowder improves with simmering time.)

6 When serving, garnish with parsley (if using). Place a small piece of butter in each soup plate before serving the chowder.

Yield: *6 servings*

Each serving *contains 437 calories, 30 grams carbohydrate, 55 grams protein, and 10 grams fat. It constitutes 5 Protein choices, 4 Milk choices, ½ a Starch choice, and 1 Fat and Oil choice.*

Contributed by: Rhonda Reid, Regional Nutritionist, Cambridge Bay, Nunavut

(Rhonda notes that "To enhance the nutritional quality, add diced carrots and corn when adding the raw char. This recipe doubles and triples well. The recipe can be adapted to other types of fish as well.")

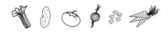

British Columbia

Oatmeal Bannock

1 L (4 cups) unbleached flour
45 mL (3 tbsp) baking powder
15 mL (1 tbsp) sugar
2 mL (½ tsp) salt
250 mL (1 cup) whole-wheat flour

125 mL (½ cup) canola or sunflower oil
625 mL (2½ cups) small-flake oatmeal (or quick rolled oats [not instant])
150 mL (⅔ cup) skim milk powder
500 mL (2 cups) water

1 Sift together first 4 ingredients.

2 Add whole-wheat flour and small-flake oatmeal.

3 Gradually add oil, mixing with a fork, to make a crumbly mixture.

4 Dissolve milk powder in water, and add to dry mixture, adding more water if necessary so that it holds together as a lump.

5 Press onto a greased cookie sheet until about 2.5 centimetres (1 inch) thick.

6 Prick with fork and bake at 200°C/400°F for 25 minutes.

7 Let cool slightly before cutting.

Yield: *50 servings*

Each serving contains 90 calories, 15 grams carbohydrate, 2 grams protein, and 2 grams fat. It constitutes 1 Starch choice, and ½ a Fat and Oil choice.

Contributed by: Esther Stevens, R.D.N., Kitimat, British Columbia

(Esther notes that "This moist loaf makes enough for a crowd. The loaf also freezes nicely; just let it cool completely first.")

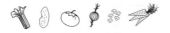

Alberta

Corn Chowder

1 large onion

2 strips bacon, diced

2.5 L (10 cups) water

8 to 10 stalks celery, diced

5 medium potatoes, diced

5 mL (1 tsp) pepper

750 mL (3 cups) milk, skim or 1%

250 mL (1 cup) flour

125 mL (½ cup) chicken base, low salt

500 mL (2 cups) corn

75 mL (⅓ cup) fresh chives or green onions, chopped

1 Cook onion and bacon in medium skillet. Drain fat.

2 In a large stockpot, bring to a boil water, celery, potatoes, onion, bacon, and pepper. Cook until vegetables are tender.

3 Mix milk, flour, and chicken base. Add to soup. Simmer gently.

4 Add corn and chives, and heat through.

Yield: 8 servings

Each serving contains 222 calories, 45 grams carbohydrate, 9 grams protein, and 2 grams fat. It constitutes 2½ Starch choices, ½ a Milk choice, and ½ a Fat and Oil choice.

Source: Mary Crier, Cook, Hobemma, Alberta

Contributed by: Heather Komar, B.Sc., R.D., Lethbridge, Alberta

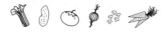

Potato Soup

500 mL (2 cups) milk, skim or 1%

1 L (4 cups) potatoes, peeled and diced

375 mL (1½ cups) celery, diced

1 large onion, finely diced

2 cloves garlic, crushed

15 mL (1 tbsp) fresh or dried rosemary

2 mL (½ tsp) pepper

25 mL (2 tbsp) margarine, non-hydrogenated

1.125 L (4½ cups) flour

1 In a 7-L (6-quart) saucepan, over medium heat, slowly heat milk to boiling. Add potatoes, celery, onion, garlic, rosemary, and pepper; cook covered over medium heat until vegetables are tender.

2 Combine margarine and flour, first with a fork and then with fingers, until crumbly. Pour in small heavy skillet and brown well over medium heat.

3 Slowly sprinkle flour mixture into simmering vegetable mixture, stirring constantly to prevent lumps. Cook until thick. Serve hot.

Yield: 10 servings

Each serving contains 305 calories, 60 grams carbohydrate, 9 grams protein, and 3 grams fat. It constitutes 3½ Starch choices, ½ a Milk choice, and ½ a Fat and Oil choice.

Source: Gertrude Strikes With A Gun, Piikani Elder, Southern Alberta

Contributed by: Heather Komar, B.Sc., R.D Lethbridge, Alberta

The Alberta recipes are reproduced, with kind permission, from the book *First Nations Healthy Choice Recipes*, published by the Chinook Health Region and the Southern Alberta Aboriginal Diabetes Coalition.

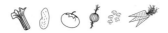

Saskatchewan

Berry Breakfast Drink

175 mL (¾cup) chopped ice
125 mL (½ cup) orange juice
125 mL (½ cup) yogurt
½ banana

125 mL (½ cup) Saskatoon berries
2 large strawberries
25 mL (2 tbsp) ground flax seed
45 mL (3 tbsp) roasted crushed almonds

1 Put all ingredients (except the roasted crushed almonds) in blender and blend for 1 minute or until smooth.

2 Stir in 45 mL roasted crushed almonds, and serve.

Yield: 1 serving

Each serving contains 535 calories, 55 grams carbohydrate, 18 grams protein, and 27 grams fat. It constitutes 4 Fruit and Vegetable choices, 1 Milk choice, 2 Protein choices, and 4 Fat and Oil choices.

Contributed by: Rachel Simonson, R.D., Regina Qu'Appelle Health Region, Saskatchewan

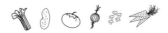

Chuckwagon Chili

¾ kg (1½ lb) lean ground beef

1 medium onion, chopped

1 398-mL (14-oz) can kidney beans and juice

1 284-mL (10-oz) can mushrooms, drained

2 medium carrots, sliced

1 284-mL (10-oz) can low-sodium tomato soup

1 mL (¼ tsp) pepper

5 mL (1 tsp) chili powder

Low-fat cheese, shredded (optional)

1 Brown beef and onions; drain excess fat.

2 Add rest of ingredients.

3 Stir and bring to boil.

4 Let simmer about 20 minutes.

5 Taste and add more seasoning if desired.

6 Top with shredded low-fat cheese (if using), and serve with salad and whole grain bread.

Yield: 4 to 6 servings

Each serving contains 346 calories, 15 grams carbohydrate, 32 grams protein, and 16 grams fat. It constitutes 4 Protein choices, 2 Starch choices, and 1 Fat and Oil choice.

Contributed by: Rachel Simonson, R.D., Regina Qu'Appelle Health Region, Saskatchewan

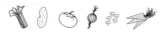

Manitoba

Manitoba Beef Kabobs

½ kg (1 lb) beef sirloin or round, cubed

25 mL (2 tbsp) canola oil

25 mL (2 tbsp) red wine vinegar

5 mL (1 tsp) garlic powder

5 mL (1 tsp) onion powder

1 mL (¼ tsp) ground pepper

5 mL (1 tsp) dried oregano

5 mL (1 tsp) Worcestershire sauce

15 mL (1 tbsp) soy sauce

½ green pepper, cut in chunks

½ yellow or red pepper, cut in chunks

8 fresh mushrooms

8 cherry tomatoes

¼ yellow onion, cut in chunks

1 In small bowl combine oil, vinegar, garlic powder, onion powder, pepper, oregano, Worcestershire sauce, and soy sauce.

2 Put meat in a large bowl or plastic container. Pour marinade over cubed meat and toss the meat well with the marinade. Cover and refrigerate for at least 2 hours or overnight for best results.

3 If using wooden skewers, soak in water. Remove from water and on each skewer alternate the meat and vegetables as desired.

4 Arrange on the barbecue, indoor grill, or broiler pan. Cook until meat is done, about 10 minutes, turning occasionally.

Yield: *8 skewers*

Each serving *contains 129 calories, 15 grams protein, and 7 grams fat. It constitutes 2 Protein choices, and 1 Fat and Oil choice.*

Contributed by: Kathryn Penner, R.D., C.D.E., Winkler, Manitoba

(Kathryn suggests that the skewers be served on a bed of rice with a mixed garden salad on the side. A fruit yogurt for dessert completes the meal.)

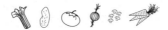

Turkey Rolls

4 25-centimetre (10-inch) whole-wheat flour tortillas

125 mL (½ cup) ultra-light cream cheese

5 mL (1 tsp) garlic powder (measure to taste)

250 mL (1 cup) chopped green and red pepper

125 mL (½ cup) chopped green onion

180 grams (6 oz) cold turkey or chicken, sliced

1 Mix cream cheese and garlic powder together and set aside. Chop up the peppers and onions. Spread each tortilla with cream cheese mixture. Arrange turkey in a single layer over the cream cheese. Sprinkle turkey with chopped peppers and green onions.

2 Roll up tightly, jellyroll style, and refrigerate in air-tight container for a least 2 hours before serving.

3 Cut each roll into 12 2.5-centimetre (1-inch) slices. Discard ends. Enjoy!

(continued)

Yield: 48 pieces

4 pieces contain 72 calories, 8 grams carbohydrate, 4 grams protein, and 3 grams fat. It constitutes ½ a Protein choice, and ½ a Starch choice.

Contributed by: Kathryn Penner, R.D., C.D.E., Winkler, Manitoba

(Kathryn notes, in reference to the turkey rolls, "Great appetizer! Fast and easy, but best of all your friends will think you spent hours in the kitchen.")

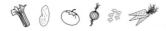

Ontario

One Pot Easy Chicken Rice

250g (½ lb) boneless chicken, cut into bite-size pieces (use a combination of breast and thighs)

5 mL (1 tsp) dark soy sauce

5 mL (1 tsp) light soy sauce

2 mL (½ tsp) sesame seed oil

2 mL (½ tsp) sugar

5 mL (1 tsp) minced garlic

5 mL (1 tsp) minced ginger

250 mL (1 cup) rice

250 mL (1 cup) stock

125 mL (½ cup) water

10 mL (2 tsp) oil

Salt, pepper to taste

Cilantro for garnish (optional)

1 Marinate chicken with the dark and light soy sauce, sesame oil, and sugar.

2 Put rice in a sieve and run cold tap water through to wash thoroughly. Let rice sit in sieve to dry.

3 In a nonstick pot, heat oil over medium heat and sauté garlic and ginger until slightly brown.

4 Add rice and continue to sauté until rice grains are coated with oil mixture.

5 Add stock and water and bring to gentle boil. Let rice boil for 1 minute.

6 Add chicken to rice, making sure that it sits on top of the rice mixture in one layer; do not stir.

7 Bring to a gentle boil again. After 1 to 2 minutes, turn heat down to low.

8 Cover pot and let rice steam for about 25 minutes or until rice and chicken are cooked.

9 Let sit for at least 5 minutes before serving.

10 Sprinkle with chopped cilantro.

11 Serve hot with plenty of green vegetables.

Yield: *4 servings*

Each serving *contains 273 calories, 30 grams carbohydrate, 18 grams protein, and 9 grams fat. It constitutes 2 Starch choices, 2 Protein choices, and ½ a Fat and Oil choice.*

Contributed by: Bin Chin R.D., C.D.E., Ajax, Ontario

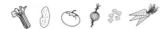

Quebec

Lentil Rice Casserole

250 mL (1 cup) dry brown lentils, boiled, unsalted

7 mL (1.5 tsp) salt

1 mL (¼ tsp) ground black pepper

2 medium white onions

15 mL (3 tsp) canola oil

500 mL (2 cups) long-grain brown rice, cooked

1 clove garlic, minced, if desired

1 Rinse lentils and soak in cold water for 30 minutes.

2 Drain and place in medium pot on stove.

3 Add 625 mL (2½ cups) water, salt and pepper.

4 Bring to boil; reduce heat and simmer about 40 minutes or until tender.

5 While lentils are cooking, chop onions and fry in 5 mL oil. Remove to a plate.

6 Drain boiled lentils, and sauté them in 10 mL remaining oil, stirring constantly until dry and crisp, about 3 minutes.

7 Add rice, half the sautéed onion, and chopped garlic (if using); continue to sauté 2 to 3 minutes while tossing carefully.

8 Place in serving bowl and top with remaining onion.

Yield: *4 servings*

Each serving *contains 320 calories, 55 grams carbohydrate, 16 grams protein, 5 grams fat and 14 grams fibre. It constitutes 2 Starch choices, 2 Protein choices and 1 Fruit and Vegetable choice.*

Contributed by: Sondra Sherman, P.Dt., C.D.E., Mavis Verronneau DES Montreal Chapter, Montreal, Quebec

(Sondra has been using this recipe for over 20 years and it's "just delicious.")

New Brunswick

Madawaska Ploye

500 mL (2 cups) buckwheat flour
250 mL (1 cup) white flour
5 mL (1 tsp) salt

425 mL (1¾ cups) cold water
550 mL (2¼ cups) boiling water
45 mL (3 tbsp) baking powder

1 Mix buckwheat flour, white flour and salt with the cold water. Mix well.

2 Gradually add the boiling water to the mixture. Mix well. Add the baking powder. Set aside for at least 1 hour.

3 In a non-stick frying pan, pour a little bit of the mixture. Cook the ploye on one side only.

(Can be eaten with non-hydrogenated margarine, molasses or maple syrup.)

Yield: *30 to 35 portions*

Each serving *contains 40 calories, 8 grams carbohydrate, and 1 gram protein. It constitutes ½ a Starch choice.*

Contributed by: Janie Levesque, R.D., Campbellton, New Brunswick

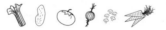

Nova Scotia

Heart-Smart Biscuits

1 L (4 cups) flour
25 mL (2 tbsp) baking powder
5 mL (1 tsp) baking soda
5 mL (1 tsp) salt
5 mL (1 tsp) sugar

325 mL (1½ cups) plain low-fat yogurt
125 mL (½ cup) vegetable oil
1 egg plus enough low-fat milk (about ½ cup) to make 175 mL (¾ cup)

1 Combine dry ingredients and mix well.

2 In separate bowl mix yogurt, oil, egg, and milk.

3 Add wet ingredients to dry ingredients.

4 Gently combine with a fork. Do not over-mix.

5 Pat dough on a floured surface.

6 Cut out 24 medium-size biscuits.

7 Place on a baking sheet, bake at 200°C/400°F for 15 to 20 minutes.

Yield: *24 servings*

Each serving *contains 132 calories, 17 grams carbohydrate, 3.4 grams protein, and 5.2 grams fat. It constitutes 1 Starch choice, and 1 Fat and Oil choice.*

Contributed by: Pamela Soley, P.Dt., Canso, Nova Scotia

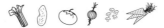

Prince Edward Island

P.E.I. Potato Chili

500 mL (2 cups) tomato juice

500 mL (2 cups) vegetable stock

3 P.E.I. potatoes, diced

1 medium onion, chopped

2 small carrots, chopped

1 celery stalk, chopped

1 green or red pepper, chopped

2 garlic cloves, crushed

1 398-mL (14-oz) can kidney beans

1 540-mL (19-oz) can chopped tomatoes

250 mL (1 cup) dried green or brown lentils

1 284-mL (10-oz) can chickpeas

25 mL (2 tbsp) chili powder

5 mL (1 tsp) dried oregano

2 mL (½ tsp) dried basil

0.5 mL (⅛ tsp) pepper

125 mL (½ cup) plain low-fat yogurt (optional)

(continued)

1 Wash lentils.

2 Drain and rinse chickpeas.

3 Combine all ingredients, except yogurt, in a heavy saucepan, cover and bring to a boil. Reduce heat and simmer about 30 minutes, stirring occasionally, until lentils are tender.

4 Dish into serving bowls and garnish with a dollop of yogurt, if desired.

Yield: *8 servings*

Each serving *contains 285 calories, 53 grams carbohydrate, 17 grams protein, 2 grams fat, and 16 grams fibre. It constitutes 1 Protein choice, 2 Starch choices, and 2 Fruit and Vegetable choices.*

Source: PEI Potato Board

Contributed by: Libby Logan, R.D., Summerside, PEI

(Libby notes that "When I first tasted this recipe, I actually had to be shown the recipe before I would believe that it didn't contain meat. It is delicious and very satisfying and filling!")

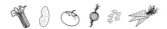

Newfoundland and Labrador

Steamed Partridgeberry Pudding

375 mL (1½ cups) all purpose flour	50 mL (¼ cup) margarine
30 mL (2 tbsp) granulated sugar	375 mL (1½ cups partridgeberries*)
15 mL (1 tbsp) baking powder	125 mL (½ cup) skim milk
1 mL (¼ tsp) salt	1 medium egg, beaten

* Cranberries or blueberries may be substituted

1 Stir dry ingredients together in a bowl.

2 Rub in margarine.

3 Fold in berries.

4 Add the milk and beaten egg, stirring lightly to make a batter.

5 Pour into a greased mould.

6 Place over boiling water and steam for 1 hour.

Yield: *12 servings*

Each serving contains 118 calories, 17 grams carbohydrate, 3 grams protein, and 5 grams fat. It constitutes 1 Starch choice, and 1 Fat and Oil choice.

Contributed by: Jocelyn Martin, R.D., St. John's Newfoundland

(Jocelyn notes that "In Newfoundland, this type of pudding is commonly served as part of the starchy food with the traditional boiled "Jigg's Dinner," similar to the English Corned Beef Dinner. It may also be served warm, with a fruit sauce or butter-scotch sauce over the top, as a dessert.")

Fish Cakes

½ kg (1 lb) Atlantic cod, cooked, deboned and flaked*

1 medium onion, chopped fine

5 mL (1 tsp) margarine

6 small potatoes, cooked and mashed**

15 mL (1 tbsp) margarine

1 mL (¼tsp) white pepper

2 mL (½ tsp) Newfoundland savory or parsley

1 medium egg, beaten

50 mL (¼ cup) all-purpose flour

15 mL (1 tbsp) margarine or vegetable oil

* Cook fish by poaching in lightly salted water.

** Cook potatoes by boiling in lightly salted water.

1 Prepare fish and potatoes as indicated.

2 Sauté onion in 5 mL of margarine until translucent.

3 Mash together fish and potatoes with 15 mL of margarine.

(continued)

4 Add onions and seasonings.

5 Add beaten egg and mix well.

6 Chill until cool and firm.

7 Form mixture into cakes, about 7.5 centimetres (3 inches) round.

8 Lightly coat cakes with flour.

9 Fry cakes in remaining margarine or vegetable oil over medium-high heat, about 2 to 3 minutes on each side or until crisp and golden.

Yield: 6 servings

Each serving contains 226 calories, 21 grams carbohydrate, 21 grams protein, and 6 grams fat. It constitutes 3 Protein choices, 1 Starch choice, ½ a Fruit and Vegetable choice, and 1 Fat and Oil choice.

Contributed by: Jocelyn Martin, R.D., St. John's, Newfoundland

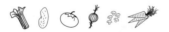

Appendix C

Straight Goods on a Tangled Web: Diabetes Web Sites Worth Visiting

· ·

In This Appendix

▶ Starting at the authors' Web sites

▶ Checking general sites about diabetes

▶ Looking at companies that make diabetes products

▶ Combining athletics and diabetes

▶ Exploring sites that address Aboriginal issues

▶ Discovering sites about children and diabetes

▶ Searching Web pages in French

▶ Finding sites for the visually impaired

▶ Sniffing out Web sites with recipes for people with diabetes

▶ Getting the lowdown on diabetes in dogs and cats

· ·

*I*n just a few short years, the World Wide Web has gone from a topic of esoteric conversation amongst "techies" to being an invaluable resource to hundreds of millions (soon to be billions) of people. It seems almost inconceivable, but a famous electronic encyclopedia didn't even have an entry for the Web as recently as the 1995 edition.

Of course, as any Web surfer knows, with the good comes the bad. One minute you are looking at a high-quality, reputable, well-maintained site like that of the Canadian or American diabetes associations and the next click you are looking at Uncle Bob's Instant Diabetes Cure. The problem is not that great information isn't out there; the problem is trying to figure out which sites have it and which just pretend to.

We discuss here sites that we have found particularly useful. You should be able to get answers to just about any questions that you have. However, you must be cautious. A Web site is offering information to many people; it does not know you and your unique needs. Therefore, you should not make any major changes in your diabetes care without first checking with your health care team. Remember also that the Web is constantly changing and growing, so the Web addresses we mention may change.

If you want to stay abreast of new, worthwhile sites, one helpful way to do this is to periodically check the "links" pages of sites that you have come to know and trust.

Ian and Alan's Web Sites

Start your search at our Web pages:

```
www.ianblumer.com
```

```
www.drrubin.com
```

You can find general information and advice about diabetes, tips, new developments, and answers to questions.

Ian's site has a list of all the Web sites listed in this appendix, so you need only click on them to see them for yourself.

General Sites

All-encompassing sites such as the following will tell you about diabetes from A to Z. In keeping with that, we list them alphabetically.

The American Diabetes Association (ADA)

There's loads of information at this helpful site, but as you might imagine, it uses American units (for glucose, cholesterol, and so on), which can make it confusing for those of us north of the 49th parallel. Also, it uses American guidelines, which at times can be quite different from Canadian ones.

```
www.diabetes.org
```

The Canadian Diabetes Association (CDA)

The CDA site is particularly helpful as it looks at diabetes issues from a Canadian perspective. Canadian guidelines are the backbone of the supplied information, and, of course, this site uses Canadian (international, actually) units. Particularly helpful is the listing of resources (including addresses and phone numbers) available in your province or territory and even within your community.

```
www.diabetes.ca
```

Diabetic Exercise and Sports Association

The Diabetes Exercise and Sports Association Web site is a place where you can find out about many different kinds of exercise and how they fit with your diabetes. You will also find others who share your interests. You can find this group at

```
www.diabetes-exercise.org
```

MEDLINEplus Drug Information

You'll find excellent information at this site, clear and well-presented, on virtually any drug you are likely to be prescribed. Highly recommended.

```
www.nlm.nih.gov/medlineplus/druginformation.html
```

Scientific Sites

These sites are geared toward health care professionals; however, if you have a good understanding of diabetes and can put up with the medicalese, you will be able to find very useful information here.

CenterWatch Clinical Trials Listing Service

Whether you are a layperson or a physician, you may find it very difficult to keep tabs on what research studies are underway. Even the Internet is only partially helpful, since there is no one site that lists all the studies that are going on at any given time. Also, many studies are run on a small scale and/or are industry-sponsored, and these studies are often not noted on the Web.

CenterWatch Clinical Trials Listing Service lists many studies that are looking for participants. If you think you are interested in being part of research (some of which is truly cutting edge), have a look at this site.

```
www.centerwatch.com
```

Medscape Diabetes and Endocrinology Home Page

Especially helpful for providing in-depth discussion on diabetes topics, this site provides current, state-of-the-art information as well as reviews of important topics. (Ian has even set his browser to use this site as his home page.)

```
www.endocrine.medscape.com/Home/Topics/endocrinology/
endocrinology.html
```

PubMed Search Service of the National Library of Medicine

Surf on over to the National Library of Medicine in the United States. It's easy to use and gives you (for free) a large number of the latest scientific papers on any medical topic of interest. Bear in mind that these are academic references and are written for health care professionals.

```
www.ncbi.nlm.nih.gov/PubMed
```

Sites about Diabetes and Aboriginal Populations

Canadian Diabetes Association (CDA)

The CDA site has excellent information on Aboriginal issues and has links to a number of additional Aboriginal diabetes sites.

```
www.diabetes.ca
```

Diabetes Close to Home

Though this site focuses on awareness and prevention of diabetes in northern Saskatchewan, the well-presented information is widely applicable.

```
www.diabetes.kcdc.ca
```

Sandy Lake Health and Diabetes Project

Read here about the innovative project that the Sandy Lake community has developed to combat diabetes.

```
www.sandylakediabetes.com
```

Sites about Diabetes and Children

Children with Diabetes

This site is the creation of a father of a child with diabetes and has an enormous database of information for the parents of children with diabetes.

```
www.childrenwithdiabetes.com
```

Juvenile Diabetes Research Foundation of Canada (JDRF)

The JDRF prides itself on its contribution to research in diabetes, and this site reflects that. You can find what you want to know about the latest government programs that emphasize finding a cure for diabetes.

```
www.jdrf.ca
```

Sites about Insulin Pump Therapy

Sites devoted to insulin pump therapy are very informative and definitely worth looking at if you are considering this treatment option. These sites, however, tend to be written by very passionate people discussing a treatment they feel very passionately about, so there is the possibility that some of the information will not be presented with full objectivity.

Insulin Pumpers Canada

This advocacy-oriented site is affiliated with a larger, international organization. They are not directly aligned with any specific pump manufacturer which helps them to remain objective about one company's products compared to anothers. This is a good place to start your reading about pumps and it offers some excellent links to further your search.

```
www.insulin-pumpers.ca
```

S.U.G.A.R.

This is the site of a charitable organization whose express purpose is to offer financial assistance to individuals who could not otherwise obtain an insulin pump.

```
www.sugarcharity.org
```

Sites for the Visually Impaired

Some excellent sites are geared specifically to the issue of visual impairment.

American Foundation for the Blind

The American Foundation for the Blind has resources, information, reports, talking books, and limitless other facts and wisdom about dealing with visual impairment.

```
www.afb.org
```

Blindness Resource Center

This site points you in the right direction for information on every aspect of blindness. It is a guide to other sites about visual impairment.

```
www.nyise.org/blind.htm
```

The Canadian Council of the Blind

This organization is an advocacy group *for* visually impaired people, run *by* visually impaired people.

```
www.ccbnational.net
```

The Canadian National Institute for the Blind (CNIB)

The CNIB is a well-known organization that serves to assist people with visual impairment. Their well-organized site details the different services they have to offer.

```
www.cnib.ca
```

Recipe Web Sites for People with Diabetes

You can find a number of excellent recipes on World Wide Web sites. Particularly good ones are noted here.

The American Diabetes Association (ADA)

The ADA has an extensive list of recipes — enough to keep you full for ages.

```
www.diabetes.org
```

The Canadian Diabetes Association (CDA)

Not as extensive as the ADA's list, but still food for thought, is the CDA's list of recipes.

```
www.diabetes.ca
```

Children with Diabetes

Here you'll find a huge collection of recipes including those submitted by their readers (which is good in that they come personally recommended; however, it also means the recipes may not have been evaluated by a professional dietitian).

www.childrenwithdiabetes.com

Diabetic Gourmet Magazine

In this online magazine you'll find many recipes and even a rating system — you can vote thumbs up or down on last night's dinner. Of course, your kids will already have voiced their opinion *without* the computer.

www.diabeticgourmet.com/

Sites of Companies That Make Diabetes Products

Are you looking for information from the companies that make the products you need to control your diabetes? If you have questions about the proper use of a drug or a device, you can usually find it answered here.

Insulin

- ✔ Aventis: www.aventis.ca
- ✔ Eli Lilly: www.lilly.ca
- ✔ Novo Nordisk: www.novonordisk.ca

Insulin pumps

- ✔ Animas Corporation: www.animascorp.com
- ✔ Deltec Inc.: www.delteccozmo.com
- ✔ Disetronic Medical Systems Inc.: www.disetronic-usa.com
- ✔ Medtronic MiniMed Inc.: www.minimed.com

Glucose meters

- Bayer: www.bayer.ca
- Becton-Dickson: www.bddiabetes.com
- Lifescan: www.lifescancanada.com
- Novo Nordisk: www.novonordisk.ca
- MediSense: www.medisense.com
- Roche: www.rochecanada.com
- Therasense: www.therasense.com

Disposable A1C devices

- Metrika Inc.: www.metrika.com

Pens and pen needles

- Auto Control Medical: www.autocontrol.com
- Becton-Dickson: www.bddiabetes.com
- Eli Lilly: www.lilly.ca
- Novo Nordisk: www.novonordisk.ca

Lancing devices and lancets

- Bayer: www.bayer.ca
- Becton-Dickson: www.bddiabetes.com
- Lifescan: www.lifescancanada.com
- MediSense: www.medisense.com
- Roche: www.rochecanada.com
- Therasense: www.therasense.com

Syringes

- Auto Control Medical: www.autocontrol.com
- Becton-Dickson: www.bddiabetes.com

Urine test strips

- Bayer: www.bayer.ca
- Roche: www.rochecanada.com

Sites in French

There are not nearly as many French language sites as there are English, but the following are particularly helpful:

- **Association Canadienne du diabète**: www.diabetes.ca/Section_Main/francais.asp
- **Association diabète Québec**: www.diabete.qc.ca
- **Section Diabète, site de Santé Canada**: www.hc-sc.gc.ca/pphbdgspsp/ccdpc-cpcmc/diabetes-diabete/francais/index.html
- **Dr. Samuel**: http://drsamuel.cyberquebec.com/index.html

Animals with Diabetes

Yes, your dog and cat and many other animals can get diabetes. Here is a site for your beloved pet.

www.petdiabetes.org/

Appendix D

Glossary

A1C: A measurement of overall blood glucose control for approximately the last 2 to 3 months. (Also referred to as the hemoglobin A1C or HbA1C).

Acarbose: An oral hypoglycemic agent that lowers blood glucose by blocking the breakdown of carbohydrates in the intestine.

ACE inhibitor: A class of drug that lowers blood pressure and that is especially useful to prevent kidney malfunction and cardiovascular disease in people with diabetes. (Examples of ACE inhibitors are Altace and Vasotec.)

Actos: *See pioglitazone.*

Amaryl: *See glimepiride.*

Amino acids: Compounds that link together to form proteins.

Antibodies: A type of protein formed when the body detects something foreign such as bacteria.

Aspart: A type of rapid-acting insulin.

Atherosclerosis: Narrowing of arteries due to deposits of cholesterol and other substances.

Autoimmune disorder: Disease such as type 1 diabetes in which the body's immune system mistakenly attacks its own tissues.

Autonomic neuropathy: Diseases of nerves that affect organs not under conscious control, such as the heart, lungs, and intestine.

Avandia: *See rosiglitazone.*

Basal insulin: The low level of insulin present in the body around the clock in people taking intermediate- or long-acting insulin or on insulin pumps. Basal insulin is generally used in combination with bolus insulin.

Beta cell: A type of islet cell in the pancreas that makes insulin.

Blood glucose meter: A small, portable machine that allows for moment-to-moment measurement of your blood glucose level.

Body mass index: A measure of whether or not you are at a healthy weight for your height.

Bolus insulin: Rapid- or fast-acting insulin given with meals or snacks to quickly raise the blood insulin levels to reduce blood glucose. Bolus insulin supplements the use of basal insulin.

Brittle diabetes: A condition of erratic blood glucose control in people with type 1 diabetes often leading to hospitalizations with ketoacidosis or hypoglycemia. With optimal diabetes management, brittle diabetes is seldom encountered.

Carbohydrate: One of the three major energy sources, the one usually found in grain, fruits, and vegetables and the one most responsible for raising the blood glucose.

Carbohydrate counting: Estimating the amount of carbohydrate in food in order to determine insulin needs.

Cataract: A clouding of the lens of the eye often found earlier and more commonly in people with diabetes.

Cholesterol: A fat-like substance that is needed in the body (for example, for the production of certain hormones), but if present in excess levels can cotribute to the development of atherosclerosis.

Creatinine: A substance in blood that reflects the approximate level of kidney function. Used to calculate the *creatinine clearance* which is a more precise measure of how efficiently your kidneys are able to purify your blood.

Dawn phenomenon: The tendency for blood glucose to rise early in the morning due to secretion of hormones that counteract insulin.

Diabeta: *See glyburide.*

Diabetes: A disease in which there it too much glucose in the blood due to insufficient or ineffective insulin.

Diabetologist: A physician who specializes in diabetes treatment.

Dialysis: Artificial cleaning of the blood when the kidneys are not working.

Diamicron: *See gliclazide.*

Dyslipidemia: Abnormal cholesterol and triglyceride levels in the blood.

Endocrinologist: A physician who specializes in diseases of the glands, including the adrenal glands, the thyroid, the pituitary, the parathyroid glands, the ovaries, the testicles, and the pancreas.

Fats: The most concentrated source of calories of the three major energy sources. Some fats come from animals and some from plants. Excess levels of certain types of fats can increase the risk of atherosclerosis.

Food Group System: A system — designed to facilitate diabetes meal planning — where foods are divided into seven groups according to the amount of carbohydrate, protein, and fat they contain.

Fibre: A substance in plants that can lower fat and blood glucose and can help prevent constipation.

Fructose: The sugar found in fruits, vegetables, and honey.

Gastroparesis: A form of autonomic neuropathy involving nerves to the stomach that results in food being held in the stomach.

Gestational diabetes mellitus: Diabetes that develops during pregnancy and goes away once pregnancy ends, but that indicates you are at increased risk of later developing type 2 diabetes.

Gliclazide: An oral hypoglycemic agent that lowers glucose by stimulating insulin release from the pancreas.

Glimepiride: An oral hypoglycemic agent that lowers glucose by stimulating insulin release from the pancreas.

Glucophage: *See metformin.*

GlucoNorm: *See repaglinide.*

Glucose: A simple form of sugar that is the body's main source of energy.

Glucose tolerance test: A test where you consume a sugar-rich drink and your glucose levels are tested several times to establish if you have diabetes.

Glyburide: An oral hypoglycemic agent that lowers glucose by stimulating insulin release from the pancreas.

Glycemic index: The extent to which a given food raises blood glucose.

Glycogen: The storage form of glucose in the liver and muscles.

Health care team: The group of people that work together to keep you healthy. You, the person with diabetes, are the most important member of the team. Other members include your family doctor, your diabetes specialist, your diabetes educator, your dietitian, your eye doctor, your pharmacist, and, when necessary, other specialists (such as a podiatrist, dentist, cardiologist, kidney specialist, neurologist, emergency room physician, and so forth).

Hemoglobin A1C: *See A1C.*

High-density lipoprotein (HDL): A good form of cholesterol that helps to protect you from atherosclerosis.

Honeymoon phase: A period of variable duration, usually no more than a few months, after the onset of type 1 diabetes when the need for injections of insulin is reduced or eliminated.

Humalog insulin: *See Lispro insulin.*

Hyperglycemia: Higher than normal blood glucose levels.

Hyperosmolar Hyperglycemic State: A dangerous condition of very high blood glucose in type 2 diabetes associated with severe dehydration.

Hypoglycemia: Lower than normal blood glucose levels.

Impaired fasting glucose (IFG): A condition in which fasting blood glucose levels are higher than normal, but not high enough to establish a diagnosis of diabetes. *Also see prediabetes.*

Impaired glucose tolerance (IGT): A condition in which the blood glucose level is higher than normal — but not high enough to establish a diagnosis of diabetes — during the post-drink phase of a glucose tolerance test. *Also see prediabetes.*

Insulin: The key hormone, made by the islet cells of the pancreas, that permits glucose to enter cells.

Insulin glargine: A new insulin that provides a constant, basal level 24 hours a day.

Insulin pump: A device that delivers insulin into the body through a small catheter under the skin.

Insulin reaction: Hypoglycemia as a consequence of injected insulin.

Insulin resistance: A condition in which the body does not properly respond to insulin. This is typically present in people with type 2 diabetes.

Intensive diabetes management: The term *typically* applied to people with type 1 diabetes who are on three or more insulin injections per day or are using an insulin pump. This term is, however, more appropriately used to refer to *any* person with diabetes, regardless of the type of treatment they are on, so long as the treatment is aimed at achieving optimal blood glucose control.

Islet cells: The cells in the pancreas that make insulin, glucagon, and other hormones.

Ketoacidosis: An acute loss of control of diabetes with high blood glucose levels and breakdown of fat leading to acid production. Much more common in type 1 than type 2 diabetes.

Ketone: A breakdown product of fat formed when fat rather than glucose is being used for energy.

Ketonuria: Ketones in the urine.

Lancet: A sharp needle to prick the skin for a blood glucose test.

Lantus: *See insulin glargine.*

Laser treatment: Using a device that burns small areas at the back of the eye to prevent worsening of retinopathy.

Lente insulin: A type of intermediate-acting insulin.

Lipohypertrophy: Area of fatty deposit under the skin from overuse of an insulin injection site.

Lispro insulin: A type of rapid-acting insulin.

Low-density lipoprotein (LDL): A bad form of cholesterol that contributes to the development of atherosclerosis.

Macrosomia: An overly big baby.

Macrovascular complications: Damage to the heart, brain or legs due to blockage of large blood vessels.

Metabolic Syndrome: A combination of several factors, typically including an overweight state, abnormal lipids, elevated blood pressure, and increased blood glucose.

Metabolism: The body's use of energy and nutrients to maintain good health.

Metformin: An oral hypoglycemic agent for diabetes that lowers blood glucose by blocking release of glucose from the liver.

Microalbuminuria: Abnormal loss of a specific type of protein, called albumin, from the body into the urine.

Microvascular complications: Damage to the retina, nerves, or kidneys due to blockage of small blood vessels.

Monounsaturated fat: A form of fat from certain vegetable sources that does not raise cholesterol.

Nateglinide: An oral hypoglycemic agent that lowers glucose by stimulating insulin release from the pancreas.

Neovascularization: Formation within the eyes of abnormal, fragile blood vessels that are prone to bleeding.

Nephropathy: Damage to the kidneys.

Neuropathy: Damage to parts of the nervous system.

NovoRapid: *See aspart.*

NPH insulin: A type of intermediate-acting insulin.

Omega-3-fatty acids: A type of fat, found in certain fish, that may protect against the development of atherosclerosis.

Ophthalmologist: A medical doctor who specializes in diseases of the eyes.

Oral hypoglycemic agent: A glucose-lowering drug taken by mouth.

Pancreas: The organ behind the stomach that is actively involved in digestion and metabolism and contains the insulin-producing islet cells.

Peripheral neuropathy: Damaged nerve fibers, typically in the feet, that cause pain and numbness.

Pioglitazone: An oral hypoglycemic agent that lowers glucose by reducing insulin resistance.

Podiatrist: A person who specializes in treating the feet.

Polydipsia: Excessive intake of water.

Polyunsaturated fat: A form of fat from certain vegetable sources that may lower HDL.

Polyuria: Excessive urination.

Post-prandial: After eating.

Prandase: *See acarbose.*

Prediabetes: A new term that includes *impaired fasting glucose* and *impaired glucose tolerance.* Having prediabetes puts you at much greater risk of later developing diabetes.

Pre-prandial: Before eating.

Protein: One of the three major energy sources, the one usually found in meat, fish, poultry, and beans. Protein is necessary for the body to maintain healthy tissues.

Proteinuria: Abnormal loss of protein from the body into the urine.

Regular insulin: A type of fast-acting insulin.

Repaglinide: An oral hypoglycemic agent that lowers glucose by stimulating insulin release from the pancreas.

Retina: The part of the eye that senses light.

Retinopathy: Disease of the retina.

Rosiglitazone: An oral hypoglycemic agent that lowers glucose by reducing insulin resistance.

Saturated fat: A form of fat from animals that raises cholesterol.

Somogyi effect: A rapid increase in blood glucose to a high level in response to hypoglycemia occurring during the night.

Starlix: *See nateglinide.*

Sulfonylureas: A class of glucose-lowering agents, which work by stimulating insulin secretion from the pancreas.

Trans fatty acids: A type of fat, formed during food processing, that may worsen cholesterol levels and contribute to the development of atherosclerosis.

Triglycerides: The main form of fat in animals.

Ultralente insulin: A type of long-acting insulin.

Index

Notes

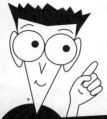

FOR
DUMMIES®

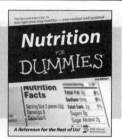

The easy way to get more done and have more fun

...LTH & DIET

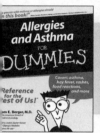

Allergies and Asthma
Covers asthma, hay fever, rashes, food reactions, and more
Reference for the Rest of Us!
0-7645-5218-X

Controlling Cholesterol
0-7645-5440-9

Nutrition
2nd Edition
Nutrition Facts
0-7645-4082-3

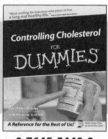

Thyroid
Reference for the Rest of Us!
0-7645-5385-2

Vitamins
Your complete A-to-Zinc guide to vitamins
Christopher Hobbs, Elson Haas, M.D.
A Reference for the Rest of Us!
0-7645-5179-5

Migraines
Manage your migraines with help from this friendly guide
A Reference for the Rest of Us!
0-7645-5485-9

Also available:

Alzheimers For Dummies
(0-7645-3899-3)

Anorexia & Bulimia
For Dummies
(0-7645-5487-5)

Asthma For Dummies
(0-7645-5487-5)

Back Pain Remedies
For Dummies
(0-7645-5132-9)

Breast Cancer For Dummies
(0-7645-2482-8)

Controlling Cholesterol
For Dummies
(0-7645-5440-9)

Depression For Dummies
(0-7645-3900-0)

Dieting For Dummies
(0-7645-5126-4)

Fertility For Dummies
(0-7645-2549-2)

Fibromyalgia For Dummies
(0-7645-5441-7)

Heart Disease For Dummies
(0-7645-4155-2)

High Blood Pressure
For Dummies
(0-7645-5424-7)

Hypoglycemia For Dummies
(0-7645-5490-5)

Menopause For Dummies
(0-7645-5458-1)

Migraines For Dummies
(0-7645-5485-9)

Nutrition For Dummies,
3rd Edition
(0-7645-4082-3)

Prostate Cancer For Dummies
(0-7645-1974-3)

Quitting Smoking
For Dummies
(0-7645-2629-4)

Weight Loss Kit For Dummies
(0-7645-5334-8)

...LTH, SPORTS & FITNESS

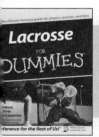

Lacrosse
The ultimate lacrosse guide for players, coaches, and fans
Reference for the Rest of Us!
1-894-41349-0

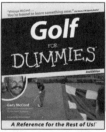

Golf
2nd Edition
Gary McCord
A Reference for the Rest of Us!
0-7645-5146-9

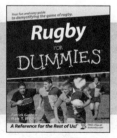

Rugby
Your fun and easy guide to demystifying the game of rugby
A Reference for the Rest of Us!
0-470-83405-6

Also available:

Baseball For Dummies,
2nd Edition
(0-7645-5234-1)

Basketball For Dummies,
2nd Edition
(0-7645-5248-1)

Curling For Dummies
(1-894-41330-X)

Fishing For Dummies
(0-7645-5028-4)

Football For Dummies,
2nd Edition
(0-7645-3936-1)

Formula One Racing
For Dummies
(0-7645-7015-3)

Golf Rules & Etiquette
For Dummies
(0-7645-5333-X)

Hockey For Dummies,
2nd Edition
(0-7645-5228-7)

NASCAR For Dummies
(0-7645-5219-8)

Sailing For Dummies
(0-7645-5039-X)

Soccer For Dummies
(0-7645-5229-5)

Tennis For Dummies
(0-7645-5087-X)

...ilable wherever books are sold.
...o www.dummies.com or call 1-877-762-2974 to order direct.

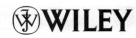
WILEY

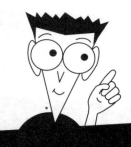

FOR DUMMIES®

A world of resources to help you grow

TRAVEL

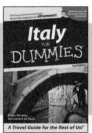

0-7645-5453-0

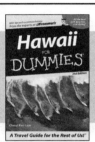

0-7645-5438-7

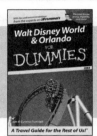

0-7645-5444-1

Also available:

America's National Parks For Dummies (0-7645-5493-X)

Caribbean For Dummies (0-7645-5445-X)

Cruise Vacations For Dummies 2003 (0-7645-5459-X)

Europe For Dummies (0-7645-5456-5)

Ireland For Dummies (0-7645-5455-7)

France For Dummies (0-7645-6292-4)

Las Vega For Dummies (0-7645-5448-4)

London For Dummies (0-7645-5416-6)

Mexico's Beach Resorts For Dummies (0-7645-6262-2)

Paris For Dummies (0-7645-5494-8)

RV Vacations For Dummie (0-7645-5443-3)

EDUCATION & TEST PREPARATION

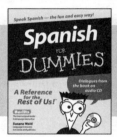

0-7645-5194-9

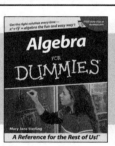

0-7645-5325-9

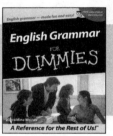

0-7645-5322-4

Also available:

The ACT For Dummies (0-7645-5474-3)

Chemistry For Dummies (0-7645-5430-1)

English Grammar For Dummies (0-7645-5322-4)

French For Dummies (0-7645-5193-0)

GMAT For Dummies (0-7645-5251-1)

Inglés Para Dummies (0-7645-5427-1)

Italian For Dummies (0-7645-5196-5)

Research Papers For Dummies (0-7645-5426-3)

SAT I For Dummies (0-7645-5472-7

Latin For Dummies (0-7645-5431-X)

HISTORY & POLITICS

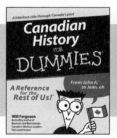

1-894-41319-9

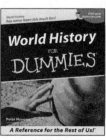

0-7645-5242-2

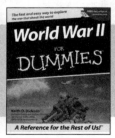

0-7645-5352-6

Also available:

British History For Dummies (0-7645-7021-8)

Canadian History For Dummies (1-894-41319-9)

The Civil War For Dummies (0-7645-5244-9)

Congress For Dummies (0-7645-5421-2)

Politics For Dummies, 2nd Edition (0-7645-0887-3)

Supreme Court For Dumm (0-7645-0886-5)

U.S. History For Dummies (0-7645-5249-X)

The Vietnam War For Dummies (0-7645-5480-8)

World History For Dummie (0-7645-5242-2)

World War II For Dummies (0-7645-5352-6)

Available wherever books are sold. Go to www.dummies.com or call 1-877-762-2974 to order direct.

FOR DUMMIES®

Plain-English solutions for everyday challenges

ME & BUSINESS COMPUTER BASICS

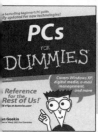

0-7645-4074-2

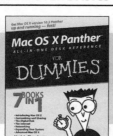

0-7645-4325-3

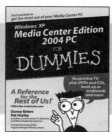

0-7645-4357-1

ERNET & DIGITAL MEDIA

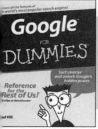

0-7645-4420-9

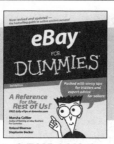

0-7645-1642-6

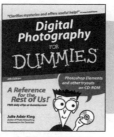

0-7645-1664-7

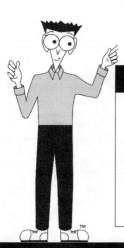

Get smart! Visit www.dummies.com

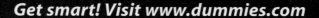

- **Find listings of even more *For Dummies* titles**

- **Browse online articles, excerpts, and how-to's**

- **Sign up for daily or weekly email tips**

- **Check out Dummies fitness videos and other products**

- **Order from our online bookstore**

Available wherever books are sold. Go to www.dummies.com or call 1-877-762-2974 to order direct.

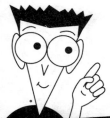
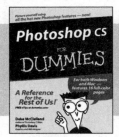
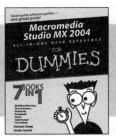
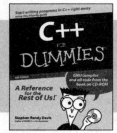
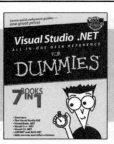
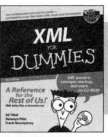
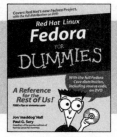
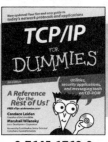
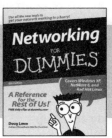

FOR DUMMIES®

The advice and explanations you need to succeed

RSONAL FINANCE & BUSINESS

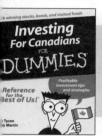

Investing For Canadians
1-794-41300-8

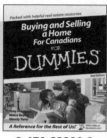

Buying and Selling a Home For Canadians
0-470-83320-3

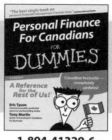

Personal Finance For Canadians
1-894-41329-6

Also available:

Accounting For Dummies
(0-7645-5314-3)

Business Plans Kit
For Dummies
(0-7645-5365-8)

Canadian Small Business Kit
For Dummies
(1-894-41304-0)

Managing For Dummies
(0-7645-1771-6)

Mutual Funds For Canadians
For Dummies
(0-470-83251-7)

Resumes For Dummies
(0-7645-5471-9)

Starting an eBay Business
For Dummies
(0-7645-1547-0)

QuickBooks All-in-One Desk
Reference For Dummies
(0-7645-1963-8)

Tax Tips For Canadians
For Dummies, 2004 Edition
(0-471-83416-1)

ME, GARDEN, FOOD & WINE

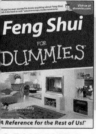

Feng Shui
0-7645-5295-3

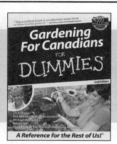

Gardening For Canadians
1-894-41337-7

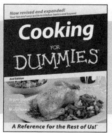

Cooking
0-7645-5250-3

Also available:

Bartending For Dummies
(0-7645-5051-9)

Christmas Cooking
For Dummies
(0-7645-5407-7)

Diabetes Cookbook
For Dummies
(0-7645-5230-9)

Grilling For Dummies
(0-7645-5076-4)

Home Maintenance
For Dummies
(0-7645-5215-5)

Slow Cookers For Dummies
(0-7645-5240-6)

Wine For Dummies
(0-7645-5114-0)

NESS, HOBBIES & PETS

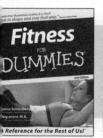

Fitness
0-7645-5167-1

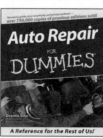

Auto Repair
0-7645-5089-6

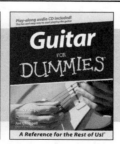

Guitar
0-7645-5106-X

Also available:

Cats For Dummies
(0-7645-5275-9)

Chess For Dummies
(0-7645+5003-9)

Dog Training For Dummies
(0-7645-5286-4)

Knitting For Dummies
(0-7645-5395-X)

Labrador Retrievers For
Dummies
(0-7645-5281-3)

Martial Arts For Dummies
(0-7645-5358-5)

Piano For Dummies
(0-7645-5105-1)

Pilates For Dummies
(0-7645-5397-6)

Power Yoga For Dummies
(0-7645-5342-9)

Puppies For Dummies
(0-7645-5255-4)

Rock Guitar For Dummies
(0-7645-5356-9)

Weight Training For Dummies
(0-7645-5168-X)

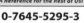